BIOETHICS AND MORAL CONTENT:
NATIONAL TRADITIONS OF HEALTH CARE MORALITY

Philosophy and Medicine

VOLUME 74

ASIAN STUDIES IN BIOETHICS AND THE PHILOSOPHY OF MEDICINE 3

The titles published in this series are listed at the end of this volume.

BIOETHICS AND MORAL CONTENT: NATIONAL TRADITIONS OF HEALTH CARE MORALITY

Papers dedicated in tribute to Kazumasa Hoshino

Edited by

H. TRISTRAM ENGELHARDT, JR.
Department of Philosophy, Rice University
and
Baylor College of Medicine, Houston, USA

and

LISA M. RASMUSSEN
Department of Philosophy, Rice University, Houston, USA

SPRINGER-SCIENCE+BUSINESS MEDIA, B.V.

Library of Congress Cataloging-in-Publication Data is available.

ISBN 978-90-481-5658-0 **ISBN 978-94-017-0902-6 (eBook)**
DOI 10.1007/978-94-017-0902-6

Printed on acid-free paper

TABLE OF CONTENTS

PART IV / GLOBAL BIOETHICS AND ITS CRITICS

H. TRISTRAM ENGELHARDT, JR.
AND LISA M. RASMUSSEN

BIOETHICS IN THE PLURAL: AN INTRODUCTION TO TAKING GLOBAL MORAL DIVERSITY SERIOUSLY

I. DIALOGUES ON DIFFERENCE

On August 15, 1979, the first author of this article presented a paper concerning the philosophy of medicine at Sophia University in Tokyo. In the audience were philosophers, theologians, and physicians – they were politely puzzled concerning the claims made about the new field of bioethics. During that trip to Tokyo, the first author also visited in passing at Kitasato University's hospital in Tokyo. In all of these meetings, it was clear that the Americans, Texans, and Japanese saw issues of bioethics from radically different perspectives. Yet, the Americans claimed that the differences were superficial. In fact, they held that all sides should come to recognize that they shared a common understanding of ethics, which was to ground the new field of bioethics.

This visit was followed by a series of meetings, again in August, this time in 1986, at Kitasato University School of Medicine in Sagamihara City. Once again, the audience was politely puzzled, although a number of the physicians voiced the view that the medical ethics of Japan was radically different from that of the United States. The response on the part of most of the American bioethicists was again to assure their Japanese hosts that the bioethics they (the Americans) were expounding reflected the common morality of mankind, whether or not the Japanese recognized this to be the case. The Americans were of the view that the critical reflective character of Western philosophy had brought them to understand the conceptual assumptions at the root of proper moral deportment. They were convinced that, with analysis and reflection, the considered judgments of Japanese philosophers and physicians would come to accord with that of American bioethics. This was the year in which the first author of this introduction published the first edition of *The Foundations of Bioethics* (Engelhardt, 1986). This author was, needless to say, skeptical of the position taken by his American colleagues, although he with his libertarian arguments appeared nevertheless strange to his Japanese hosts. He recognized, among other things, that American and Japanese bioethicists were attempting

H.T. Engelhardt, Jr. and L.M. Rasmussen (eds.), Bioethics and Moral Content: National Traditions of Health Care Morality, 1–14.

somewhat similar but still essentially different undertakings under the rubric of bioethics.

These encounters have been followed by a number of important meetings with Japanese scholars over the years. One of the most significant was the meeting with Kazumasa Hoshino and his colleagues. Through him and the Liaison Society of Ethics Committees of Medical Schools in Japan, the first author came to recognize both how similar and how different ethics committees and ethics consultations functioned in Japan versus the United States. Over the years, through numerous interchanges, this became even clearer. This encounter with the differences between Japanese and American approaches took further shape over the years at various conferences, including the very significant conference the proceedings of which appeared as *Japanese and Western Bioethics: Studies in Moral Diversity*, edited by Kazumasa Hoshino (Hoshino, 1997). Japanese bioethics distinguished itself from American bioethics by the former's focus on deeply developed senses of moral virtue and character, which were understood to guide the harmonious interaction of physicians, patients, and their families, and by the latter's focus on individuals, their autonomy, and their good. This peculiarly fragmented American approach has obvious roots in the ways in which religious and moral pluralism have structured the American experience. Physicians, patients, and their families cannot presume a common understanding of human virtue, character, and flourishing. Indeed, the American experience has involved creating space for the peaceable expression of moral difference.

The differences among moral perspectives and their implications for the practice of bioethics became clear to the authors of this introduction as they explored the nature of practical bioethics. At the bedside, physicians, patients, and their families often possess radically different expectations regarding the role and functions of bioethicists. Even within the same culture, at least within the same Texan and American culture, there is a significant range of expectations from bioethicists.

II. DIFFERENCES IN BIOETHICS: A CRITICAL ASSESSMENT

The authors of the essays in this volume honor the work of Kazumasa Hoshino in many different ways. Robert Veatch, David Thomasma, Lisa Rasmussen, and Michael Fetters and Marion Danis focus on differences between Western bioethics and Japanese bioethics, illustrating both similarities and differences between the two cultures. Tangjia Wang, Fabrice Jotterand, Ho Mun Chan, Mark Cherry, Ruiping Fan and Kurt Bayertz and Kurt Schmidt give accounts of disagreement between cultures regarding bioethics, impressing upon us the importance of Hoshino's insights concerning the implications of cultural diversity for bioethics. Finally, Hans-Martin Sass, Jonathan Chan, and Corinna Delkeskamp-Hayes tackle the possibility of a global ethics directly, and Ruiping Fan offers a defense of bioethics grounded in a Reconstructionist Confucian account of moral probity.

A. Section One: Physician Virtue and National Traditions

Section One addresses the question of the role of the physician. Robert Veatch begins by taking us on a conceptual tour in "The Physician: Professional or Entrepreneur?" Western bioethics is confronted with these two views of physicians, and Veatch points out the problems with each. Viewing doctors as belonging to a noble profession with its own special requirements (such as making house calls, providing free service for the poor, and behaving as a pillar of the community) is appealing in many ways, not least because it is how they have been seen historically. However, such a view is at odds with the physician as self-interested. According to Veatch, therein lies one of the problems: this model requires physicians to be supererogatory. It also ignores the fact that conflicts of interest cannot be removed simply by forbidding physicians to own laboratories to which they can send specimens from their patients. Any choice that involves pay to the doctor involves a potential conflict of interest; however, a physician must earn a living.

As for the entrepreneurial model, which construes physicians as businessmen, it too has problems. *Caveat emptor* requires the patient to be a more informed "buyer" than the doctor might be able to help him become. A sensible patient/buyer might want to know the doctor's economic incentive structure, utilization rates, investment interests and so on. In addition, Veatch argues, the more patients regard physicians as entrepreneurs, the less reason they have to trust them. In time, with sufficient information, rigorous outside regulation would become necessary. Veatch does not draw conclusions from these observations, leaving readers to make up their own minds. However, he does look briefly at Japanese culture, asking whether Japanese face the same choice between physician models. He concludes, following Unschuld (1979), that rather than the professional/entrepreneur dichotomy, Japanese may face a different choice: physician as professional vs. physician as family member. There are tensions between these models as well. Veatch leaves it to others to pursue the implications of and arguments for each of them.

In "The physician-patient relationship and individualization of treatment from the view of traditional Chinese medical practice," Tangjia Wang describes different approaches to the physician-patient relationship. He outlines four models of this relationship (beneficence, entrustment, partnership, and autonomy), and argues that each one, taken by itself, has limitations. He then diagnoses some problems with current physician-patient relationships, among them the alienating effects of technology, the marketing of medicine, and the increase in medical specialization. Wang recognizes that many of these recent developments might prove beneficial to patients; what he suggests, then, is that there is a way in which to ameliorate the troublesome aspects of these developments. He advocates a return to a beneficence model in response to what he sees as an over-reliance on respect for patients' autonomy as a guide for the physician-patient relationship. However, he does not favor a rejection of autonomy completely. Rather, he claims,

> the traditional strong beneficence model should be changed into [a] weak one by introducing the autonomy of the patient into clinical life. That is to say, in the majority of cases the patient's right of self-determination should be respected, but if there is conflict between respect for life and the right of autonomy, we should value the former over the latter (p. 38).

Surely the ongoing debate between proponents and critics of the autonomy model shows that this is far from being a settled question. In his criticism of the autonomy model, Wang himself exhibits the reluctance to accept Western bioethics, a viewpoint that Hoshino has long discussed.

B. Section Two: Medical Technologies and National Bioethics

In "Medical technologies and universal ethics in transcultural perspective," Hans-Martin Sass discusses the possibility of a universal or global ethics and advocates its creation. According to him, "most moral communities of world religions and other systems of belief definitely are preconditioned to support the visions and mission of universal ethics" (p. 71). Just as we share a common need for shelter, Sass argues, we also share some basic human values and virtues. Extending the comparison, he views a world of "different moral houses": all provide commonly needed shelter, but may be radically different in structure, appearance, and decoration. What makes us different and enables us to respect each other's differences is what is on, so to speak, the "upper floors" of our moral houses. On those upper floors, there is room for different communities' providing different "interior design" regarding choices of procreation, health care, the end of life, etc. As he puts it,

> Certain principles, primary virtues ... such as personal integrity, reliability, punctuality, professional expertise and professionalism, truthfulness, politeness, kindness, decency, listening and understanding, openness, fairness, loyalty and trustworthiness will be indispensable for all *structural aspects* of the buildings, even though some constructions might differ from others in regard to this form of stability and reliability. On the *ground floor*, all houses share the principle of vehemently fighting the starvation, killing and torturing of all fellow humans, whether from this house or others, and of providing care and support for the sick, poor, and others who cannot care for themselves. But on the *higher floors* different houses will hold different opinions (p. 55).

Along with the observation of these shared values, Sass also recognizes that it is important to respect individual choice. The model suggests that we may share some values and not others. Undoubtedly, there is much more to say about whether the model shows that at the foundations we share one morality.

In "Brain death, pregnancy and cultural reluctance toward scientific rationalism," Kurt Bayertz and Kurt Schmidt provide a concrete example of the lack of consensus both internationally and intra-nationally. The Erlangen baby case of 1992, in which an 18-year-old woman with a 14-week pregnancy was deemed brain-dead after an automobile accident in Erlangen, Germany, provoked an unanticipated amount of public involvement and outrage. Due to press accounts of the case (both accurate and inaccurate), the public became divided over the issue of brain death in a way that it had not previously appeared to be. According to Bayertz and Schmidt, four separate sets of concern help to explain this reaction.

As in any developed country, there is a deep divide between the lay public's understanding of science and the understanding necessary to comprehend fine-grained arguments about medical technology. First, this divide stems from simple misunderstandings about such issues as the definition of brain death, the prognosis for brain-dead individuals, and the explanations for the apparent continuation of life (for example, respiration, circulation, and gestation). Second, our failure to find a language appropriate to such novel situations causes us to feel uncertain. In this case, there was no clear term applicable to mother or fetus: was the mother dead? How was it possible to be born from a dead mother? If the mother was dead, how was she still "alive" to gestate the fetus? Was the fetus simply incubating in a corpse? Or was the mother not actually dead, despite medical consensus on the status of brain-dead patients? As Bayertz and Schmidt illustrate, it is not simply the fact that it was unclear what terms to use that divided and outraged the public, but it was also the circumstance that none of the choices was value-neutral.

Third, there are conflicting values and principles at stake in alternative definitions. Did the fetus and the brain-dead mother have equal, competing claims for consideration, or did one trump another? As they summarize the matter, "each conceivable decision [in the case] would have represented a provocation for at least one of the various groups" (Bayertz and Schmidt, p. 83). Finally, there were legal problems (not least of which, but interestingly practical in its scope, was the question of inheritance were the baby to be born to a mother for whom a death certificate had been completed prenatally).

In many different ways, Bayertz and Schmidt's paper is an illustration of moral pluralism and the clash between cultures. These issues were brought up quite clearly within Germany in the Erlangen case. But even more can be drawn from this case as it concerns international cultural clashes. They point out that just days before the Erlangen case broke, Kasumasa Hoshino explained to an audience at the Inaugural Congress of the International Association of Bioethics why brain death was not generally accepted by the Japanese people. It is important for many Japanese actually to see the dead person as *dead*, and as Hoshino states, "[for the Japanese, brain death] is a foreign concept and [they] are far from being able to witness the death themselves visually at the bedside of the deceased" (Hoshino, 1993, p. 238, as quoted in Bayertz and Schmidt, p. 89). Just as it seems clear to many Western bioethicists that there is a consensus on brain death,[1] it is clear to others that there is no such thing.

Maurizio Mori, in "Bioethics in Italy up to 2002: An overview", gives a history of the development of bioethics in Italy. Its interest goes beyond mere historical reporting, however: Mori shows the tension between Roman Catholic and secular influences that has been active in Italian bioethics since its inception. He also describes the deep political tenor of bioethics in Italy. As he points out, in Italy "an 'intellectual contribution' is often valued not on the basis of academic criteria (originality, clearness, etc.), but on other criteria, such as possible social or political consequences, etc." (p. 97). It is because of this tendency of Italians that Mori is careful to distinguish, in Italy, between "*bioethics as a cultural movement* (or *intellectual debate*), devoted to the critical evaluation of received opinions and elaboration of new ideas to be advanced by scholars and people; and *bioethics as an institutional setting* aimed at influencing public opinion or controlling social change in the field of health care and issues concerning living stuff" (p. 98).

According to Mori, in the 1970s and 1980s, bioethics in Italy was mainly a cultural movement. Scholars debated the philosophical and bioethical concepts. A tension emerged between proponents and opponents of 'applied' ethics. They were also the beginnings of the formulation of a secular bioethics. The Roman Catholic church became more involved as well. In 1985, Pope John Paul II opened the *Centro di Bioetica*, and Roman Catholic scholars began to formulate positions on various bioethical issues. Mori points out that at this point in history, scholars in bioethics were both trying to persuade their colleagues of the legitimacy of bioethical inquiry and simultaneously trying to determine exactly what bioethics was about – an experience that will certainly sound familiar to most readers. This stage ended when the Roman Catholic church began to put limits on theologians' freedom of research and public expression of opinion. Bioethics began to become institutionalized.

The second stage Mori discusses is bioethics as political, in its institutional setting. Early in the 1990s, bioethics was absorbed into university departments where Roman Catholics held power. As a result, a monsignor was the first tenured bioethics professor in Italy. As Mori summarizes, "in the first part of the '90s, Catholics had a complete monopoly on the teaching of bioethics in the universities" (p. 105); they also controlled most of the political commissions. Recent developments give Mori reason to suspect that Italy is on the verge of a third stage, one less influenced by the Roman Catholic church. However, it is certain that tensions between Roman Catholic and secular views (not to mention the views of many other religious groups) will continue to dominate discussion in Italy.

Fabrice Jotterand treats the history of and cultural influences on bioethics in Switzerland in "Development and identity in Swiss bioethics." Switzerland is, as Jotterand points out, extraordinarily diverse in its cultural, linguistic and religious makeup. This is not simply the case of a country with a "melting pot" of citizens, though it is that as well. In Switzerland there are in addition deep, historical differences separating Swiss-Germans, Swiss-Italians, and Swiss-French, each of which looks back to its "linguistic representative" (i.e., the home country of its language and culture), as Jotterand puts it. Add to this the circumstance that Switzerland has tried both to secularize and to respect its citizens' religions, and it is patent that Swiss bioethics must contain within itself a sizeable diversity of views.

Jotterand divides the history of Swiss bioethics into two periods: 1943-1988 and 1988 to present. In 1988, the Swiss Society of Biomedical Ethics was formed. This was the first time that "outsiders" (i.e., non-physicians) began reflecting on medical ethics. Interestingly, Jotterand notes in Swiss bioethics something that Mori noted in Italian bioethics: an initial struggle for academic support and recognition, followed by increasing involvement in national examinations of bioethics. While Jotterand acknowledges that there may be agreement on a few core issues in bioethics, he also cautions against a simple accession to a global – or even European – bioethics. Differences among countries may be far more significant than similarities.

C. Section Three: Death, Culture, and Moral Difference

Michael Fetters and Marion Danis open this section by reporting on their fascinating empirical study of the differences between Japanese and American views on cardio-pulmonary resuscitation in their article, "Death with dignity: Cardiopulmonary resuscitation in the United States and Japan." In the United States, advance directives are relatively common, and decisions about cardiopulmonary resuscitation (CPR) at the end of life occur in the context of patient wishes either as expressed in an advance directive or via family or surrogate reports about what the patient would have wanted. As Fetters and Danis point out, in the United States all such decisions focus on the patient's autonomy. In contrast, Japanese physicians make decisions about CPR in the context of the *family's* desires – *not* because they are considered the best historians of the patient's wishes for the end of his life, but because of the primacy of the family in Japanese life.

One physician in their study voices a cultural commonplace: "[in Japan] it is said that death is something you should see" (p. 153). Because the goal of CPR in Japan is to enable the patient's family to witness the death of the patient, CPR might continue for 24 hours if it takes that long for a family member to reach the bedside, though physicians might be convinced that there is no chance for actual resuscitation. In the United States, some might consider this an affront to a patient's dignity; in Japan, on the other hand, it is (among other things) considered a way in which a family shows love to a patient by not letting him die alone. Indeed, as Fetters and Danis point out, it is so important to be at the bedside at a family member's death that there are specific socially accepted exceptions to the requirement. It is not hard to imagine the possible resulting difference in policy and resource allocation decisions between Japan and the U.S.

Ho Mun Chan focuses on the influence of cultural differences on a Hong Kong euthanasia policy in "Euthanasia, individual choice and the family: The case of Hong Kong." The contrast Chan draws is between the individualism of societies that depend heavily on the notion of autonomy and societies in which the family authority is overriding. He first carefully delineates various circumstances in which euthanasia might be considered an option, and the moral differences between various situations, invoking a distinction between cessation of treatment and euthanasia. In cases of cessation of treatment, he points out the different ways in which justification for such a decision might be obtained. As he argues, "[i]n the liberal model, such a decision is justified in terms of the self-determination and the best interests of the patient, whereas in the model of familialism, which is a popular model in Eastern societies, e.g., Japan, Mainland China, and Hong Kong, the justification is coined in terms of the autonomy and the interests of the family" (Chan, p. 166).

Chan recognizes that familialism is vulnerable to the charge that families can easily hurt one of their members, intentionally or unintentionally, and that autonomy is a reasonable safeguard in this case. He thus proposes "a moderate version of familialism." According to this model, a patient can be asked in what manner decisions regarding his or her care are to be made. This respects autonomy in a thin sense, but also leaves sufficient room for a society with a familial tradition to maintain that tradition. The problem comes, Chan points out, when a patient is incompetent and has not previously expressed wishes regarding treatment decision making. In this case, he argues, the default should be that families make decisions for patients. The onus is on the patient to declare wishes to the contrary. Given the cultural context in Hong Kong that Chan highlights, this seems the most reasonable default position in Hong Kong (though as Chan also discusses, this may be changing, albeit slowly). On the other hand, it may be the wrong approach in the United States. However, one should note that the reliance on family reports of the patient's past wishes imports in an often clandestine fashion a strong salience of family authority.

Corinna Delkeskamp-Hayes closes this section with "Dissensus in the face of a passion for consensus: How the Japanese and the Germans could still understand one another." She traces the many divergence points between cultures that on their surface appear similar. She begins by summarizing what she calls the "Western propensity to universalize ethical claims," a tendency rooted both in Christianity and "pagan rationalism". The merging of the two views (instigated by Aquinas) has resulted, she argues, in a generic ethical view that both holds ethical truths to be universal and holds reason to be sufficient to discover them. However, she points out, there is no depth to this generic ethics: its integrity fails when confronted with deep differences. For example, she points out that many believe in the "sanctity of life", but find that their understandings of this sanctity vary widely. Germany refused to sign the *European Convention for the Protection of Human Rights and Dignity of the Human Being with Regard to the Application of Biology and Medicine* over just such differences of opinion: the *Convention* permits interventions into the structure of the human genome, while Germany forbids it. Further differences include views concerning the early human embryo and medical research. At least part of this conservatism on Germany's part is due, Delkeskamp-Hayes argues, to its history of National Socialism and the medical experiments conducted in World War II. As she makes clear, it is not merely old cultural traditions that create a cultural context; significant historical events can leave a deep, shared impression on an entire country. Even such a profound historical influence does not guarantee unity. As she argues, "Germans are in the process of learning that even within Germany there are no longer universally acknowledged, content-rich moral principles that could justify enforcing of what some hold morally obligatory for all on those of a different moral creed" (p. 200).

D. Section Four: Global Bioethics and its Critics

Finally, Section Four focuses directly on moral diversity and global bioethics. Lisa Rasmussen addresses the impact of cultural context on clinical bioethics consultation in "Moral diversity and bioethics consultation". Though bioethics – and bioethics consultation in particular – is becoming increasingly popular in the United States, Rasmussen points out that there has been no concomitant increase in clarity regarding the job of the bioethics consultant. Existing accounts are vague and fail to give concrete guidance. Bioethics consultants are often in the position of playing many different roles (she has identified at least 12), both individually and in combination. What guides a bioethicist when performing these roles? Which take priority, and why? Rasmussen points out that to answer these questions, we must look at roles and the justifications for them carefully. As these roles become more defined, it is clear that in varying cultural contexts, some roles simply would not be included in the job of a bioethics consultant. The American model cannot become the global model. Moral diversity does not manifest itself simply in individual situations; at times it can radically change the very behavior of the participants and the roles they take themselves to play.

The next contribution is one made by the recently deceased (April 25, 2002) bioethicist and moral theorist David Thomasma, who in his work explored with rich imagination and analytic skill the challenges of contemporary bioethics. In "The challenge of doing international bioethics," Thomasma investigates impediments to a global bioethics. The first difficulty that strikes him, as it must strike many, are the everyday differences that become obvious upon exposure to different cultures. He gives the example of the perception Japanese have of Americans: "Western culture can look like a post-adolescent uninvolvement with the common good" (p. 221). To Westerners, on the other hand, the Japanese focus on obedience and family loyalty might look retrograde or hidebound. Deeper differences only complicate matters. Thomasma argues that "international bioethics will depend upon at least two major actions. First, a respect for persons as enculturated with their own value systems; and, second, a baseline arrived at through international dialogue about fundamental human rights in health care, much as the UN Charter does for broader human rights issues" (p. 224).

Thomasma endorses a communitarian ethics, which among other things corrects "an overemphasis on individualism"; such an ethics should recognize the cultural context of values; allow for the exploration of cases via narrative; give preference at times to the common good over individual good; and be "led away from the purely personal and rational will (freedom of choice), to qualities or instincts of compassion and empathy with all living creatures" (p. 228). As applied to international bioethics, Thomasma suggests a number of conditions that ought to be coupled with the communitarian theory he outlines. In the main these involve mutual understanding and appreciation – or at least dialogue – about foreign cultures. Most interesting is his suggestion that "discourse about biomedical ethics must have some *a priori* commitments present on the table. These are 'experiential conditions' because they may not be metaphysically defensible, *per se*. Instead they arise from the past experience of a culture whose history demonstrates the evil effects of ignoring these commitments" (p. 231). What these *a priori* commitments might look like is for the reader to ponder.

In "Taking moral diversity seriously: A discussion of the foundations of global bioethics," Jonathan Chan addresses the theoretical possibility of a global bioethics. He argues that essentialist theories, convergence theories and contract-based theories are all flawed and cannot support a global ethic, but that this does not yet preclude the possibility of a global ethic based on other sources. He discusses Confucianism as a flawed essentialist theory (and holds that other essentialist theories such as Natural Law are likewise flawed), for it claims that there is something essential about a given morality. His claim is that any such argument begs the question, assuming without proof that such an "essence" exists, in the face of the obvious fact of pluralism of moral values. Convergence theories assume either that there is or should be a convergence on moral principles (this type of theory is well represented by the principlism of Beauchamp and Childress). Chan argues that as a descriptive thesis, this type of theory fails on the empirical evidence of deep disagreement, while as a normative thesis, it begs the question by assuming what it sets out to prove (namely, the universality of certain moral principles). The final option, contractarianism, fails, according to Chan, over the question of side-constraints on a justified agreement. If a theory fails to provide such side-constraints, it invites and legitimates agreements reached by any means, including coercion and manipulation. If it succeeds in providing side-constraints, it assumes moral content, thus belying the motivation for contractarianism in the first place, which is the side-stepping of the question of conflicting moral values. Chan lingers on contractarian theories to discuss Baker's new version of this type of theory, which specifically aims at finding an international, interculturally valid ethic. In the end this, too, fails, according to Chan, leaving the question of the viability of a global ethic open.

Mark Cherry's paper, "Coveting an international bioethics: Universal aspirations and false promises," takes an extended look at some of the deep differences between Western cosmopolitan liberalism and traditional cultures and religions. Similar to the differences that Hoshino has highlighted between Japanese and Western Culture, Cherry identifies differences between "western culture" writ large and the many culturally and religiously diverse communities that thrive within that culture while preserving their own way of life (for example, the Amish, Orthodox Jews, and Orthodox Christians, etc.) However, as he points out, the hegemony of Western cosmopolitan liberalism renders it difficult (if not impossible) for many such cultures to practice their beliefs as they see fit. One solution to this problem, Cherry argues, is to found our societies on the principle of permission and the institution of private property. As he concludes,

> Respecting the freedom of persons defaults to protecting liberties of association, contract, conscience, and religion, and thereby to protecting the possibility of substantial moral diversity. Freely chosen, market-based health care financing, procurement, and distribution, respect the liberty of persons to pursue their own deep moral commitments. Unlike the cosmopolitan lip-service paid to the value of moral pluralism, freedom as a side-constraint carves out and protects social space for the possibility of moral diversity in health care (Cherry, 2002, pp. 271–272).

Within the latter understanding of society, a plurality of peaceable communities with their divergent bioethics could flourish.

Finally, Ruiping Fan supplies a vibrant example of an ethics embedded in an Asian cultural context. In 'Reconstructionist Confucianism and bioethics: A note on moral difference', he addresses Confucianism's content-rich approach to the issues of bioethics. First, he argues that it helps to explain the way in which bioethics in the Pacific Rim, influenced in part by Confucianism, differs from Western bioethics. Second, it is part of an ongoing response by a small but growing group of authors to the anti-Confucianism that began in the early 20th century and continues today. Finally, he offers it as a normative position worthy of consideration and adoption even by non-Confucians. The Confucian position on family and the moral life (as it concerns both patients and their families and physicians) suggests a different approach to, for example, informed consent than is assumed in the West. In his reflections on the differences, Fan articulates the kinds of differences that Hoshino has brought to light.

III. THE PERSISTENCE OF DIFFERENCE

Despite the strengthening economic forces of globalization, which are binding humans together in a market compassing the world, real moral difference remains. This difference is in part religiously based. Different religions ground radically different approaches to issues such as abortion, euthanasia, and stem cell research, to identify only three issues. Differences also are grounded in deeply culturally embedded understandings of moral probity that have profound implications for bioethics and health care policy. In the Pacific Rim, for example, there is, as some of the authors of these essays indicate, a resurgence of interest in Confucian thought. Ruiping Fan's project of Reconstructionist Confucianism embraces the goal of articulating a vigorous Confucian view for the 21st century. He among other voices speaks to the need to avoid assimilation by the dominant American-Western European vision of bioethics and health care policy. Moral difference will not go away.

This volume and the essays it compasses offer the reader an opportunity to explore some of the roots of moral difference, challenging aspirations to a global bioethics. These essays are richly in debt to the work both written and personal of Kazumasa Hoshino. The strength of his intellectual insight and the virtue of his commitment to exploring the moral differences that enrich the human condition have proved the source for the energies that have fashioned this volume. We the editors and the field remain enduringly in his debt for his insight and dedication.

NOTE

1. See the discussion in Bayertz and Schmidt on Wikler's presentation at the 1993 conference, p. 88, this volume. As they observe, "[h]ere, the brain death criterion appears to be the product of a context-free rationality; its metaphysical and cultural foundations are simply ignored" (p. 88).

PART I

PHYSICIAN VIRTUE AND NATIONAL TRADITIONS

ROBERT M. VEATCH

THE PHYSICIAN: PROFESSIONAL OR ENTREPRENEUR

By May of 1990 when I first traveled to Kyoto and met Dr. Kazumasa Hoshino, he was already organizing his Third International Bioethics Symposium (Hoshino, 1991). He was, by then, not only a distinguished physician of Kyoto University, he was also an internationally recognized leader in the study of bioethics. He has been particularly insightful in recognizing the national uniqueness of the conceptualization of the roles of patient and health care provider and the various bioethical traditions that surround them. Perhaps it is because of his experience with and understanding of the traditions of Western medicine that he has been so helpful in articulating the uniqueness of Japanese medical relations.

While recognizing and expressing some degree of empathy with the American patients' rights movement, he understands and helps Westerners understand why the individualism, self-determination, and demands for bluntness in communication, which are consistent with the American ethos, do not fit the core values of Japanese culture. His sympathetic exegesis of the Japanese concept of *was* – which he associates with the terms *conciliation, concord, unity, harmony, submission,* and *reconciliation* – has helped Westerners understand a very different cultural foundation for a patient-physician relation (Hoshino, 1995a; 1995b; 1997, p. 19).

In an effort to continue the international comparative work that he has stimulated, I would like to examine the emerging controversy over the health care provider's role. In particular, I would like to examine the recent debate over whether the physician is best thought of as a *professional* or as an *entrepreneur.* I hesitate to do so since I have learned just enough of the Japanese culture in my study of and visits to Dr. Hoshino's land to understand that those very terms probably do not pose the issue properly for the Japanese mind.

I. PROFESSIONAL AND ENTREPRENEUR: THE CONCEPTS

It is common in English-language writing on health care in Japan, as well as in the United States and other countries in which English is the primary

H.T. Engelhardt, Jr. and L.M. Rasmussen (eds.), Bioethics and Moral Content: National Traditions of Health Care Morality, 17–33.

language, to refer to the physician as a medical *professional*. Increasingly, however, we are recognizing that health care is big business and that the physician must also be a master of the business of his or her practice. While *profession* is sometimes used as a synonym for occupation, those who worry about the moral and conceptual relations of "physicianing" usually have something narrower in mind when they call the physician a professional. A *profession* is distinguished from the world of *business* by several characteristics. Sociologists of the professions identify these characteristics as including the possession of a systematic body of theory, authority to define problems and their treatment, community sanctions to admit and train its members, and a culture including institutions for carrying out its function (Brieger, 1995, p. 1688, citing work in the 1950s by Ernest Greenwood). From the point of view of biomedical ethics, however, the definitive characteristics of a profession are the responsibility for generating and enforcing its own code of ethics and an essential altruism. These are symbolized in both Western and Eastern traditions by the physician's moral commitment to the welfare of the patient. This core ethic is seen in both the Hippocratic Oath (Edelstein, 1967, p. 6) and the Japanese "Seventeen Rules of Enjuin" of the sixteenth century (Veatch, 1989, pp. 140-41; Bowers, 1970). The Japanese code, for example, specifies that the physician should not strain to become famous and should not rebuke the patient even if he does not compensate the physician with money or goods. He should be delighted if another physician succeeds in treating the patient after he has failed.

This altruism is central to the professions – the priest, the teacher, as well as the physician. Hence the Japanese term often used for the collectivity of physicians is *seishoku* or "sacred profession". The primary objective of the professional is not self-profit, but service to others. Of course, professionals, like all humans, must receive compensation, but their primary focus is on promoting the welfare of the patient.

As the economics of medicine have become more conspicuous and health care costs have become a more dominant concern, the entrepreneurial aspect of the practice of medicine has become much more visible. Of course, physicians who survived in their profession always had to pay some attention to the economic dimensions of their small businesses, but recently in the West, especially in the United States, physicians have come to be perceived (and sometimes to perceive themselves) as business people or entrepreneurs, running financially lucrative commercial operations with self-interest as a legitimate part of the agenda.

I am not knowledgeable enough to do anything more than make suggestions and raise questions about the Japanese conceptualization of the physician's role. Dr. Hoshino would be far better at addressing the question of whether this professional/entrepreneur distinction also applies in Japan. I have heard it said, however, that some social critics have suggested that "physicianing" has become more an art of mathematics (*san-jyutsu)* than an art of humaneness (*jin-jyutsu*), implying that the physician's economic calculations are sometimes gaining a more central spot in Japan as well as the West (Kimura, 1991, p. 239). The famous mid-twentieth century leader of the Japanese Medical Association, Taro Takemi (1994, pp. xxv-xxvii), has even suggested that these concerns go back into the Edo era. In honor of Dr. Hoshino, whose *jin* is never to be confused with *san*, I want to explore this shift from the role of professional to that of entrepreneur, focusing primarily on the practice of medicine in the United States and its Western precursors, but also raising some questions about how Eastern traditions conceptualize this role.

II. FROM CRAFT TO PROFESSIONS TO BUSINESS: WESTERN CONCEPTIONS OF THE HEALING ROLE

While many assume that the Hippocratic ideal constitutes the origins of medicine as a profession in the West, there is much evidence that Hippocratic medicine was much more of a craft or trade. The famous physician/historian Ludwig Edelstein begins his essay on "The Hippocratic Physician" by stating, "The Hippocratic physician is a craftsman" (Edelstein, 1967, p. 87). He continues:

> As a craftsman, the physician of antiquity is classified socially as a businessman. While the modern doctor, in spite of the payment he receives, is not on the same social level as the other craftsmen who, like him, are paid for their services, the ancient physician is the equal of the other craftsmen and thereby occupies a low position in society (Edelstein, 1967, p. 87).

The Hippocratic writings advise the physician to refrain from taking on patients with hopeless, incurable conditions. This advice is given, at least in part, to avoid having blame attach to him for the failure, thereby tarnishing his reputation (Edelstein, 1967, pp. 97-98). Thus, the sharp dichotomy between professional and businessman or entrepreneur does not emerge until more modern times.

By the Middle Ages of Western history medicine began to assume more of the trappings of a profession, but even as late as the nineteenth century, John Shaw Billings could divide physicians into three classes: a small group interested in patients mainly as material for their scientific studies, a larger group mainly interested in "money, or rather the social position, pleasures and power, which money only can bestow," and a majority who were not well-educated, clearly stretching the limits of the concept of professional (John Shaw Billings, 1876, cited in Brieger, 1995, p. 1693). None of the three seem to come close at all to qualifying as medical professionals in the sense of showing the mastery of a body of theory and dedication to patient welfare that we would associate with the moral notion of professional.

Clearly there are lines in the ancient Hippocratic literature that would support the concept of the medical professional as altruistic, patient-centered care-giver. That is the core of the Hippocratic ethic, with its appeal to the duty of the physician to benefit the patient according to his ability and judgment, but neither ancient Hippocratic nor modern Western physicians are devoid of more self-interested motivation. By 1986 the physician analyst of the *New England Journal of Medicine*, John Iglehart, could conclude that the medical "profession [in America] is increasingly being seen as more nearly a commercial enterprise with vested economic interests than a calling of professionals whose foremost concern is the well-being of the patient" (John Iglehart, cited in Brieger, 1995, p. 1694). The *Journal's* editor, Arnold Relman (1980, cf. Engelhardt and Rie, 1988), and others were attacking medicine as being too much a part of the "medical-industrial complex".

III. THE MODERN PHYSICIAN AS BUSINESS PERSON

The contrast between the physician as altruistic professional and the physician as more self-interested entrepreneur came to a head in the recent American debate over whether physician ownership of outside laboratories, diagnostic and imaging centers, and other for-profit business ventures poses a conflict of interest that is incompatible with the more altruistic role of the physician as patient-centered professional.[1] This debate raises fundamental questions about our understanding of the profession of medicine, its purpose and mission. Before we can know whether physicians engaged in clinical practice ought simultaneously to be owners or investors in outside facilities to which they might refer patients, we really need to know how we – the members of the profession and the broader society – understand what it means to be a physician. Before contrasting these images with Japanese understandings of the physician, we need to clarify alternative images of the physician in contemporary Western society and what the implications of those images are for the question of physician ownership and investment in profit-making facilities whose income can be influenced by the physician's clinical decisions.

I believe that much more is at stake than simply the risk that physician self-interest will occasionally influence patient decisions about the use of diagnostic and imaging centers. Our very conception of what it means to be a physician will be shaped by the policy decisions facing us.

This portion of this paper sets out, in broad brushstrokes, two alternative conceptualizations or models of the physician's role. By deciding how closely each of these fits with what a culture wants the physician to be in the twenty-first century, a framework for setting conflict of interest policy will be provided. Of course, as in any modeling exercise, it is unlikely that a culture will see itself as purely in one of these models or the other. Some elements of each may seem appropriate. Moreover, we are not suggesting that one or the other of these models is necessarily right – morally or legally. For this analysis, we are not addressing either the question of what is the most ethical understanding of the physician's role or what is currently legal. Once the models are set out and their implications understood, we believe society will be able to determine for itself what its policy regarding conflict of interest ought to be. Only when that decision is made will it be possible to ask the legal question of what the law ought to be and whether changes need to be made in current law to make the practice of medicine morally consistent with our image of a medical practitioner with ethical integrity.

IV. MODEL ONE: THE 'PROFESSIONAL' MODEL

Traditionally, medicine has been seen as a profession, a calling, in which its members have a set of responsibilities that are thought, in their core, to be essentially non-economic. The Hippocratic Oath, the traditional moral summary of the physician's ethic, pledges the physician to work only for the benefit of the patient according to the physician's ability and judgment. It places the morality of medicine in an almost religious context.

In fact, in its origins, the Hippocratic Oath almost certainly represents a quasi-religious philosophical-scientific cultic group, which, according to recent scholarship, was associated with the Greek philosophical school of Pythagoreanism. Thus the Hippocratic Oath does not grow out of the Judeo-Christian heritage that has come to so dominate the West. (In fact, some argue that there are many provisions in the Oath that are incompatible with Judaism and Christianity.) Nevertheless, the profession of medicine has roots that are related to religion-like responsibilities. The physician, like the priest, is expected to be what sociologists call "collectivity-oriented", that is, the professional is committed to the interests of the other party, not to self-interest. In fact, this is one characteristic that has traditionally separated true professionals from mere business people.

Of course, physicians, like priests, must have some material means of support. It would be naively romantic to assume that they could totally divorce themselves from some form of income. But, according to this traditional model, the profession of medicine should be as separate as possible from the business of medicine. Investing in the businesses to which one sends one's patients would be hard to justify. This is one of the reasons why physician ownership of pharmacies and physician dispensing has been controversial in Western culture. According to the model that views the practice of medicine as a calling, there should be no economic arrangement that could have any bearing on the physician's commitment to the patient's welfare. According to this view physicians should no more have ownership interests in the business of medicine than priests would have ownership in the business of marketing Bibles, choir robes, or other religious paraphernalia.

Problems with Viewing Medicine as a Profession

This understanding of the nature of medicine almost certainly will not be maximally lucrative. Still, it is not without its advantages. For example, it seems to place medicine on the moral high ground. While it treats the practice of medicine as something of an obligation calling for certain sacrifices, not the least of which might be financial, it also treats medicine as something ennobling. That is, in part, why some of the most respected practitioners of American medicine – people like Arnold Relman and Edmund Pellegrino – have spoken so forcefully in favor of this model.

Still there are potential problems with viewing medicine as an altruistic, patient-centered calling. Perhaps the most serious is the radical implication of the model if it were fully applied. One serious question is what the imperative to divorce the practice of the calling from any arrangements that could serve self-interest would mean for other practices of physicians. For example, physician ownership of or investment in hospitals would seem to raise similar questions to those raised by their involvement in practice-related joint ventures in laboratories and diagnostic centers.

More critically, what would be the implications for procedures within the physician's own office? Ordering of tests, x-rays, physical exams, follow-up appointments, or any other procedure that could generate income for the physician seems to raise the same issue as involvement in outside profit-making facilities. So do all compensation arrangements that make physician income related to the decisions made in the clinical setting. Not only all fee-for-service medicine, but also all managed care arrangements making physician income dependent on clinical practice decisions would be called in to question. Certainly, staff model HMOs and IPAs that reward physicians with bonuses if care is provided frugally link the practice of medicine to physician self-interest just as outside ownership of facilities does.

It has been argued that these conflicts of interests arising within the physician's own practice are different because they are more limited; physicians can only do so many physical exams a year while they can refer for unlimited diagnostic tests. This is not an entirely satisfactory response, however. For one, if the economic incentive is designed to limit care rather than provide it, the only limit of the influence is the point at which nothing is done for the patient. Moreover, even for traditional fee-for-service, there seems to be virtually no limit for procedures that would be done by office staff rather than by the physician him- or herself. Most significantly, it is not a very comforting argument to claim that in-office financial incentives should be permitted to continue within the model of the profession as a calling just because there might be limits to the abuse that can occur. If medicine is really understood by the profession and by society as a calling engaged in solely out of commitment to the patient, then the extent of the abuse does not seem relevant.

There are other problems in viewing the profession of medicine as a calling in which one is devoted solely to the welfare of the patient. If one is to act as a physician solely out of commitment to the patient, then logically one can never morally act out of self-interest or even out of the interest of others important to the physician, such as the physician's family. That, however, seems unrealistic. It is not even clear that morally that is what we should ask of physicians. Surely, at some point, physicians are entitled to incorporate their own interests and those of their family into their decisions. In the United States we assume that they must be expected, for example, to go on vacation, use answering services, and participate in coverage arrangements, even if those are not fully in accord with the patient's best interest. This model of medicine as a profession devoted solely to the welfare of patients seems romantic and unworkable.

The model of the physician as one engaged in an altruistic calling, if taken to its logical conclusion, makes the physician out to be superhuman. Even priests cannot live up to that high of a standard. In fact, the most radical critics of the profession of medicine are watching the current conflict of interest debate carefully. Some are hoping physicians will overstate their altruism, thus undercutting their credibility, while others are hoping physicians will proclaim their business mentality publicly, thus reducing them to the status of other self-interested entrepreneurs.

V. MODEL TWO: THE ENTREPRENEURIAL MODEL

This suggests the alternative model, to which Western culture has turned to base its response to the current conflict-of-interest debate. As we have seen, at times in its history, medicine has been conceptualized more as a craft than as a profession. Norms for the group existed, but there was no expectation that the patient or client would always be served at the expense of self-interest.

By the middle ages this notion of the physician as a craftsman was being replaced with the more professional model, complete with the characteristics of the profession including autonomy in setting internal norms, self-regulation, and, most critically for our purposes, the idea that service to the patient took priority over self-aggrandizement.

Still, there have been times at which more entrepreneurial interests have manifested themselves. The American ethos is one that condones, indeed savors, a rugged individualism. Individual achievement and pursuit of self-determined ends has been linked to American culture from its origins (Veatch, 1997). Whether as part of the Protestant pursuit of certainty of salvation or as a more secular ideology of the invisible hand, individual accomplishment has found a way to emerge as consistent with the more communal goals of advancement of a more social ethic. This has always permitted the physician to behave as if he were, in some sense, engaged in a small business.

However, even when physicians have behaved more like business people, there have been limits. Even ordinary business people have moral and legal limits placed on their behavior: they are not supposed to lie, deceive, or misrepresent their product. They must respect certain legal protections of trade secrets, etc. There is, if you like, an entrepreneurial ethic as well as a professional one.

Physicians have tended to become more entrepreneurial in the last decade or two. Flat prohibitions on advertising have been replaced by more limited prohibitions of false and misleading advertising, a requirement fitting for any business person. Concerns about market share, cost containment, pricing, and other market concepts have crept into the vocabulary of physicians. Outside non-physician ownership of the basic institutions of health care delivery has solidified the image that medicine is more like a business.

Nevertheless, clear differences are still perceived between entrepreneurial medicine and other businesses. Most critically, the buyer cannot always be expected to be in a position to evaluate what he or she is buying. Hence in the West, particularly in the United States, external standards are imposed on the conduct of physicians that are more severe than those imposed on other businesses. It is seen in the rules of informed consent, but also in the requirements of strict disclosure – a standard well beyond that applied to other, more ordinary business people.

Disclosure in the case of the more professional model of medicine as a calling, if it existed at all, served the purpose of presenting options to patients so that they could participate in the choice among reasonable alternatives. As long as the professional remained essentially patient-centered, disclosure was normally not necessary to protect the patient against possible conflicts of interest.

In the more entrepreneurial model, however, disclosure serves a more central, controversial role. As with research involving human subjects, entrepreneurial physicians are expected to disclose extensive information to patients precisely because a potential conflict of interest exists. Disclosure becomes one of the strategies for patient protection against abuse growing out of the economic self-interest of the provider, a function not normally necessary in the more professional model. The concern that the physician is losing professional altruism and adopting a more entrepreneurial spirit is one of the reasons that American patients are demanding more information and more control over their critical medical decisions (Veatch, 1995).

Problems with the Entrepreneurial Model

Just like the professional model of medicine as a calling, the entrepreneurial model poses difficult problems for medicine. Precisely because of the risk of conflicts of interest, there is a much higher standard of disclosure. Anglo-American law refers to the reasonable person standard as the standard now largely replacing the professional standard. Under it, clinicians must disclose all that the average, reasonable person would want to know (or find material) before deciding how to participate in a treatment plan. The key question is just what patients would want to know. The American Medical Association has long recognized the duty of the entrepreneurial physician to disclose any financial interests in outside facilities to which patients will be referred. But once the physician is conceptualized as having multiple agendas that are potentially in conflict and once informing patients is advocated as a means of protecting patients from the risks of conflicts of interest, surely much more needs to be disclosed. Patients would want to know the names of alternative facilities in which their physician has no business interests. Patients would plausibly want to know not only of the economic interests and alternative facilities; they would seemingly want to know what the economic incentives are that could influence their clinician (any special terms that make referral attractive to the physician, how rates of return compare to other investments, etc.). They would reasonably want to know how their physician's utilization rate compares to other physicians who do not have such investment interests. They would want to know whether other patients in similar situations would be exposed to similar risks. They would want to know what limits are placed on Medicare and

Medicaid patients, for instance. They would want to know the results of studies showing the effect of ownership on usage patterns. By the time patients are told all they would reasonably want to know about such entrepreneurial arrangements, it is possible that it would make referral of patients to facilities in which their primary physician has an ownership interest impossible.

There is no reason why the disclosure requirements should be limited to outside economic interests. The requirement plausibly would extend to in-office procedures, ordering of exams, tests, recommendations for surgery, etc.

There are more problems with the entrepreneurial model clinicians should consider. If patients begin to conceptualize physicians as part business people/part care givers, the arousal of patient suspicion could be much more pervasive. Trust in the patient/physician relation could be expected to decline – not only for those patients referred to physician-owned facilities, but also to all other patients who begin to learn of the new physician agenda. Once physicians are entrepreneurs, the lifestyle of the entrepreneur seems appropriate. Advertising would take on new meaning and new proportions. With a decline in trust, there is reason to believe that malpractice will increase still further. The result could be demeaning for the practitioner – a lowering of expectations of both patients and physicians. Physicians will gradually be thought of as business people, a special class of business people to be sure, but business people nonetheless. They would have agendas having nothing to do with service to patients.

There is a final problem with the emergence of entrepreneurialism in medicine. To the extent that multiple agendas are present that lead to the protective device of extensive disclosure requirements, outsiders are naturally going to begin to insist on increased regulation and protection. The safe harbor rules (government rules that specify ownership patterns that are presumed safe from criticism) would appear to be only the tip of the iceberg. Even if the substantial majority of physicians can be trusted, the adoption of the entrepreneurial model, in which multiple interests can be in conflict, over the one viewing the practice of medicine as a calling devoted exclusively to the welfare of the patient, means that the potential for abuse is present. An increase in outside regulation would seem inevitable. In its full form the entrepreneurial model could eventually lead to a market conception of medicine in which physicians no longer make decisions. Rather they market products and services while consumers shop and buy.

VI. THE RESOLUTION IN WESTERN CULTURE

This seems to leave the practice of medicine between a rock and a hard place. If we opt for the old, romantic view of medicine as a calling in which physicians are devoted solely to the welfare of the patient, physician ownership of outside medical services seems excluded in principle. But other entrepreneurial efforts such as hospital ownership, fee-for-service medicine, and financial incentives in managed care also seem to be called into question. This requires of physicians almost superhuman altruism, more than we have a right to expect. The professional model has radical implications, carrying far beyond the issues of outside ownership interests.

On the other hand, if physicians adopt a more modest strategy, they are faced with disclosure requirements that seem to go far beyond what even new and relatively enlightened defenders of the entrepreneurial model would seem to require. They lower society's image of the physician to a special kind of business entrepreneur. They invite further outside regulation. Potentially they destroy the reputation of the medical practitioner.

It would be tempting to strive for some kind of compromise between the views of the physician as a single-minded noble servant of the patient and as a special kind of business person, an entrepreneur who will try to avoid sacrificing the patient's interests to the physician's other projects. However, a compromise runs the risk of building medicine of the twenty-first century into the worst of both worlds – neither a noble, almost priest-like servant, nor a realistic entrepreneur bound by the morality of an honest business person. Before society can assess its policy regarding financial interests in outside medical facilities, it may first have to choose which image of medicine it wants to project in the new century.

VII. THE ROLE OF THE PHYSICIAN IN JAPANESE CULTURE

One who takes Dr. Hoshino's work seriously would be wary of assuming that this controversy over the entrepreneurial and professional models of the physician role can be transferred to other countries such as Japan. On the other hand, contemporary world cultures are sufficiently interdependent that one would expect that this tension between business and professional conceptualizations would raise recognizable issues. At the same time, one would expect that the problem may have a very different history and would take on a very different character. Unfortunately, my knowledge of Japanese culture does not permit a full analysis; it, at most, lets some questions be raised.

The questions that appear to need attention include whether a business/professional distinction can be found in Japanese culture that is comparable to that found in the United States, in which business people are expected to pursue self-interest within a set of moral constraints while professionals are expected to altruistically serve patients while receiving compensation for their work. Dr. Hoshino has on a number of occasions given an account of the traditional paternalism of Japanese medicine and the absence of an emphasis on autonomy or self-determination of patients (Hoshino, 1992, pp. 379-80; 1995a; 1997; see also Tsuchida, 1992; Ishiwata and Sakai, 1994, pp. 61-62, 64). It would appear that this combination of reliance on physician judgment and reluctance of patients to assert their own choices would heighten the responsibility of the physician to act with a sense of duty to the patient. Dr. Hoshino has pointed out that the Japanese Criminal Code requires physicians to act "so as not to cause possible disorders or adverse effects in their patients" (Hoshino, 1992, p. 380). All of this seems to suggest a duty to benefit the patient that fits what Westerners would consider the professional rather than the business conceptualization.

While Western, especially American, culture struggles with the relation between the business and the entrepreneurial spirit, Japanese culture may find professionalism in tension with a different norm. For Japanese medicine, the dynamic that strikes an outside observer is the problem of the relative authority of the physician and the patient's family. While professionalism implies autonomy of the professional as an independent, if paternalistic, decision-maker, Western students of Japanese culture are told that it manifests a "mutual dependency" (Tanida, 1996, p. 202; see also Tsuchida, 1998). According to Tanida (1996, p. 202), "the personality of Japanese people is not something that belongs to an individual, but rather something which belongs to the family, community, or society" (See also Tsuchida, 1998, and Ohi, 1998). Thus Dr. Hoshino, in his commentaries on the Japanese concept of *was*, shows how the family emerges as the collective decision-maker. The patient, he suggests, will defer to the family, reflecting the connotations of the Japanese term best expressed in English as conciliation, concord, unity, harmony, or submission (Hoshino, 1995a, pp. 71-72). The Japanese concept of *amae*, best expressed in English as *dependence*, is frequently cited as a central characteristic of the Japanese personality (Doi, 1981). What strikes an outsider as puzzling is the apparent tension between this pervasive *amae* or mutual dependence and the assertive, authoritarian dominance that is associated with the professional as paternalistic decision-maker. Could it be that the traditional Japanese rejection of individualism and self-determination minimizes the significance of the alternative of the entrepreneurial model while posing the traditional ideal of family healer as the model that contrasts with the physician as autonomous professional?

VIII. FROM FILIAL DUTY TO MERE PROFESSIONAL: CONFUCIAN CONCEPTIONS OF THE HEALER

The influence on Japan from China of both Confucian and Buddhist thought has often been noted (Kimura, 1994; Takemi, 1978; Kitagawa, 1995). A provocative study of ancient Chinese medical ethics by the German social historian Paul Unschuld suggests a pair of alternative models for the physician's role: the healer as family member and the healer as professional. With the greatest of hesitancy as an outsider, I suggest that this tension may pose to Japan a set of alternatives that is analogous to the Western contrast between the physician as professional and as entrepreneur. Unschuld (1979, pp. 232, 109) claims that classical ancient Confucian medicine was a resource managed within a family. According to Unschuld:

> In Confucian society the attempt was made (although it did not become reality) to give each individual so much medical training that medical care within the family would be guaranteed, and beyond this to put medical practice outside the limitations of the family into the hands of civil servants, who were to practice only on the basis of a service orientation and not on the basis of profit maximumization (1979, p. 116).

Hence one of the classical Confucian medical ethical virtues – in addition to humaneness (*jen*) and compassion (*tz'u*) – was filial piety (*hsiao*) (Unschuld, 1978, p. 200). The idea of a virtue for the physician based on familial relations is incomprehensible in Western culture. Indeed, in the West it is considered inappropriate for a physician to practice medicine on a family member. The emotional involvement is considered too intense to permit the proper detachment needed for the healer's role.

Unschuld claims that only when the familial practice of medicine proved impossible did the patient have to make do with a "mere professional", that is, one who practiced medicine as an occupation outside of family ties with the necessary requirement that it generate an income. The impact of Confucian medical ethics was to give an account of how physicians could be trusted with medical wisdom even though they were not part of the family structure.

Is it too much of a stretch to say that Japanese medicine is still struggling with this ambiguity of the relation between the family and the professional physician who is not part of the family? It is remarkable to an outsider that the acceptance of the role of the patient as passive, dependent personality leads to acceptance of the authority simultaneously of the family and the physician without raising what appears to a Westerner to be the obvious question of what should happen when family and physician disagree.

It seems clear that the concern of autonomy and paternalism leads Westerners to be concerned about authority relations in the roles of patient and physician. While the professional role with its commitment to altruism commits the physician to the welfare of the patient, increasingly we acknowledge that physicians, like all other human beings, must pursue self-interest. The mere fact that the welfare of the patient is the announced concern of the physician does not satisfy the concern about paternalism. Some more radical critics have even gone so far as to prefer the entrepreneurial model in which any guise of altruism is supplanted with an openly-admitted economic self-interest. At least then the patient knows where he stands and has a more forthright basis for insisting on adequate information to make personal choices about medical treatments.

It seems that to the Japanese mind, with its relative disinterest in autonomy and its greater concern for relations of *was* and *amae*, the collective cooperation of family and physician can embrace the professional and familial perspectives with only the very recent hint that medicine is mathematics rather than humaneness, *san-jyutsu* rather than *jin-jyutsu*. We can only hope that we have minds as wise and as cosmopolitan as Kazumasa Hoshino's to help us understand the proper role of the physician in these times in which family, professionalism, and entrepreneurship are posing such difficult challenges.

Georgetown University
Washington, D.C., U.S.A.

NOTE

[1] I served as a consultant to the American Medical Association during its review of this debate. With their permission, in this paper I draw on some of the conceptual analysis done for them.

REFERENCES

Bowers, J. Z. (1970). *Western Medical Pioneers in Feudal Japan.* Baltimore: The Johns Hopkins University Press.

Brieger, G. H. (1995). 'Medicine as a profession.' In: W. T. Reich (Ed.), *Encyclopedia of Bioethics*, Vol. III, (pp. 1688-1697). New York: Macmillan.

Doi, T. (1981). *The Anatomy of Dependence.* Tokyo: Kodansha International Ltd..

Edelstein, L. (1967). 'The Hippocratic physician.' In: Owsei Temkin and C. Lilian Temkin (Eds.), C. Lilian Temkin (Trans.), *Ancient Medicine: Selected Papers of Ludwig Edelstein* (pp. 87-110). Baltimore: The Johns Hopkins Press.

Engelhardt, H. T. Jr., and Rie, M. A. (1988). 'Morality for the medical-industrial complex: A code of ethics for the mass marketing of health care.' *New England Journal of Medicine* 319(16), 1086-1089.

Hoshino, K. and Saito, T. (Eds.) (1991). *Taiji no Seimei to Songen [The Life and Dignity of the Fetus].* Tokyo: Sokyusha. [In Japanese and English]

Hoshino, K. (1992). 'Bioethics in Japan: 1989-1991.' In: B. Andrew Lustig, Baruch A. Brody, H. Tristram Engelhardt, Jr., and Laurence B. McCullough (Eds.), *Bioethics Yearbook. Vol. 4., Regional Developments in Bioethics 1989-1991* (pp. 379-387). Dordrecht: Kluwer Academic Publishers.

Hoshino, K. (1995a). 'Autonomous decision making and Japanese tradition.' *Cambridge Quarterly of Healthcare Ethics* 3, 71-74.

Hoshino, K., assisted by Tomoaki Tsuchida and Akira Akabayashi (1995b). *Shi no Songen - Nichibei no Seimei Rinri* [*Dignity of Death - Bioethics in Japan and U.S.A.*], Kyoto: Shibunkaku Shuppan.

Hoshino, K. (1997). 'Bioethics in the light of Japanese sentiments.' In: Kazumasa Hoshino (Ed.), *Japanese and Western Bioethics* (pp. 13-23). Dordrecht: Kluwer Academic Publishers.

Ishiwata, R. and Sakai, A. (1994). 'The physician-patient relationship and medical ethics in Japan.' *Cambridge Quarterly of Healthcare Ethics* 3, 60-66.

Kimura, R. (1991). 'Fiduciary relationships and the medical professional: A Japanese point of view.' In: Edmund D. Pellegrino, Robert M. Veatch, and John P. Langan (eds.), *Ethics, Trust, and the Professions* (pp. 235-245). Washington, D.C.: Georgetown University Press, Washington, D.C.

Kimura, R. (1994). 'Bioethics and Japanese health care.' *Washington-Japan Journal* 2 (No. 4), 1-8, 12.

Kitagawa, J. M. (1995). 'Medical ethics, history of: Japan through the nineteenth century.' In: Warren T. Reich (Ed.), *Encyclopedia of Bioethics*, 2nd ed (pp. 1491-1496). New York: Macmillan.

Ohi, G. (1998). 'Advance directives and Japanese ethos.' In: Hans-Martin Sass, Robert M. Veatch, and Rihito Kimura (eds.), *Advance Directives and Surrogate Decision Making in Transcultural Perspective.* Baltimore: Johns Hopkins University Press.

Relman, A. S. (1980). 'The new medical-industrial complex.' *New England Journal of Medicine* 303 (17), 963-970.

Takemi, T. (1978). 'Medical ethics, history of: Traditional professional ethics in Japanese medicine.' In: Warren T. Reich (Ed.), *Encyclopedia of Bioethics,* Vol. III (pp. 924-926). New York: The Free Press.

Takemi, T. (1994). 'Human survival science and bioethics.' In: *Ethical Dilemmas in Health and Development* (pp. xv-xxxii). Tokyo: Japan Scientific Societies Press.

Tanida, N. (1996). 'Bioethics is subordinate to morality in Japan.' *Bioethics* 10, 201-211.

Tsuchida, T. A. (1998). 'Yet ambivalent about advance directives.' In: Hans-Martin Sass, Robert M. Veatch, and Rihito Kimura (eds.), *Advance Directives and Surrogate Decision Making in Transcultural Perspective.* Baltimore: Johns Hopkins University Press.

Tsuchida, T. (1992). 'From ethos to ethics: Japanese views on life and death.' In: Institute of Medical Humanities (Ed.), *Toward a New Replenishment of Medical Education and Hospital Service* (pp. 319-325). Tokyo: Kitasato University.

Unschuld, P. U. (1978). 'Confucianism.' In: Warren T. Reich (Ed.), *Encyclopedia of Bioethics* (pp. 200-204). New York: The Free Press.

Unschuld, P. U. (1979). *Medical Ethics in Imperial China: A Study in Historical Anthropology.* Berkeley: University of California Press.

Veatch, R. M. (Ed.) (1989). *Cross Cultural Perspectives in Medical Ethics: Readings.* Boston: Jones and Bartlett.

Veatch, R. M. (1995). 'Hikakubunkateki Shiten karamita Shumatsuki-Iryo no Rinri' ['Ethics of terminal care from a comparative-cultural point of view']. In: Kazumasa Hoshino (Ed., assisted by Tomoaki Tsuchida and Akira Akabayashi), *Shi no Songen - Nichibei no Seimei Rinri [Dignity of Death - Bioethics in Japan and U.S.A.]* (pp. 179-190). Kyoto: Shibunkaku Shuppan.

Veatch, R. M. (1997). 'Autonomy and communitarianism: The ethics of terminal care in cross-cultural perspective.' In: Kazumasa Hoshino (Ed.), *Japanese and Western Bioethics* (pp. 119-129). Dordrecht: Kluwer Academic Publishers.

TANGJIA WANG

THE PHYSICIAN-PATIENT RELATIONSHIP AND INDIVIDUALIZATION OF TREATMENT FROM THE VIEW OF TRADITIONAL CHINESE MEDICAL PRACTICE

I. INTRODUCTION

Behind every system of medicine hides a set of ethical values that immanently dominate persons' attitudes toward disease and death, and exert a subtle influence upon both the physician-patient relationship and paradigm of medicine in society. With the development of increasingly sophisticated technology, the specialization of modern medicine and the rise of the civil rights movements, we increasingly fall into ethical dilemmas concerning the physician-patient relationship. Now, we should open our eyes to a usually neglected fact that "modern medicine suffers from the loss of the authentic personal relationship crucial in medicine and medicine care" (Hui, 1996, p. 5).

Obviously, the possibilities of rational orientation for a harmonious physician-patient relationship lay neither in a sophisticated technology itself, nor in the specialization of medicine, but rather in the development of a new paradigm of medicine, and in communication, understanding and coordination between physician and patient, and in intercultural, multicultural or transcultural dialogue and cooperation of different systems of medicine.

I believe modern medicine might draw some inspiration and wisdom from traditional Chinese medicine and thereby recover the importance of the relational dimension intrinsic to the clinical encounter between physician and patient. I shall proceed in this paper by first demonstrating the limitations of four models of the physician-patient relationship. Then I shall state the main problems with the physician-patient relationship in society. Finally I shall clarify the principle of individualization in traditional Chinese medicine and its meaning for the paradigm of modern medicine.

H.T. Engelhardt, Jr. and L.M. Rasmussen (eds.), Bioethics and Moral Content: National Traditions of Health Care Morality, 35–46.

II. THE LIMITATIONS OF THE AUTONOMY MODEL

Generally speaking, there are four possible models of the physician-patient relationship: beneficence, entrustment, partnership, and autonomy. Despite this generalization, there is not always a very clear demarcation among them in actual clinical practice, and sometimes several models co-exist, probably depending on the concrete situation (Wolff, 1994).

Hippocratic medicine has been treated as the beneficence model in which some kind of ethical paternalism is involved. On the beneficence model, a physician should regard it as a "categorical imperative" to maximize the patient's medical benefits regardless of what kind of demand the patient has made on him. At the same time, "the patient should obey the doctor's commands and even must place himself in the physician's hand" (Beauchamp, 1990), since the well-being of the patient takes precedence over everything else. Before the ideas of a right-based ethic gained worldwide dissemination in the 1960s, the beneficence model played a dominant role in almost every society.

In traditional Chinese medicine, it is the highest principle for a physician to help patients rid themselves completely of their ailments and to help seriously ill patients to take a turn for the better. Until now, "conscientious in medical treatment and miraculously bringing the dying back to life" has been the highest praise for a physician. Confucian ethics of virtue emphasizes that a physician should first have the heart of benevolence and the sense of duty of a noble man. This conception was completely kept even if other ethical values were destroyed during the Cultural Revolution of the 1960s and 1970s.

The entrustment model states that the physician-patient relationship is something like the relationship between lawyer and client, where the physician autonomously offers special diagnosis and treatment, such as laboratory tests, local anesthesia, general examinations, etc., without the special permission of the patient. On this model, the interests of both sides are considered at the same time. From the beginning, the patient transfers his right of decision-making to the physician; the physician by himself decides how to serve the patient. This model, which is usually employed only by those patients who are not severely ill, is characterized by a balance between the right of the patient and the objective of the physician, based on the trust, honesty and autonomy of the patient. The ethics of entrustment may provide the foundation for this model.

The partnership model states that the physician acts as an advisor-expert to the patient, who is an active partner, responsible for himself. But generally the model is only applied to cases where the patient hopes to get advice from the physician about how to prevent, limit or improve various chronic diseases such as heart disease, hypertension, diabetes, etc. Under this model, the responsibility of the physician is mainly to help the patient to help himself, but the patient's self-orientation, self-determination and self-responsibility always take priority over other considerations in the physician-patient relationship. To make an important contribution, the patient must have some experience with self-observation and self-examination of the main symptoms such as blood pressure, blood sugar, pulse and so on, in order to adopt further effective measures to control the illness. The success of the partnership between physician and patient depends on the intelligence, medical knowledge, life experience and meticulousness of the patient. Discourse ethics in Habermas' sense may provide foundation for this model.

The autonomy model states that mentally competent patients have the right to make the final decision on treatment plan or surgery when there is a conflict between the patient's wishes and the physician's advice about the best possible treatments. On this model, the physician has a duty to present all information and to act on the patient's wishes even when the patient refuses some treatment (for instance, the refusal of blood transfusion by some Jehovah's Witnesses). In this case, the physician can tell the patient all kinds of advantages and disadvantages of treatment and then wait for the patient to make the decision. The physician need not be morally responsible for any failure of treatment (including the death of the patient) derived from the false or foolish autonomous choice of the patient. Therefore, to follow the dictate of the patient seems to be the ethical imperative for the physician. Here, we could find that the autonomy model deals with the physician-patient relationship only in light of the patient's wishes, so we would call it the subjective model. On the contrary, the beneficence model deals with the physician-patient relationship in light of the best results of treatment, so we would call it the objective model. In comparison with the beneficence model, the autonomy model is mainly concerned with the rights of the patient. This explains why the autonomy model could not play a dominant role in medical practice before the right-based ethic began to dominate in Western society. As Thomas Murray said, "autonomy sometimes appears to be regarded as a kind of universal moral solvent" (Murray, 1994).

However, the uncritical acceptance of the autonomy model in any case is leading to the crisis of the physician-patient relationship (Hoshino, 1997), which is a symptom of the trust crisis in modern society. On the one hand, faced with the crisis, modern medicine needs self-reflection and self-criticism; physicians should ask themselves what destroyed patients' trust in physicians. On the other hand, we should ask if we have lost the ethical value of respect for life, which is, in my opinion, the highest value of human beings and the final reason for the existence of medicine. What kind of choice is rational when respect for the life of a patient and respect for the right of a patient clash? In a developing society with terrible shortages of medical resources, allowing unlimited autonomy can sometimes harm the common good, because the physician lacks time and energy enough to explain every detail of all treatment alternatives again and again. Suppose that the physician had to treat 100 patients one day; if one patient takes too much of the physician's time, many other patients would not get treatments immediately. Therefore, in a society short of medical resources, the beneficence model is still the only realistic choice, but it should not exclude the possibility of patients participating in the decision-making of treatments. It should be admitted that this model has its problems, especially in a society with increasing emphasis upon the right to individual self-determination. When a skillful physician does not know what kind of treatment is best for the patient, the patient must know if a possible treatment is worth the expense.

Clearly, it perhaps increases unease and anxiety to set aside the wishes of the patient. Once the patient becomes a passive object without any subjectivity in the beneficence model, we could not rule out the possibility that a few physicians use patients as objects of experiments for the purpose of personal academic achievements. As is now known, some physicians under the Nazi regime even carried out involuntary euthanasia on deformed persons under the pretext of beneficence. For these reasons, the traditional strong beneficence model should be changed into the weak one by introducing the autonomy of the patient into clinical life. That is to say, in the majority of cases the patient's right of self-determination should be respected, but if there is conflict between respect for life and the right of autonomy, we should value the former over the latter. Since society forbids drivers to drink alcohol, forces motorcyclists to wear helmets, and prohibits drug-taking or smoking, why does society not go so far as to allow the physician to save patients who ignore his wishes when it certainly means death for the patient to refuse some kind of treatment?

In fact, we need a kind of autonomy grounded in the respect for life, which is the starting point and the highest goal of all systems of medicine. At any rate, we should ask ourselves what kind of autonomy is rational and what kind of autonomy is irrational. If autonomy were rational in any case, drug takers would have good reason to say that ingesting cocaine is rational. In contemporary society, autonomy is often abused. Etymologically, the term autonomy is derived from Greek *autos* (self) and *nomos* (rule, law, or governance), which means self-determination as well as self-limitation based on some universal principle. As Confucius said, "Do as you please, but not beyond limits of rule" (Confucius, 1996, p.31).

As inheritors of the Greek spirit, Westerners should understand this point. Only acting freely on a universal moral imperative can be classified as real autonomy as opposed to heteronomy in the Kantian sense. Regrettably, some people separate absolutely the two aspects of autonomy. In other words, they try to keep the "self-determination" part of the meaning, but exclude the "self-limitation on the basis of a universal rule" part, so that acting on one's own will becomes an overwhelming value to some people.

However, there can be no harmonious and fruitful physician-patient relationship if the physician and patient act only on their respective wills without commonly recognized ethical principles, among which the respect for life, I think, is the first. The crisis of the contemporary physician-patient relationship is the crisis of both the traditional beneficence model and the autonomy model, whereas total autonomy is a radical reaction to strong paternalism. Among a number of factors related to the crisis, the most important are the rise of civil rights movements, the marketization of medicine, the specialization of medicine and the wide use of high-tech equipment.

The rise of the civil rights movement awakens the consciousness of self-determination in people and thus makes patients unsatisfied with simply following the commands of physicians. In this way, "When applied to the practice of medicine the idea of a right-based ethic clashed with the Hippocratic model of beneficence. The dawn of the patient autonomy movement changed the paradigm of ethics from a physician-based model of beneficence to a patient-based model of autonomy" (Voth, 1996). For this reason, the feminist movement is a strong challenge to the traditional conception of abortion. Similarly, voluntary euthanasia seems to be a realization of the so-called "right to death" for some people. Because mercy killing is morally unacceptable in Hippocratic medicine as well as traditional Chinese medicine, some physicians who believe in the holiness of life feel themselves trapped in ethical dilemmas which confront the alternatives of respect for life and respect for the wish to die.

The marketization of medicine greatly changed the face of the physician-patient relationship. On the one hand, physicians seem to become a special interest group whose motivation to work is the acquisition of social wealth (although they still keep some nominal professional ideals of the past). In its pursuit of interest, medicine as a profession is approaching other profit-oriented professions. Correspondingly, the physician-patient relationship is becoming an interest relationship. As a result, the beneficent image of the physician is eroded and the patient's trust in the physician is naturally threatened, especially when, for example, the patient has to pay very high expenses caused by unnecessary examinations. On the other hand, with the prevalence of commercialism in the medical field, the patient comes gradually to understand the physician-patient relationship as a relationship between service-giver and customer. Hence, patients always have to protect themselves against any possible infringement of their rights of autonomy.

Specialization in medicine brought the separation of diagnosis from the treatment of disease and thus changed the traditional one-to-one relationship between the physician and the patient into the relationship between a patient and the community of physicians. When a patient must encounter many unfamiliar faces in order to have his serious illness treated, long waits for test results will reinforce the patient's unease, anxiety and helplessness. It is particularly obvious when the diagnosis and treatment of some diseases must be done with the coordination and cooperation of several departments of a hospital. In modern medicine, the independence and authority of physicians is limited due to the fiscal and practice surveillance by government, public opinion and law. When the physician takes double responsibilities for the patient and society, he would rather become a functionary and focus his mind not on how to deal with his personal relation to the patient but on his specialized activities. This is why the patient sometimes finds physicians to have icy manners.

The autonomy model is a result of the wide use of high-tech equipment and various new medicines with side effects. No doubt the patients benefit much from the development of medical technology, but the demand for standardization and conformity of treatment associated with the use of high-tech equipment discourages the physician from developing a personal connection to patients with anxieties, fears, dreams and the desire to be cared for. The various machines and equipment seem to become a barrier between the physician and patient. In a factory-like hospital, patients tend to be treated as if they were products on the line, and the physician becomes, as it were, a white-coated technician or engineer. Patients hope to have a connection with the physician when they anxiously wait for the examination of an x-ray, CT, etc., when they are objectivized in the examination, or when they are regarded as a diseased object. Today, patients face many more choices in diagnosis and treatment and more uncertain factors (including more or less potential harm to them) than in the previous era. Patients' worries about side-effects increase in proportion to this uncertainty, and may have a negative impact on the credibility of medicine and the physician. Against this background, the patient's autonomy becomes a means of self-protection against potential harms, whether or not any physician actually intends to harm a patient.

III. A LESSON FROM TRADITIONAL CHINESE MEDICAL PRACTICE

How can we overcome the crisis of the physician-patient relationship in contemporary society? Maybe nobody can provide a completely satisfactory solution to the problem once and for all, but it is possible for us to develop a mutually edifying relation between the physician and the patient. First, we should recognize the limitations of the above-mentioned models among which the physician-based model and the patient-based model are not reliable enough to form a harmonious relationship because of their imbalance. Second, we need to reestablish the mutual trust of the physician and patient for the sake of a creative solution to the above problem. Third, we should recognize a hierarchy of principles in the face of irreconcilable differences. Finally, we should construct a healthy system of modern medicine conducive to the formation of an authentic personal physician-patient relationship by critical adoption of the principle of individualization maintained by traditional Chinese medicine.

In clinical practice, traditional Chinese medicine (TCM) attaches great importance to treatment individualized to the patient, season and locality. The treatment individualized to patients is characterized by respect for individual differences in many aspects such as age, sex, constitution, mental state, way of life, etc. Based on the categorical identification of disease, the compatibility of Chinese herbs must always be changed according to the individual situations of patients, even if they suffer from the same disease in Western medicine's opinion. So, strictly speaking, there is no standard prescription in TCM, although one could find the so-called basic prescription for many diseases in some textbooks of medicine. According to *Internal Classical*, the Bible of TCM, persons should be divided into 25 types and the same prescription is not appropriate to different patients with the same disease. It is for the purpose of treatment individualized to patient that even in the 2nd Century B.C., Chun Ruyi, physician of the Western Han Dynasty, made case histories in the modern sense.

Treatment individualized to the season takes the position that the compatibility of herbs should be adjusted to the features of the changing climates of different seasons. *Internal Classical* formulated this principle as follows: "the use of cold medicine should be far from cold climate, the use of cool medicine far from cool climate, the use of warm medicine far from warm climate, the use of heat medicine far from heat climate" (Huang Ti Internal Classics, 1963, p. 461). (Here, cold, warmth, and heat refer to the character of medicines; they do not mean temperature in an ordinary sense.)

Treatment individualized to locality means that the physician should take account of the features of different localities when he prescribes for the patient. For example, in the cold and dry area, moist herbs are generally given to the patient, whereas in the rainy area, herbs reducing dampness should be used to treat diseases.

The principle of individualization has its origin in classical Chinese philosophy. According to this philosophy, the human body is an open system communicating with the universe and disease is related to six excessive atmospheric factors, the deficiency of vital energy, and seven emotional factors. As a miniature of the universe, the human body is something like Leibniz's monad--everybody seems to be a micro-universe different from each other, but each commonly reflects the larger universe. In the world, no patients are identical, just as no leaves are identical. Therefore, respect for individual differences is fundamental to the treatment of patients in TCM as opposed to the standardized treatment emphasized by Western medicine.

The principle of individualization demands that an authentic personal physician-patient relationship be formed to promote a harmonious cooperation between physician and patient, which proves to be an important condition of successful treatment. TCM emphasizes the mutuality of the physician-patient relationship which doesn't arise from the convention of both sides, but rather from the ethical requirements of society as whole, because physician and patient, as members of a social community, are subjected to universal ethical values such as honesty, integrity, compassion, benevolence, respect for life, etc. Substantially, the ethical values of TCM are only a concretization of the universal Confucian ethic. The moral requirements of the society to the physician are also the moral requirements to all social members including the patient.

Since the physician-patient relationship is an interaction, only mutual efforts can create a harmonious atmosphere conducive to fruitful cooperation. Therefore, traditional Chinese society proposed ten rules for the physician and the patient respectively, which were admirably summarized by Paul U. Unschuld (1974, S.352-355). The following are the rules for the patient:

1) Choose a skillful physician.
2) Be willing to take medicine.
3) Go to see the physician as early as possible.
4) Do not have sexual intercourse until you are restored to health.
5) Do not be angry.
6) Eat and drink rationally.
7) Do not be troubled with terrible ideas.
8) Do not believe in heresy.
9) Reduce social contact and go to sleep on time.
10) Pay for the physician.

In many respects, Chinese moral requirements to the physician are similar to the ideas that the Hippocratic oath and Geneva Declaration of WMA formulate. For instance, they emphasize that the physician should respect life, act as a benevolent person, give priority to the patient's interests, keep the patient's secrets, and treat all patients indiscriminately.

With regard to the last point, Sun Simiao, a famous Chinese physician of the 7th Century, formulated it most completely: "All patients asking for treatments should be treated equally without discrimination as if they were your intimate persons, whether they are poor or rich, noble or lowly, old or young, beautiful or ugly, hostile or friendly, Chinese or foreigner, intelligent or foolish" (Sun Simiao, 1955, p. 1).

Considering the close connections between emotions and diseases, TCM asks the physician to become a physician of the soul, an understanding interlocutor, a listener who really knows the anxiety, hopes, fears, and wishes of the patient, in order to make the patient experience heartfelt care from the physician. In other words, the physician should not regard the patient as an object or a machine. For this reason, the authentic personal relation between physician and patient is morally encouraged in TCM.

However, the model of the physician-patient relationship in TCM is not simply the beneficence model but a mixture of several models, although the beneficence model plays the main role in most cases. After all, for lack of special medical knowledge, a patient has to place himself on the passive side. The patient has almost no alternatives when he has an acute or serious illness. In this case, it is just best for the patient's interests if we give priority to the beneficence model. On the contrary, the patient's total autonomy here would quickly reduce the effectiveness of the treatment and the physician's enthusiasm to a stalling point, thus putting the patient in a dangerous situation.

In fact, the autonomy model is not only a product of rights-based ethical trends, it is also the result of a cold impersonal relationship between physician and patient in modern society, as well as the by-product of the patient's worry about possible side effects of the treatments and medicine. If the treatments are safe and reliable, it is unnecessary for the patient to focus his mind on the autonomous decision of treatments. Therefore, developing effective treatments and medicines without side effects promotes harmonious physician/patient relationships.

One of the problems plaguing Western medicine has been side-effects. TCM is regarded as a good way to reduce side effects. Therefore, in almost every large hospital in China, there is a special department of TCM in which not only are many chronic and complicated diseases effectively treated, but also herbal medicine is used to reduce the side effects caused by radiation and chemical treatment. It is said that for several hundred types of medical and surgical problems, the coordination of TCM with Western medicine is better than either one used alone. In this case, the patient's trust in the physician is easily formed due to the herbal medicine's ability to blunt side effects.

In treatment individualized to the patient, face-to-face communication enables the patient to know everything he wishes from the physician. At the same time, the patient is more ready to express his ideas, anxieties, hopes, fears and wishes, which helps naturally to reduce his mental stress. On the other hand, the physician needs to know the emotion, food, drink and daily life of the patient in order to treat the disease effectively. The patient usually must know what kinds of foods he should avoid. So, while the physician seems to be an advisor-expert, the patient becomes an inquirer. In addition, the patient or his family must prepare medicinal herbs following the physician's instructions, which can reinforce the patient's sense of self-responsibility. That is why we assert that the physician-patient relationship in TCM is a mixture of the partnership model, the beneficence model and the entrustment model, including the autonomy of the patient.

How is individualization of treatment possible under the conditions of modern medical technology? On the one side, modern medicine, characterized by standardization and specialization, should continue to adopt the conception of holistic and dialectical treatment proposed by TCM and focus much more energy, money and technology on prevention of diseases following the principle, "prevention is preferable to treatment," suggested by TCM more than two thousand years ago. On the other side, indeed, we should transform more radically the traditional bio-medical paradigm into a bio-psycho-socio-environmental paradigm of medicine, which demands a new way of medical education and professional training suitable to this change. Moreover, we should change the present situation in which people one-sidedly emphasize the effectiveness of medical means, including medicine but neglecting its side effects, in order to bring a sense of security to patients when they face many treatment alternatives. Reducing side effects, in the holistic view of TCM, is a more effective treatment. I believe modern medicine will move to an era of individualized treatment, just as modern industry is changing from mass manufacturing to somewhat more individualized production of goods.

Fudan University
Shanghai, China

REFERENCES

Beauchamp, T.L. (1990). 'The promise of the beneficence model for medical ethics.' *Journal of Contemporary Health, Law & Policy* 6, 145-155.

Confucius (1996). *The Anelects of Confucius,* with a commentary by lai Kuohong. Shanghai: Fudan University Press.

Hoshino, K. (1997). 'Bioethics in the light of Japanese sentiments.' In: K. Hoshino (Ed.), *Japanese and Western Bioethics* (pp. 13-24). Dordrecht: Kluwer Academic Publishers.

Huang Ti Internal Classical (1963). Beijing: The Press of People's Health.

Hui, E. (Ed.) (1996). 'Introduction of editor.' *Christian Character, Virtue & Bioethics.* Vancouver: Regent College.

Murray, J.J. (1994). 'Individualism and community: The contested terrain of autonomy.' *Hastings Center Report* 24, 32-33.

Sun Simiao (1955). '*Da Yi Jin Chen.*' In: *Invaluable Prescriptions for Ready Reference.* Beijing: Press of People's Health.

Unschuld, P.U. (1974). 'Medizin und Ethik. Sozialkonflikte im China der Kaiserzeit. Wiesbaden' Steiner. Cf. Anhang in *Medizin und Ethik,* Hrsg von Hans-Martin Sass. Phillip Reclam jun, Stuttgart. 1994, S.352-355.

Voth, A. (1996). 'Physician beneficence, patient autonomy and Christian values.' In: E.C. Hui (Ed.), *Christian Character, Virtue & Bioethics* (pp. 199-217). Vancouver: Regent College.

Wolff, H. P. (1994). 'Arzt und Patient.' In: H.-M. Sass (Ed.), *Medizin und Ethik* (pp. 184-212). Stuttgart: Philipp Reclam jun.

PART II

MEDICAL TECHNOLOGIES AND NATIONAL BIOETHICS

HANS-MARTIN SASS

MEDICAL TECHNOLOGIES AND UNIVERSAL ETHICS IN TRANSCULTURAL PERSPECTIVE

> "It would be extremely difficult to change the ethos of a country by invoking theoretical arguments or rational approaches."
>
> (Kazumasa Hoshino)

I. RESPECT FOR PERSONS: A EUROPEAN NARRATIVE ON UNIVERSAL ETHICS

Controversies over the moral and cultural properties of medical technologies are rooted in differences of individual and collective values and wishes, systems of belief and reference, and in traditions towards medicine, life, the preservation of life and the acceptance of death. These controversies shape the self-understanding and the self-determination of educated individuals as well as the course of transcultural dialogue and the evolution of cultures and attitudes. Discourse, understanding, controversy, and tolerance are the life and blood of peaceable and free societies, based on the respect for persons, the recognition of individual conscience and the risks, obligations and rights associated with choice and error. The alternative to our post-enlightenment and post-modern discourses and quarrels over values and visions would be hierarchical systems of heteronymous domination, torture, and ideational exploitation and tutelage – systems developed by self-proclaimed philosopher-kings and priest-czars for the exploitation of their fellow humans, beginning in pre-historic times, successful from the times of the pharaohs through the dark ages and middle ages of humankind to the Hitlers, Stalins, Pol Pots, Bin Ladens and Saddam Husseins of our times.

It was Spinoza who, in 1670 in his *Tractatus Theologico-Politicus*, observed that peace and the fabric of society would not fall apart when individual freedom and liberty are granted; rather peace, respect for persons and all other treasured values of a society rich in cultural and ethical values would fall apart if individual freedom were *not* granted

H.T. Engelhardt, Jr. and L.M. Rasmussen (eds.), Bioethics and Moral Content: National Traditions of Health Care Morality, 49–75.

(Spinoza, 1670). In his *Foundations of Bioethics*, Tristram H. Engelhardt, Jr., gives a wealth of arguments and information in support of Spinoza's enlightened vision (Engelhardt, 1996). And for those who do not read books, the deeds of the McCarthys, Hitlers, and Bin Ladens of our times are evidence enough that the "people's power" recipe is superior to the "leader's power" model of yesterday.

There is a story of a travelling merchant who was robbed, badly beaten, and left half-dead. Various people passed the crime scene thereafter – orthodox theologians, experts in ethics, and a moral and religious stranger to this area around the Jordan River in Palestine. The stranger was from Samaria, a not well-educated or respected group among the neighboring cultures and communities. Everyone saw the beaten man in his misery, but no one stopped, no one cared, no one helped. Reasons for this unethical behavior might have been (a) fear that the robbers were still around, (b) no feeling of moral obligation to the stranger, or (c) a discrepancy between ethical theory and factual moral practice. Only the man from Samaria stopped, provided first aid, brought the victim to the next hotel, paid for his care and left. Who was the merchant's neighbor?

In Western civilization this narrative of the "good Samaritan" is a well-known case study in universal ethics, first told by Jesus (Luke 10:29) when asked by his enemies, fundamentalist Jewish theologians in Jerusalem, how he would define neighborhood ethics and solidarity. In this story there are three features important to universal ethics and to Hoshino's thesis that "it would be extremely difficult to change the ethos of a country by invoking theoretical arguments or rational approaches" [8:74]:

(1) *Moral principles of universal acceptance and validity must be and will be understood immediately* and without any further theoretical explanation or legal or ethical instruction.

(2) *There are conflicts between ethical theory and moral practice.* In real-life situations, there is a difference between ideology or academic theory on one side and factual care and practice of solidarity on the other. Moral attitudes are not necessarily based on explicit ethical theories and some edifices of moral theory even neglect to recognize the moral stranger as a fellow human being.

(3) *There are a small number of ethical principles evident to every human being and universal to all moral communities.* Some *prima facie* moral obligations seem so basic and universally shared by the

majority of cultural, ethical and religious traditions, that they need no further argumentation and may be called *a priori* universal ethics (Sass, 1994).

From the perspective of European philosophy and moral reasoning, I will discuss several aspects of universal ethics in more detail: (1) arguments supporting visions of universally shared basic principles of ethics, (2) value conflicts between universal ethics and moral traditions, (3) the relationship of universal ethics to communitarian values, human rights and civil rights, (4) conflicts between individual criteria and quality standards or objective norms, (5) the organ transplantation controversy, (6) the design of an ethically acceptable model of human genotyping, and (7) the role of education, cultural diversity, creativity, and the dignity of the individual's conscience as prime factors for the establishment and protection of human dignity, rights, obligations, and networks of moral communities.

II. KANT AND THE *A PRIORI* EVIDENCE OF UNIVERSAL ETHICS

Kant made an epistemological distinction between *a priori*, i.e., what is evident to everyone without prior empirical experience, and *a posteriori*, i.e., what becomes knowledge only after experiments and various kinds of experiences (Kant, 1787). If we transport that distinction from the fields of epistemology and metaphysics to the fields of ethics, culture, and education then moral principles, values, and attitudes which should be evident to all reasonable people and shared by individuals and communities independently of their particular systems of belief or orientation could be called universal ethics. Kant held that all humans are born with an inherent respect for the '*sittengesetz*', i.e., respect for the rule of morality. In arguing that all humans, independently of culture and experience, are naturally endowed with properties to distinguish good and evil, virtues and vices, he follows the Western natural law tradition, holding that basic norms of ethics are inherently present in human nature. But he differs from the natural law tradition in as far as he questions whether a particular custom or morality or the rules of one particular moral community can be argued for by reference to nature and natural laws. Specific rules of moral communities have to be questioned whether or not they embody what in Kant's vision was universal to all humans: *respect for human dignity* and *respect for rules* and principles that support the respect for human dignity rather than neglecting or degrading it (Kant, 1788).

Kant made it quite clear that no system of positive law should be regarded as the authoritative model for all, while others have suggested that such an authoritative model could be developed (Logmans et al., 1998). His approach to ethics has been called formalistic, as he does not call for specific civil rights and obligations except for respect for human dignity and a process of ethical assessment, which, if generalized, would provide good rules for everyone and could be accepted by everyone. This formalism has *a mission and vision of content*: maxims in ethics, moral attitudes, moral communities and traditions must be analyzed and assessed in how far they respect and support the dignity, liberty, and security of fellow humans. It is this communication-in-trust and cooperation-in-trust model of natural law philosophy that envisions responsibility and responsiveness, discourse, mutual aid and care as *a priori* evident essential characteristics of human nature.

Human solidarity in situations of extreme danger is such an essential principle, universally recognizable by all well-minded individuals and in all moral communities, independently of religious belief, race, gender, social position, specific personal advantages, gifts, and disadvantages. A review of cultural traditions, contemporary worldviews and moral communities shows support for principles of solidarity, in particular with the vulnerable, sick, poor, and dying. Even anarchism cannot live without the notion of solidarity, as Kropotkin's book '*Mutual Aid*' (1902), one of the classical readings in anarchism, demonstrates.

This European pretext for assessing some ethical principles and visions universally, based on the vision of a natural respect for human dignity, but still needing to find the most adequate expression of such a vision in a particular situation or moral community, and critical to questionable particular cultural traditions or customs, supported by different metaphysical or fundamentalist forms of reasoning or low-theory common-sense attitudes, might understand the Taoist saying "the world is a sacred vessel, which must not be tampered with or grabbed after. To tamper with it is to spoil it, and to grasp it is to lose it. In fact, for all things there is a going ahead, and a time following behind" (Lao Tzu, 1989, p. 29). While the Taoist position seems to be more accommodating to traditional conduct and customs, but ready to go ahead if the time is right or if great imbalances have developed, the post-enlightenment European approach is more active, sometimes not ready to appreciate rich moral and cultural traditions and communities. But both modes of reasoning reject fundamentalist ideologies as the bases for moral or legal attitudes or requests; both are post-conventional in as far as they discuss, reason, and argue. Kant's model of emancipation and the Chinese concept of the Tao are visions and mission statements, not scientific interpretations of natural or social data. In this regard, they share the view of recent statements on human rights by UNESCO and other international bodies such as the United Nations' 1948 Universal Declaration of Human Rights that "all human beings are born free and equal in dignity and rights" (United Nations, 1948, art. 1).

Both positions also seem to share a common understanding that so-called systems of ethics, abstract rules, laws or regulations are written on paper only and are powerless if not embodied in real-life virtues and action. Therefore, universal ethics should not focus on the content of rules alone, but on the *process* of envisioning, protecting, supporting and developing them as well. Rules in themselves are nothing, and are sometimes even counterproductive. As the Tao says, "the more taboos and inhibitions there are in the world, the poorer the people become" and "the more articulate the laws and ordinances, the more robbers and thieves arise" (Lao Tzu, 1989, no 57).

III. UNIVERSAL ETHICS VERSUS CULTURAL TRADITIONS

The richness of cultural traditions and positions, of creativity and innovation, of diversities in moral and social communities, and the varieties of the arts, crafts, and sciences suggest that human properties, gifts, ambitions, successes, and their priorities in vision, hope, fear, care, and concern are quite different. The common human *global cultural heritage* finds its expression in *diversity and creativity*, and even in often extreme forms of self-expression and eccentric customs and attitudes. All cultural communities are proud of their specific cultural achievements, and organizations such as UNESCO have taken pride in and accepted responsibility for recognizing, protecting and supporting cultural diversity, thus recognizing, protecting and supporting human dignity and creativity in the variety of its expressions. Cultural goals and visions are not universally shared, and some are rejected, abhorred and quite controversial even within a given culture.

At first glance, the vision and mission of universal ethics seem to be different from the vision and mission of culture. They concentrate on and demand something that is universal, definite, reliable, trustable, whatever the cultural trends or traditions, or the priorities and modes of development or concern. The historian Jacob Burckhard once said: more often than not human rights have to be protected against the fads of culture and politics, not along with them. Some cultural communities accept, have no problems with, or actively support abortion, promiscuity, forms of slavery or dependency, different cultural and moral status based on gender or age, or any other distinctions differentiating between people and attaching values of human or social worth accordingly on fellow humans. These attitudes and practices are unacceptable to universal ethics. But if we want to undo all differentiations and distinctions of individual cultures, we have to build a world society unfavorable to cultural extravagances and eccentricities, superior individual achievements, individual visions, callings, and missions. In consequence, we would have to dispense with the respect for the individual human being, her "right to life, liberty, and security" (United Nations, 1948, art. 3), and we would have to reject the notion that humans are "endowed with reason and conscience and should act towards one another in a spirit of brotherhood" (United Nations, 1948, art. 1). Those who feel obligated to disregard cultural diversity in the name of universal norms, rules, and ethics consequently will install a global totalitarian machine in which individuals are parts only to keep it running according to rules of efficient social engineering. Nobody, except totalitarians, fundamentalists, sadists, and egoists, wants to do that.

But how do we address the conflict between cultural diversity and violations of the human dignity of individuals and groups of individuals? We have to differentiate between *fundamental and supplementary ethical principles*, based on basic and non-basic human needs, fears, visions and hopes. Basic needs, even prerequisites for life itself, not just for a good life, include being free of hunger and thirst, free of pain and disease, free of torture and exploitation, free of being made an object rather than being treated as a fellow person. Whenever an individual's cultural or moral community violates these needs or supports such a violation, they do not contribute to the respect, protection, and support of human dignity, even though they themselves might claim to be virtuous within their own system of value reference. Fundamental ethical principles would be those that, according to Kant, are self-evident to all reasonable people and can be based on social contract or religious or humanist vision. The difference between fundamental and supplementary ethical principles itself depends on ethical decisions which will not be shared by all positions, as disagreement will arise as to whether or not certain maxims are fundamental or non-fundamental.

While the *foundation of all cultural edifices* has to be built on the strong base of the vision and mission of a limited number of basic human rights and obligations and of networks of civil rights for the protection of human dignity, the *upper levels of culture and creativity, values and virtues* in various religious, social, cultural or national houses will differ in floor plan and layout, priority of use, interior decorations and properties. Some might not want to live in the houses the other people or communities have build according to their vision and mission, and they might want to leave their home and join the neighbor's house in a global village rich in different styles of houses, customs, systems of reference, and openness to other people's interests, priorities and cultures. Therefore, ethics, which can universally be shared, must define and support a small number of ethical principles and processes, fundamental for the recognition and promotion of human dignity and the protection of fellow humans from inhuman or degrading treatment. But universal ethics has no right to paternalize, manipulate or destroy differences in cultural attitude and moral assessment among reasonable and responsible people and within and among moral communities holding different views on specific ethical challenges.

This model of different moral houses, owned by individuals, families or moral communities in a global village, needs further explanation, architectural review and construction expertise. Certain principles, primary virtues (in traditional European Philosophy unfortunately called 'secondary' virtues) such as personal integrity, reliability, punctuality, professional expertise and professionalism, truthfulness, politeness, kindness, decency, listening and understanding, openness, fairness, loyalty and trustworthiness will be indispensable for all *structural aspects* of the buildings, even though some constructions might differ from others in regard to this form of stability and reliability. On the *ground floor*, all houses share the principle of vehemently fighting the starvation, killing and torturing of all fellow humans, whether from this house or others, and of providing care and support for the sick, poor, and others who cannot care for themselves. But on the *higher floors* different houses will hold different opinions. In one house people will discuss what constitutes natural means of contraception and which ones would be acceptable or tolerable by this community, while the house next door has no moral problem with individual reproductive choice and might discuss limits to abortion based on gestational development of the embryo; and the house down the road holds that the "fruit of the womb", as a part of the female body and in her discretionary care only, becomes a subject of societal and communal concern and care only after birth and sustained breathing. Of course, residents of different houses disagree on visions and convictions held in the upper levels of their neighbors' conscience and concern, but they will refrain from destroying their neighbor's house or degrading her values. The houses may have interactive groups of study and assessment or build bridges between the houses. They will allow inhabitants, unhappy with the living and believing conditions in one house, to *move to another house*. The *top floor* on most houses sees ongoing debates on such peculiar things as resurrection or reincarnation after death, liberty or destiny in human life, never-ending theological and philosophical disputes of various sort and controversies among artists, schools of art, vision, belief or ideology, and their followers. It will be the designers (Sass, 1986, 1994) of these houses that make them comfortable for their inhabitants, open to the community, and with windows and doors. There are certain unquestionable structural requirements without which no house will stand and last; these are the various forms of secondary virtues. But as the Taoist remarks, good design is not good enough; good deeds are done by people, not by well-designed rooms. People need space for decisions and actions: "we make doors and windows for a room, but it is these empty spaces that make a room liveable" (Lao Tzu, 1989, p. 11).

IV. COMMUNITARIAN VALUES, HUMAN RIGHTS AND CIVIL RIGHTS

While most cultural traditions and individual and social ethics are based on community values, some of these values are in direct conflict with universal ethics and need to be dealt with in order to protect human dignity. Depending on the severity of the conflict between questionable community values and human rights, different strategies must be employed, starting with dialogue and education, and ending with restricting, forbidding and punishing cruel and degrading cultural activities: (1) discourse and education within a given community; (2)

information and communication between communities; (3) protection and support of the liberty principle, more precisely the "informed consent among educated adult" principle, if dignity or rights of others might be at risk or harmed; (4) protection of human rights through civil rights, criminal persecution and punishment.

Traditional gender roles or different moral and cultural attitudes toward children or the old, which might have had economic, political, or social benefits in the past, will have to be addressed by open cultural dialogue within societies, their particular moral communities, and among individuals. There is strong evidence that the support of education for everyone, public dialogue, and economic development will change gender roles and age related roles into the new scenarios of a future world of democratic, culturally and socially responsible civilizations. Moral decisions within the family, family planning and care for the children and the elderly best would be kept in the family, as the smallest and most intimate moral community; only in the most severe cases of cruel or degrading abuse should moral or legal communities get involved. The global moral community has already expressed moral visions and defined moral missions in declarations against racism (1963), for children (1959), women (1967), and the human genetic heritage (1997). An influx of information, education, and communication to cultural and moral communities which had little or no contact before and where there is no established culture of recognizing the moral status of a moral or cultural stranger, seem to be better instruments for modifying attitudes and practices than laws or regulations. If the global village respects individual human dignity, then the villagers and their moral and political leaders must also respect the dignity and rights of established moral and cultural communities in the support of education, communication-in-trust, and cooperation-in-trust, rather than paternalism or manipulation from the outside.

Certain cultural attitudes are unhealthy, harmful and potentially degrading, but as long as well-informed and educated adults agree to those activities and no great harm is done to others or the community, these activities have to be respected as they represent the wide variety of what people find enjoyable, beautiful, good, or worthwhile. But certain acts, even supported by cultural traditions and moral concepts, such as *female genital mutilation* on non-consenting children or juveniles, are not acceptable to *a priori principles of human dignity and rights* because (a) the process is cruel and painful, (b) the subject is not in a position to agree or disagree, (c) it might be unhealthy or even deadly, (d) it will deprive the subject of her future potential of sexual and personal development, and (e) it violates the subject's natural property of being "born free and equal in dignity and rights" (United Nations, 1948, art. 1). Foot binding as a cultural value and attitude would fall into a similar category. But whenever national or international laws or declarations promoting universal ethics make it necessary to intervene into traditional cultural activities, legal and rhetorical intervention is not enough. Moral communities, and their representatives and leaders, have to engage in dialogue and reasoning (Chadwick, 1994; Sass, 1998). Hegel, in his *Philosophy of Right* (1817), made it clear that at some point visions of human dignity have to *become civil rights* protected by legal and political authorities.

Different opinions are voiced in social and political ethics on how to support universal ethics in a future world of highly developed biomedical and communication technology. While some favor *international bioethical declarations* and guidelines in order to translate human rights issues into the specialized field of biomedicine (Sass, 1994), others argue that national law and national regulatory cultures should be given time to understand ethical and legal implications of new technologies and that the ethical and political principle of *communitarianism* "suggests that there is wisdom in examining the possibilities and extent of national regulatory mechanisms prior to the development of international ones" (Chadwick, 1994, p. 224). These are strong arguments supporting and protecting moral communities, but communally shared values and principles can only be respected as far as they themselves do not violate basic human rights, e.g., the right to think, judge, and decide in self-determination, not to be degraded or treated cruelly.

There also are *inconsistencies and imbalances within moral and cultural communities* and within national legal and regulatory frameworks. The German legal scenario, in which the zygote is better protected from being diagnosed than the fetus is from being aborted, is such a case (Sass, 1994). The Council of Europe's 1997 Convention on Human Rights and Biomedicine addressed complicated issues such as clinical research on the retarded or demented, which would much better be taken care of by expert bodies and oversight bodies, but did not address issues more crucial to all moral communities such as abortion, euthanasia, and access to health care and pain management. There also are scenarios in which individuals, groups, churches, lawyers, legislators and regulators have fought, criminalized and even killed people for generations in the name of forging consent, rather than allowing dissent. These are the scenarios where *conscience clauses* in national laws and *individualization rather than generalization* of moral judgement and moral responsibility will be the best instruments of conflict resolution and the recognition and protection of human dignity (Sass, 1996).

V. INDIVIDUAL CRITERIA, QUALITY STANDARDS AND OBJECTIVE NORMS: THE CASE OF FUTILITY

Many controversies in academic bioethics and societal and cultural clashes over values are based on unsuccessful and, I should add, sometimes totally unnecessary and unwarranted attempts to provide objective solutions for what basically are not objective, but personal and private matters. This is particularly true for most moral challenges associated with the beginnings and ends of human life: issues of contraception, abortion, the criteria for death, meaning of suffering, and criteria for quality of life. Of course, there are issues that warrant societal consensus and legal protection, but their number is smaller than assumed by many. And, where *consensus in content* cannot and should be achieved, *consensus in methods* of how to deal with dissensus and how to protect obligations and rights of individual value-based decision making becomes the preferred means of protecting all three: individual conscience, trust-based provider-client interaction in the professional setting, and peace in society. What are the controversial normative issues addressed by Advance Directives that are more appropriately resolved on a subjective rather than an objective level (Sass, 1996)? I see the following: (1) the criteria for the *salus aegroti* maxim; (2) the risks and benefits of advance medical care planning and of giving directives in advance; (3) the authorization of a trusted surrogate decision maker; (4) the risks associated with definite directives for situations not yet fully understood or experienced.

The emphasis of contemporary American bioethics on the principle of *autonomy* has identified the principle of self-determination as the prime reason to introduce model legislation in support of advance directives. The Patient Self-Determination Act (1991) of the U.S. Congress intends to allow for the translation of a patient's autonomy into the processes of clinical decision making by giving legal authority to advance medical instructions and directives. Because we are ordinarily the best judges of our own interests in terms of our own values and goals, the extension of patient autonomy also promotes patient well-being. But there is another line of arguments, not primarily based on patient autonomy and more likely to be accepted by more traditional modes of reasoning in paternalistic physician's ethics of *benevolence*. The argument is that given the post-modern diversity in values and visions in a pluralistic society, a benevolent physician cannot define the "good for the patient" based on her own values, but needs to have information on the patient's values, visions and wishes in order to incorporate the patient's criteria for "good" into differential diagnosis, prognosis and intervention (Sass et al., 1998). The need to have advance directives for medical care is based not only on the principle of autonomy, but also on the principle of benevolence, as respect for patients as persons does not allow the physician to base diagnosis and intervention on medical-technical criteria alone but requires the introduction of the patient's individual values, wishes and visions into individualized treatment decisions.

There is risk associated with making predictions prior to fully understanding the parameters and forces of future situations, in particular when the person has (a) no prior experience with those situations, (b) an incomplete understanding of decisions made in a highly technical and professional setting, and (c) no knowledge of future technical or other developments beyond her control or not foreseeable. All three risks influence advance medical directives by lay persons. We rarely have prior personal or existential experience with situations of death, dying, dementia, severe suffering or coma; we don't understand the complex technical risks and uncertainties associated with medical procedures we might refuse or request and their consequences; we do not know the non-medical circumstances of situations for which we have made distinct directives, nor do we know about the professional and technical expertise and options at that future time, some of which might be the result of future clinical research or the lack thereof. In regard to advance health care directives, we know that medical experts, physicians and nurses are quite reluctant to give very specific and inflexible directives which in a future situation might not be in the best interest of a patient to follow and might actually be counterproductive to their "good". Risks associated with designating surrogate decision makers are risks well known in all areas of personal and professional life. Such a designation requires personal prudence, experience-based trust, the competence and trustworthiness of the trustee, the exclusion of conflict of interest as much as possible, and some legal or other protection against abuse which in itself carries the risk of reducing the much needed authority of the proxy or producing other additional forms of risk, conflict or uncertainty.

The "old" and the "new" person. There is an extended debate over whether previous directives should be honored or the "presumed actual will" of the patient at the time of intervention should guide intervention decisions. The normative conflict can best be illustrated by the German situation in which a Chamber of Physicians guideline for the care of the dying requests that previous oral or written directives only be taken as a clue to determine the presumed actual will of the patient, while a Supreme Court decision holds that previous directives are binding and that so-called objective criteria of futility may only be used as a default position in the clear absence of the expression of individual preference. A possible conflict between the previous and actual person is real, but the controversy seems to be somewhat artificial and will have to be discussed in different scenarios.

As long as competent persons have not changed oral or written statements and directives, those statements should be taken as their true position and others should act accordingly in respect for persons. It is the right and obligation of competent persons who change their views and preferences to let others know, and if they do not do so they carry the risk of being misunderstood and mistreated.

If someone falls into a state such as a deep and prolonged coma, this person will have no new experience on which a change of values or wishes could be based and therefore should be treated according to wishes and values previously expressed.

Patients suffering from chronic and progressive illnesses and persons suddenly confronted with physical disabilities will or will not adapt to new and quite different parameters of quality of life. Clinicians are very aware that many chronically ill patients and also those suddenly in situations which they might have thought previously would not be worth living in, do in fact adjust to new challenges over and over again. As long as these patients are competent, they have ample opportunity to accept or reject treatment. For these patients, the use of advance directives is not indicated, and they, if they so choose, may adjust their previously stated preferences according to their new experiences of and visions for life.

Severely demented patients, not knowing who they are, where they are, and unable to recognize friends and loved ones, who, while fully competent, have executed advance directives refusing or requesting certain interventions in given situations, should be honored as the persons they were when they made those decisions which they then felt would be the most appropriate expression of their visions and values.

Hard cases, however, seem to be those where patients are semi-competent, where patients are in psychiatric confusion, or where incompetent patients request forms of comfort care which would contradict previous instructions. These are situations in which the process of making the most appropriate benevolent clinical decision is full of ambiguity and often the care for the "good" as presently expressed by the patient probably should be honored over previous statements. Advance health care documents are the only valid expression of a patient's wishes, values, and visions as long as they have not been changed or invalidated. The recognition and execution of these forms answers the question of "who shall decide" in regard to the application of highly advanced medical technology at the limits of life the answers will be different form culture to culture and from individual to individual.

VI. NEO-ORGANS, XENOGRAFTS, AND ORGAN TRANSPLANTATION

Highly advanced medical devices and procedures cause great controversies among individuals and between religious and moral communities. From an ethical point of view, it does not seem that neo-organs, xenografts, and the transplantation of organs are the result of pure scientific curiosity or the exercise of scientific freedom and liberty. Rather, they are the direct result of what I call the *therapeutic imperative*, which drives the health care expert to professionally improve the means and ways of fostering the good of the patient. Some of these new avenues seem to be more acceptable within different cultures and systems of religious belief than human organ sharing. Nevertheless, the design of biomaterial research must always take into account cultural and religious factors that might influence the acceptability of new technology as much as social and financial preconditions. For some, neo-organs might be more acceptable than xenografts; for others, xenografts might be more acceptable than living donor or human cadaveric organ donation. Cultural traditions and personal attitudes will influence the directions of future research and of highly advanced medical technologies.

There are additional ethical issues related to utilizing biomaterials and breeding *transgenic animals*: respect for animals as co-creatures and patenting. Is it immoral to breed transgenic animals or plants that carry human genetic material for the purpose of studying diseases, experimenting with treatments, or producing drugs or biocompatible organs? I do not think that these animals or plants deserve greater respect simply because they carry human genetic material than do those cultivated plants and animals that we have bred for millennia for companionship or food supply. Rather, all animals deserve respect as co-creatures who may suffer pain or otherwise feel uncomfortable.

Are genetically recombined drugs, cells, tissues, or organs *patentable*? Traditionally, forms of cultivated animal life and plant life were not patented in the same way that machines or processes are patented. Breeders were protected by different forms of "breeder's privileges". This seems to be the right way to provide for innovations and investments, to address issues of liability, to strengthen the forces of the market and to provide competition in delivering the best quality at the best price.

Or is organ or tissue donation among humans ethically preferable to neo-organs or xenograft? Very few people carry a *donor card* indicating that they have chosen to be cadaveric donors after their death. Some choose to refrain from carrying a card for very good personal, religious, or philosophical reasons, some because they have not thought about it or do not want to think about what they consider a taboo: the harm done to one's own body in the gray zone between life and decay. Many religious and philosophical visions do not conflict with giving and receiving organs; on the contrary, the Samaritan ethic of neighborly love, or the virtue of doing good to the other far beyond the realm of duty, is embedded in many religions. Would a policy requesting that every citizen have an *information card* expressing one's decision to donate or not to donate or to leave the decision to family or physicians at a later point in time be an invasion of privacy? I do not think so as long as there is no discrimination against those who decide in a way that is different from the norm. I do not see a moral harm in the possibility that national legislation might decide to instate a policy of presumed decision, either pro or contra donation, as a default position, as long as the prospective donor or non-donor has the right to opt otherwise and the opportunity to have his decision registered or otherwise made valid and available.

Would a policy of *reciprocity* in which those who carry a donor card receive higher points in a lottery system be ethically acceptable? Based on the principle of solidarity, this policy might actually increase the quantity of potential donors. The policy would also make clear that those who refuse to donate or to receive donated organs have very personal reasons for doing so, and that those commitments should be honored. The principle of reciprocity might also serve as a means to encourage decisions now rather than later, given the understandable reluctance to make commitments and venture into an area considered a taboo.

Even more complicated are ethical issues associated with living donors. We have empirical and anecdotal information regarding pressure on family members to donate. Considering recent progress in immune suppression, even kidney donation by spouses and friends has been reported to be relatively successful. However, the possibilities of conflicts of interest, discrimination, exploitation of familial relations, and even outright pressure and force, cannot be excluded from any moral assessment of the new technical probabilities of intrafamilial donation and donation by friends. Considering that the risk of such harms differs among individual cases, living donation may represent either a moral problem or a moral good.

Much greater moral and medical risk is associated with *black market payment* for organ sale. Black markets in general are inefficient economically, medically, and ethically. We have more than anecdotal evidence of exploitation of the sellers of organs, which often results in harm to their health and financial wellbeing. The World Health Organization (WHO) and most civilized countries have made the financial or other type of compensation for the exchange of organs illegal; nevertheless, there seems to be an active trade in human organs that benefits the rich and harms the poor. The selling of organs is unfair and unjust and should be punished harshly. However, if black markets thrive whenever there is high demand and a simultaneous prohibition against honoring the request, would it not be better to think about a highly regulated market as an alternative to the black market?

Could there be a *societal gratuity model* for living donors who do not want to donate an organ while being exposed to serious health risks with no compensation at all? Many societal gratuity schemes for various types of service have been developed around the world: special services and benefits for veterans of war in most countries, free use of public transportation for German members of parliament, preference in governmental or semi-governmental jobs for veterans in Canada, tax-free salaries for teachers and policemen in some countries, and active discrimination against those who do *not* have a special disorder such as blindness for certain jobs such as medical massage. So it would not be new to think about societal recognition of those who donate organs to suffering fellow humans.

What might count as a societal gratuity for those who want to donate organs to those in need? Excluding, of course, money, a list of compensations would definitely have to include health benefits such as free and safe organ removal, many years of free follow-up health care, highest priority on the list of potential recipients of organs, based on the principle of reciprocity, and life-long basic health care if such care is not provided to everyone. Other societal expressions of gratuity might include services that are not generally available or are intended for the rich only such as education for the donor and/or family members and access to loans, property sold by the government, and jobs in high demand within a quota reserved for these donors. Becoming a living donor would have to be a highly regulated process requiring a physical examination, determination of competency for prudent and autonomous decision making, and other social and personal requirements. In short, a national government would need to instate any safeguards deemed necessary to guarantee that decisions are made freely and out of a sense of solidarity and benevolence. The political and moral community would then react to such acts of benevolence and charity with their own gifts of gratuity and moral recognition.

I am not sure whether such schemes of highly regulated markets can or should be implemented or whether they would even work. But I am sure that societal gratuity schemes would be morally far more acceptable than the black market in organs of exploited people, which can be justified neither morally nor medically and has developed as such only as a direct result of the criminalization of the giving of organs for compensation. The Indian government and the governments of many other countries, for example, rightly criminalized all forms of black market organ trade and tried to reduce deception and fraud (India, 1995). But no country has yet ventured into the idea of a highly regulated market that would protect donors and serve recipients. In contrast to this reluctance, other markets that pose high risks to vulnerable populations, such as therapeutic and nontherapeutic medical research, have been developed and are highly regulated; as a result, transactions such as clinical experimentation on humans are not criminalized and driven into black markets. As transplantation of human organs does not seem to be the best and final medical or moral solution, the organ donation debate might be transitory for those involved in the discussion (but still essential and immediate for those who today are in desperate need of donor organs). But from an ethical point of view, the details and the direction of the debate are also signals of the degree of commitment that individuals, cultures, and societies feel toward those unfortunate enough to be forced to depend on their healthy fellow citizens for the very organs necessary to keep them alive.

VII. CROSSCULTURAL BIOETHICAL DESIGN OF GENOTYPING

As with all new designs in concepts and production, the risks vary over time and are related to (1) individual and collective acceptance of new concepts and new machinery, (2) the adaptability of existing legal and social cultures to new ways of thinking and working, and (3) the flexibility of new products and concepts and their supporters to adjust to or transform existing customs, procedures, and expectations. There is no clear-cut right or wrong answer to the question of how to handle the *moral risk and moral design of introducing new products and procedures* which will change existing attitudes and customs, and which will only succeed if, indeed, some attitudes and customs will change while others which I would call individual and cultural *value essentials* - will have to be protected and promoted. While the evolutionary change from traditional medicine toward gene-based medicine seems to be well established and inevitable, the cultural, moral, and legal assessments of genotyping are still controversial. In the absence of real and factual results which could be assessed more precisely and appreciated more easily, the differences between the pro and contra camps are still very wide. For some, the "genome" is a new mantra, for others, the outmost eschatological evil which will finally destroy the globe (Chadwick, 1994; Hoshino, 1997; HUGO, 1996; Lane et al., 1996; Sass, 2001).

On one side there are the *risks* that (1) new forms of social discrimination and labeling based on genetic status will occur, (2) jobs and health insurance will be refused to those with specific genetic characteristics, (3) genetic predispositions will make some susceptible to criminality, or unruly or unsocial behavior, and (4) heteronymous lifestyle regulation in the name of cost reduction or health status care will be put on those whose hereditary risks can be managed by lifestyle modification. On the other side there are the *benefits* of information, education, and knowledge. They include (1) a better understanding of individuality, i.e., that each of us has her or his very personal mixture of genetic predeterminants, some favorable and some nonfavorable, which translate into (a) the individual's personal health care challenge and (b) a stronger concept of solidarity in health care and solidarity in general, (2) better and steadily improving predictive and preventive information for individual health literacy, (3) better self-understanding one's own food and drug metabolism, and (4) better risk recognition and risk prevention in environmental and occupational health care. Being an ethicist who believes in the right and obligation of self-determination and self-responsibility, I see that there are still clouds of ambiguity around which we will never be able to totally push away. But, progress in genotyping and subsequent predictive, preventive, and therapeutic medicine will initiate the second step in the Age of Reason's vision of individual self-determination and autonomy, as it will give individuals the necessary means to "know yourself", the second step to liberating man and woman from the unknown, unpredictable, and often cruel fates and tempers of nature, polymorphism, and genetic disorders. But there are specific moral issues in genotyping which need new biomedical and bioethical harm-benefit calculations.

Autonomy and self-determination, basic principles of modern political philosophy and public policy, appear already in somewhat modified forms in the health care setting due to dependency, weakness, pain and suffering of the patient. Therefore, special features such as informed consent and surrogate decision making have been specifically developed for the health care setting, and more rigidly for the human research setting. Autonomy includes (1) informational autonomy, i.e., the right to give or withhold information freely and without pressure, (2) the right to control the fate and use of generated information for oneself and for what others, e.g., researchers and research institutions, use the information for, (3) the control over information in yet unknown scenarios which might be brought about by the use of information given to others or developed by others based on that information, and (4) the mental and contractual capacity to protect autonomy in all three mentioned circumstances (Powers, 1994).

On the other hand, social interaction, cultural achievements, and quality of life depend on information sharing, and mutual respect for *cultivated forms of use and proliferation of information.* So, autonomy over individual information is not an absolute principle, rather one which has to be valued and protected in combination with principles of exchange, truth-telling, confidentiality, trust, education, solidarity, and the right to contract freely. Also, the withholding of information regarding one's health status quite often is medically counterproductive as it will disallow the expert to diagnose, make prognosis, consult, and treat. Traditional clinical research and epidemiological studies have found ways to reasonably gather data while protecting the autonomy and health interests of probands and patients. Additional problems in genotyping arise because of the sheer limitlessness of information which possibly can be gathered, the unlimited timeframe of availability of samples once gathered, and the incapability of even experts in the field today to determine which information in the not too distant future ought to be withheld rather than communicated or acted upon for reasons of self-determination. But if, and how much, a patient wants to be involved in genotyping research and services is primarily an issue to be decided by the educated citizen herself rather than by paternalistic researchers who ask for consent. In genotyping services like bloodtyping services, the contract model is much more appropriate than the consent model and a better protection as well as expression of the patient's autonomy.

Harm and risk in genotyping research is quite different from other forms of risk and harm, such as phase I cytostatica trials. Future generations probably will understand genotyping as a routine part of physical exams, for which generic consent is given by making a doctor's appointment and for which risks are similar to those of sharing private and personal information with others in a private or workplace setting. Possible harm in genotyping can be compared to the harm of discrimination by blood-typing, which is unheard of even though some fellow humans have a more rare blood type and therefore might be less well off in certain situations. Typing blood made blood transfusion feasible; it would be harmful, unethical, and unprofessional to transfuse blood without proper bloodtyping. It is similarly harmful, unethical, and unprofessional to prescribe medication to individuals with different features of metabolism without prior appropriate cytochrome P450 genotyping and enzyme testing. Adverse effects of an individual's genetic setup in drug metabolizing enzymes include poor bioavailability, drug toxicity, drug-drug interactions, food-drug interactions, and other idiosyncratic drug reactions due to polymorphism. There is a special medical responsibility towards poor drug metabolizers and individual dosage prescription must be based on oxidation phenotyping or genotyping of patients. Not only individualized treatment, but also the allocation of scarce resources might improve by drug research and drug delivery research based on genotyping and people having individual *health status cards* as their informational property.

Other medical records, such as blood tests and imaging pictures of a person's "interior" properties, can be used in ways to harm the individual, but common sense and the active requests by patients by far outweigh considerations of harm. Also, medical customs, self-regulation, and laws protect data and records everywhere and mostly quite successfully. We read more about harm occurring from breaks in data protection of credit cards, access to unlisted phones, and mail and e-mail fraud. In the former situations, the individual is fully involved in making decisions, contracting or refusing services, and accepting risk to one's autonomy and privacy if expected associated benefits seem to outweigh harms or risks. The more actively the proband is involved in genotyping, the better for her autonomy and perception of harm, risk and self-determination. The patient's active request, rather than passive consent, would be most appropriate for genotyping research and for including genotyping with blood-typing in clinical research and routine medical diagnosis. The strong autonomy principle, as expressed in a model of "informed contract", seems to be better suited to handle genotyping than the soft-paternalism principle which involves asking for informed consent.

But given medical, cultural, and personal uncertainties over individual and collective responses to large-scale genotyping, it seems prudent to learn more about people's feelings about protecting or giving away autonomy and about the perceived harm of "typing" and being typed. If patients understand that genotyping research and services are beneficial to them, they will request involvement, better drug care delivery, and respect for their self-determination regarding information and being told the results of genotyping, including cross- and multi-purpose genotyping and the simple gathering of samples for determining future typing or modifying (Hoeffner, 1993). The scare among individuals and collectives regarding the abuse of genetic information will only go away over time and when successes are visible; only then will the media and the public calmly differentiate between the real and perceived threats and harms of genotyping to individual autonomy and self-determination. Even the HUGO ethics committee still discussed genotyping within the traditional informed consent model, not recognizing (a) a major impact on and interest in pedigree and (b) different parameters of harm as compared to traditional clinical trials.

Privacy and confidentiality issues already appear in quite modified versions in the research setting, in particular in epidemiological studies. Double blind studies, placebos, cracking the code, distribution of data in multicenter studies and among team members, publication of results, and the form and content of informed consent already contain quite complex ethical issues in traditional randomized clinical research. Long term storage for yet undetermined use, large scale cross-purpose and multipurpose analysis carry additional ethical and bioethical risk. Issues of privacy and confidentiality are addressed if results have major epidemiological or individual-patient positive or negative impact in drug development and drug delivery. Here again, the best protection and implementation of principles of privacy and confidentiality is to play decisions back to the patients. They have to see clear and convincing evidence that genotyping is in their best interest, whatever risk to privacy and confidentiality might be associated with being diagnosed.

Because the probability of benefits from cross-purpose genotyping and future yet to be specified re-testing and new-testing is of great moral importance for the individual patient, patient groups and progress in health care, it is bioethically acceptable to ask for generic consent, under the condition that the specifics of generic consent are shared with the proband: "Genetic testing on information and properties which might or might not be associated with your disease, how they are associated with it, and how we can treat you better; this might take a long time and we might look for information we don't know yet." Similar to respect for autonomy in clinical trials, the proband should have the right to withdraw consent and request that specimens be destroyed. In the U.S., the Health Omnibus Programs Extension Act (1988) proposed, as a special feature for the protection of research subjects, the so-called Certificate of Confidentiality, issueable by the DHHS for research on alcohol and drug abuse and on mental health, but then broadened it to include other forms of research (Hoagwood, 1994). The format of these CoC's might give some helpful insight into the privacy issues which have to be covered in genotyping. Research in the U.S. might benefit from a CoC, as it protects researchers and probands from disclosure of information to courts, employers, insurers, in-laws, neighbors, media, and pedigree.

Genotyping will have, much more than traditional family anamnesis and medical history, a direct effect on all members of the proband's pedigree. It can be welcome or unwelcome information depending on the presence or absence of more or less severe genetic predispositions, the results of yet to be interpreted findings, and inaccurate testing. It will come, as we know in particular from traditional as well as DNA-based diagnosis of individual and pedigree ADPKD testing, to unpredictable conflicting positions and choices among family members, which cannot be reconciled by the diagnostician, and which have to be carefully communicated and assessed beforehand by the clinicians and with the proband, preferably already within the family. But genotyping will have a major, yet culturally to be digested, influence on family relations, guilt-feelings, shame, accusations, self-denial, divorce, suicide, pattern of lifestyle decision making, carrier decisions, and family planning. Even if individuals choose for themselves the right not to know or the duty to know, others will directly or indirectly be influenced by those individual decisions. Expected successes in genotyping will provide for a second step of humans understanding themselves, following the first steps originated in the Age of Reason, when domination by nature, kings, and priests was proudly announced to be replaced by a first round in self-understanding, self-determination, and self-responsibility. Here, we have the definite steps toward the self-understanding of the individual's true biological makeup, its challenges, risks, limitations, and gifts. New obligations and rights resulting from these developments are the individual's business, not that of doctors, lawyers, politicians or the media (Kielstein & Sass, 2002).

VIII. UNIVERSAL ETHICS, THE TAO, AND THE INDIVIDUAL CONSCIENCE

Discrepancies within legal systems and ethical deficiencies in moral traditions and communities are nothing new. But most moral communities of world religions and other systems of belief definitely are preconditioned to support the visions and mission of universal ethics. *Taoist* reasoning would provide strong arguments for supporting and allowing harmony and individual and communal life while fighting or avoiding disorder, harm, or various forms of imbalance. *Buddhist* thinking centers around avoiding suffering and giving and supporting life with a minimum of suffering, if possible. *Christian* traditions of care, love, and protection from harm also request the respect of human dignity and the formulation of human rights. Universal ethics therefore can best be supported by those values and virtues of religious traditions teaching respect for human dignity, in particular the dignity of the individual conscience in making moral choices (Sass, 2002).

Controversies and conflicts in part are rooted in the dignity and the right of individual choice. Societies and cultures, religious positions and moral intuitions assess good and evil, virtues and vices, differently, therefore one should leave complex decisions regarding good and evil to the smaller moral community, i.e., the family and neighborhood, only thereafter with decreasing authority to act as moral agents, societies, politicians, and judges (Locke, 1689). For example, if a young girl, having lost her virginity, requests surgical reconstruction of her vaginal introitus, that request is of no business to society or any moral community, only a matter of her personal choice in response to certain expectations in some communities and a matter of a truthful relationship with a trusted surgeon (Logmans et al., 1998) and a matter of professionalism in surgery as a structural element in providing expert service, a so-called secondary virtue specific to a specific profession. *Subsidiarity* (Vatican, 1931), first developed as a principle for direct and individual care of the socially needy by individuals and moral communities and targeted against totalitarian welfare programs, in its universalized version, can be presented this way: Whenever and as long as philosophers, ethicists, theologians, politicians, church and state bureaucrats, physicians, groups in society, and educated citizens disagree on principles of ethics, they must agree on respecting the dignity of individual moral choice and responsibility.

European cultural traditions, honoring human dignity in the respect for the individual's conscience, are not only based in the Age of Reason concept of self-determination, but also in religious teaching calling for following one's conscience, as a recent encyclical confirms: "Like the natural law itself and all practical knowledge, the judgment of conscience also has an imperative character: man must act in accordance with it. If man acts against this judgment or, in a case where he lacks certainty about the rightness and goodness of a determined act, he stands condemned by his own conscience, *the procimate norm of personal morality*" (Vatican, 1993, art. 60). Except for the sexist language, the wide majority not only of European cultural and ethical traditions would agree to this statement.

The prime principle of conflict resolution in value clashes between individuals and within free societies is "respect for persons" and for the values and visions of the moral communities for which these humans stand. In the words of papal encyclical *Quadrogesimo Anno* (Vatican, 1993, art. 79), it is the principle of *subsidiarity*, i.e., the right of the individual or the small and primary group to do good based on their individual conscience and calling, and requests that secondary groups or society in general honor individual conscience and withhold their own action and judgment when morally acting individuals accept their challenge. Josef Hoeffner has observed that the subsidiarity principle has two edges, one targeted at the limitation of ever-growing bureaucracies and conceptual tutelage, and the other aimed at supporting and strengthening the individual's conscience and her self-responsibility and responsibility in the care of others (Hoeffner, 1997). It is not necessary to quote the philosophical masters of the Age of Reason in support of the "respect for individual conscience" principle; those of us who rather cling to traditional natural law models than to normative or utilitarian models of transcendental hermeneutics or discourse-and-contract models find evidence for the principle in the encyclical *Veritatis Splendor*. This "respect for persons" principle as phrased in European culture is not foreign to the Confucian and Buddhist teachings or the medical ethics of the Taoist physician Sun Simiao and the Confucian papers of doctor Gong Tingxian.

But religious, communal, political, or cultural pressure in the name of universal ethics, except in the most evident and rare cases, would be counterproductive to recognizing and supporting human dignity and rights. It was Spinoza (1670) who observed that peace and the fabric of society would not fall apart if individual freedom and liberty were granted, rather on the contrary, that peace, respect for persons and all other treasured values of a society rich in cultural and ethical values would fall apart if individual freedom were not granted.

Visions of universal ethics, declarations on human rights, legal systems of civil rights, institutions of education, science and technology, access to work, care, culture, and social interaction are the vessels and houses we build for the support, respect and promotion of human dignity and rights, but the way we use these products is problematic. "We make a vessel from a lump of clay; it is the empty space within this vessel, that makes it useful," as the Tao says (Lao Tzu, 1989, no 11). Universal ethics, creating and supporting a small number of these instruments, such as the principles of solidarity, subsidiarity, and respect for human dignity in the protection and promotion of "life, liberty, and security" (United Nations, 1948, art. 3), will use education, communication, and toleration as processes. There are times to educate, times to fight, and times to rule, but more often than not there are times to refrain from paternalizing people and from manipulating moral communities in order to respect the dignity of their choice. No European thought has said it better than the Tao: "You govern a kingdom by normal rules; you fight a war by exceptional moves; but you win the world by letting alone" (Lao Tzu, 1989, no. 57).

Georgetown University
Washington, D.C., U.S.A.

REFERENCES

Atsumi, K. (1992). 'Japanese view of life and organ transplantation.' In: C. M. Kjellstrand and J. B. Dossetor (Eds.), *Ethical Problems in Dialysis and Transplantation* (pp. 193-188). Dordrecht: Kluwer Academic Publishers.

Chadwick, R. (1994). 'Germ-line therapy, autonomy, and community.' *Politics and the Life Sciences* 13, 223-225.

Council of Europe (1997.) *Convention for the Protection of Human Rights and Dignity of the Human Being with regard to the Application of Biology and Medicine*, European Treaty Series, 164.

Engelhardt, Jr., H. T. (1996). *The Foundations of Bioethics*, 2nd ed. New York: Oxford University Press.

Hoagwood, K. (1994.) 'The certificate of confidentiality at the NIH: Discretionary considerations in its applicability in research on child and adolescent mental disorders.' *Ethics and Behavior* 4(2), 123-131.

Hoeffner, J. (1983). *Christliche Gesellschaftslehre*. Kevelaer.

Hoshino, K. (1995.) 'Autonomous decision making and Japanese tradition.' *Cambridge Quarterly of Healthcare Ethics* 4, 71-74.

Hoshino, K. (Ed.) (1997). *Japanese and Western Bioethics: Studies in Moral Diversity*. Dordrecht: Kluwer Academic Publishers.

HUGO, Ethics Committee (1996). 'Statement on the principled conduct of genetic research.' *Euroscreen* 6.

India (1995). *Transplantation of Human Organs Act 1994*. New Delhi: Jain Book.

Kant, I. (1787). *Kritik der Reinen Vernunft*, 2nd ed.

Kant, I. (1788). *Kritik der Praktischen Vernunft*.

Kielstein, R. & Sass, H.-M. (2002). 'How much do we want to know? Genetics in kidney disease.' *American Journal of Kidney Disease* 39(3), 637-652.

Lane, S.D. and Rubinstein, R.A. (1996). 'Judging the other. Responding to traditional female genital surgeries.' *Hastings Center Report* 26(3), 31-40.

Lao Tzu (1989). *Tao Teh Ching*, J. C. H. Wu (trans.). Boston: Shambala.

Locke, J. (1689). *Letter concerning Toleration*. London.

Logmans, A. *et al.* (1998). 'Ethical dilemma: Should doctors reconstruct the vaginal introitus of adolescent girls to mimic the virginal state?' *British Medical Journal* 316, 459-462.

Powers, M. (1994). 'Privacy and the control of genetic information.' In: M. S. Frankel and A. Teich (Eds.), *Genetic Frontiers* (pp. 77-100). Washington: AAAS.

Sass, H.-M. (1986). 'The moral a priori and the diversity of cultures.' *Analecta Husserliana* 20, 407-422.

Sass, H.-M. (1995). 'Some cultural and ethical reflections on moleculargenetic risk assessment.' *Proceedings of the International Bioethics Committee 1994*, vol. II. Paris: UNESCO.

Sass, H.-M. (1996). 'Moral risk assessment in biotechnology.' In: G. K. Becker and J. P. Buchanan (eds.), *Changing Nature's Course. The Ethical Challenge of Biotechnology* (pp. 127-144). Hong Kong: Hong Kong University Press.

Sass, H.-M. (1998). 'Why protect the human genome?' *Journal of Medicine and Philosophy* 23, 227-233.

Sass, H.-M. (2001). 'A "contract model" for genetic research and health care for individuals and families.' *Eubios Journal of Asian and International Bioethics* 11 (Sept.), 130-131.

Sass, H.-M. (2002). *Menschliche Ethik im Streit der Kulturen*. Bochum: Zentrum Medizinische Ethik.

Sass, H.-M., Veatch, R. and Kimura, R. (1998). *Advance Directives and Surrogate Decision Making in Health Care: United States, Germany, and Japan*. Baltimore: John Hopkins University Press.

Scheler, M. (1973 [1913]). *Formalism in Ethics and Non-Formal Ethics of Values*, M. S. Frings and R. L. Funk (Trans.). Evanston: Northwestern University Press.

Spinoza, B. (1670). *Tractatus Theologico-Politicus.*

United Nations (1948). *Universal Declaration of Human Rights*. New York: UNESCO.

Vatican (Pius IX) (1931). *Quadrogesimo Anno*. Rome: Vatican.

Vatican (John Paul II) (1993). *Veritatis Splendor*. Rome: Vatican.

Whitbeck, C. (1996.) 'Ethics as design: Doing justice to moral problems.' *Hastings Center Report* 26(3), 9-16.

KURT BAYERTZ AND KURT W. SCHMIDT

BRAIN DEATH, PREGNANCY AND CULTURAL RELUCTANCE TOWARD SCIENTIFIC RATIONALISM*

I. APOLLONIAN ABILITIES

A long time ago, as the gods were still descending from Mount Olympus, it so happened that Apollo found great favor with Coronis, the daughter of the King, and begot a child with her. Yet Coronis, with child, chose to betroth the mortal Ischys, son of Elatus, and everyone believed him to be the father of the godly child. When the raven, which at that time was still white, brought the news of the forthcoming betrothal to Ischys to the god Apollo, it was struck by that god's initial anger; and, ever since, the bird has been black. Beside himself with rage, Apollo dispatched his sister, Artemis, to the home of Coronis. Artemis drew her arrows and killed the unfaithful Coronis and then brought a great affliction over the land, causing many to die. As the corpse of Coronis was to be burned and the flames were already blazing, Apollo regretted his action and cried: "It defies my patience that my son is to perish with his mother!" He took the child from within the womb of the dead mother, named his son Asclepios (lat. Aesculap), taught him the art of healing and brought him to the centaur Chiron, from whom he would learn the art of surgery (Kerényi, 1966, pp. 114f.).

Thanks to modern medicine, what used to be the privilege of the gods is today within the realm of human capability: the saving of a child from the womb of its dead mother. The international literature has reported approximately ten cases over the past few years, where the organism of a brain-dead, pregnant woman has been successfully kept functioning until the birth of the child.[1] Ethicists have also taken note of this phenomenon (cf. Fletcher, 1988, p. 3), and have used it in the teaching of biomedical ethics (cf. Brody and Engelhardt, 1987, p. 380; Mappes and Zembaty, 1991, p. 635). Germany has also witnessned cases of attempting to save the fetuses of brain-dead, pregnant women: as early as 1976, the anesthetist Hartmut Menzel reported the treatment of a 22-year-old, brain-dead woman who was more than 20 weeks pregnant. At that time, "frontiers were crossed for surgical intervention" in order to "carry out one of two linked medical tasks" (Menzel, 1976, p. 62). One week later,

H.T. Engelhardt, Jr. and L.M. Rasmussen (eds.), Bioethics and Moral Content: National Traditions of Health Care Morality, 77–95.

complications arose, a Cesarean section was carried out and a girl weighing 940g was brought into the world and transferred to intensive care. Another case occurred in July 1991. Here, unbeknownst to the public, a 33-year-old brain-dead woman in the 19th week of pregnancy underwent intensive care in a Stuttgart hospital until the birth of a healthy child (cf. IV.). When one year later another case of "brain death and pregnancy" occurred, however, public reaction revealed that – at least in Germany – human beings did not feel comfortable with their new Apollonian power.

II. THE ERLANGEN CASE

On October 5, 1992, at 3 p.m., 18-year-old Marion Ploch had an accident on her way home from working as a doctor's receptionist in southern Germany. Her car crashed into a tree. As the ambulance arrived, she was still breathing spontaneously, yet had lost consciousness. She was flown by helicopter to a hospital in Erlangen, arriving intubated and artificially respirated at 3:25 p.m. At 4.25 p.m., because of her serious brain damage, she was transferred first to the neurosurgical clinic for diagnostics (CT of the skull), and later to the intensive care unit. Various diagnostic measures confirmed an existing pregnancy (approximately 14 weeks) and, at this stage, brain death was unconfirmed. "Normal intensive care treatment" then began, although the prognosis offered by the responsible neurosurgeon was unfavorable (Scheele, 1993, pp. 12f.). The patient's clinical situation stabilized exceedingly quickly, but three days later, on October 8, she was diagnosed as brain-dead.

Since the fetus seemed to be unimpaired and the dead woman's remaining bodily functions were stable, artificial respiration and feeding were continued. An attempt was made to save the life of the fetus. Whereas the organism of a brain-dead (compared to that of an apallic) human being can only be maintained artificially for a few days, the somatic functions of a pregnant, brain-dead woman seem to be able to be maintained a great deal longer, due to the fetus taking over a basic regulation of certain pituitary hormones (Scheele, 1993). On November 16, however, in approximately the 19th week of pregnancy and after 40 days of treatment, the baby was spontaneously aborted, dead on arrival. Artificial respiration of the mother ceased. It remained unclear exactly what had caused the fetus' death. The parents refused permission for an autopsy to be carried out on their daughter or their grandchild.

This refusal was preceded by a very heated public debate, lasting weeks and initiated by an article featured in the German tabloid newspaper "Bild". A great many opinions were expressed in the media, ranging from repugnance to approval. Different professional circles also expressed different opinions. Even those who condoned the physicians' behavior were uneasy and apprehensive. The German government was asked whether artificial maintenance of the bodily functions of a brain-dead, pregnant woman did not represent a violation of the dignity of human beings as guaranteed in Article 1 of German Basic Law (An, 1992). A floodgate effect was feared: people spoke of the instrumentalization of the dead woman as an "incubator", of an infringement of her human dignity and of "corpse desecration". Most of the public seemed repulsed and outraged. The occurrence was said to be "totally perverse", "macabre" and "a scandal"; it was condemned as being "outrageous, inhuman and an insult to women." Rejection was particularly widespread and extreme amongst women, partly as a result of incorrect reports in sections of the press. On November 10, the *Ärztinnenbund* [Association of Women Physicians], the *Grünen* [Green Party] and the *Evangelische Frauenarbeit* [Protestant Women's Group] submitted a petition containing 7000 signatures from all over Germany to the Minister for Women's Affairs, Angela Merkel, in Bonn, demanding that the "experiment" in Erlangen be stopped. They appealed to the Minister to make sure that now, and in the future, this kind of "medical experiment" be prohibited. They called for "official powers" to become involved; the Court responsible did not, however, take legal reprisal against the physicians in Erlangen. The reproaches continued far beyond November 16th. The Erlangen case or 'Erlangen baby' are catchwords still used today to summarize the "perversity" of modern medicine, or at least its "problematic" nature.

At first sight, this heated public reaction must come as a surprise. Firstly, it was not the first case of brain death and pregnancy in Germany, nor had any of the previous cases caused such public uproar; indeed the public had seemed to take no notice of them. Secondly, the "brain death criteria" had long been accepted by the German medical profession, about which there had never been a controversial public debate either; both the media and the public had more or less ignored any objections that were raised by individual persons regarding the concept of brain death.

However, this all changed abruptly when the media presented the public – sometimes in the form of sensational lead features – with the case of the "Erlangen baby". Contrary to appearances, a social and cultural acceptance of the concept of brain death had not yet taken place after all. Quiet doubts, which many had obviously harbored but never articulated, seemed to be confirmed by the Erlangen case. Can a woman really be "dead" when a fetus continues to grow inside her? Is the ability to deliver and give birth to a child not the best proof that the brain-dead woman is still alive, or at least not "completely dead"? A dead woman becoming a mother: is this not totally incomprehensible?

III. PROBLEMS AND PERPLEXITIES

These questions may seem naïve, the expression of insufficient medical knowledge. Likewise, the protests mentioned above may appear as an irrational reaction from a public which is always poorly informed, and which in the case in question was additionally irritated by often one-sided press reports. This impression is certainly not wrong, but it oversimplifies the situation. Even in well-informed, specialist circles – especially those of physicians, lawyers and bioethicists – the Erlangen case provoked controversial debates and vehement reproaches. It would not be an exaggeration to say that the Erlangen case posed problems for the professions involved which were just as great as those with which the public was confronted. Instead of dismissing these protests as the *mere* expression of sketchy knowledge and irrationality, we believe it to be more productive to try to understand them and identify their causes. Indeed, it is possible to identify four problem complexes which together elucidate the negative reaction of the public and the difficulties for the professions involved.

A. Common Experience Versus Scientific Findings

In cases of brain death, the phenomenological impression contradicts the medical finding. The artificially respirated brain-dead patient seems not really to be dead, but rather just sleeping. The existing pregnancy and the possibility that the brain-dead woman could still be capable of giving birth to the fetus confirmed the public impression that the brain-dead woman could not be "all that dead". Even the mother of the brain-dead

Marion Ploch stated that she never ceased to believe "that Marion was still alive. In the hospital I spoke to her, did her hair, caressed her" (Wedemeyer, 1992).

This case was also unique for the nursing staff. Although there was no doubt that Marion Ploch was brain-dead, it was also clear that life existed within her; it was "almost as if that 'life' were visible." For this reason, the brain-dead woman was not treated as dead; the staff "talked to her like they would to a normal patient" (Bockenheimer-Lucius and Seidler, 1993, p. 36). Members of the nursing team offered a further explanation for why this experience was not felt to be an unbearable burden: the intensive care therapy was practiced at the lowest level, while the nursing care (their real task!) was uppermost (Bockenheimer-Lucius and Seidler, 1993, pp. 35, 40).

B. Linguistic Limitations

The limitations of our everyday language led to additional and considerable difficulties in comprehending just exactly what was going on. The main difficulty was that we did not know which terms to use to describe the two principals involved. *Who* or *what* – as a magazine article put it – was in intensive care: "A mother-to-be? A corpse in which a child is alive? A collection of organs forming a biological incubator? Or an (...) object with which ambitious scientists are experimenting?" (Bräutigam, Kruse and Rückert, 1992, p. 17). Even the physicians involved found this a problem. The brain-dead woman, as Prof. Johannes Scheele, responsible physician in the Erlangen case, aptly put it, is like a stone that has petrified whilst falling: "We do not have the words to describe this state (…). It did not exist when language was invented" (Bockenheimer-Lucius and Seidler, 1993, p. 17). And *what* was inside Marion Ploch: an unborn life, a fetus, a child, a human being? One of the professors involved in the Erlangen decision was later reproached for often referring to the rights of the "child", thus suggesting a preliminary decision regarding the "moral status" of the fetus; it would have been more precise to have used the term "*Ungeborenes*" (*unborn life*) (Schöne-Seifert, 1993, pp. 16ff.).

The answers to these terminological questions are of some significance in an evaluation of the entire case. On the one hand, a *psychological* problem arises. Where not even language is able to cope, our well-adjusted sense of emotional orientation is very unlikely to cope: a situation provoking uneasiness and repulsion. Some of the severe reactions to the Erlangen case are the result of such revulsion and disapprobation. And yet the terminology used also has *ethical* implications. Depending on whether one speaks of a "mother" or a "corpse", of a "fetus" or a "child", differing values are signaled, influencing the actions of the physicians. Moreover, we do not have objective criteria by which to decide whether a "mother" or a "corpse" is at stake. The choice of terminology determines which *aspects* of the case one wishes to take into consideration. These aspects have to be kept separate, as the current discussion shows, if a sensible debate is to take place and confusion avoided. Yet what happens if *several* terms are accurate? If Marion Ploch is a "mother" *and* a "corpse"? Is an *overall view* of the various aspects then still possible?

C. Ethical Dilemmas

This brings us to a third reason why this case is so difficult to evaluate: various claims and interests are in conflict. If the woman had not been pregnant, it would have been a medically "standard situation". Organ removal was ruled out, so intensive care would have been stopped. But Marion Ploch was pregnant, and the fetus survived her death. It is then obvious that not *one* claim, *one* interest is at stake, but *two* – potentially competitive – claims and interests. Abortion represents a similar situation, the difference being that the woman is alive and claiming her right to self-determination. And there are good reasons for believing that this right weighs "more" than the claims of the fetus. Yet here this was obviously not the case. Marion Ploch was dead. Even those not prepared to accept the brain death definition cannot argue that the claims of the fetus in this case weighed "less" than the mother's right to self-determination. Marion Ploch was unable to act autonomously. A dead person is more than just "biological substance" which can be disposed of at will; he or she has, for example, a right to remain free from slander (Feinberg, 1974), to have his or her declared wishes respected, and his or her body treated with dignity. These rights should be balanced against competing claims and interests. It makes a difference whether somebody refuses to donate their organs or insists on taking an unborn to the grave with them. The different – and sometimes competing – interests and values were obviously evaluated differently, reflecting conflicts among the various groups involved. One solution that would have satisfied all sides did not exist. In the absence of a morality binding everybody equally, *each* conceivable decision would have represented a provocation for at least one of the various groups. Even bioethical analysis that expects to come up with an unambiguous verdict – each naturally expecting it to be in favor of whichever view he/she happens to support – could only disappoint in this respect.

D. Legal Problems

Since the physicians recognized that they were also incapable of deciding on each relevant matter for the brain-dead mother, they applied to the appropriate district court for the allocation of a *Pflegschaft* (guardianship), in order to have a direct conversational partner (proxy) make further decisions. This in turn revealed that not only had the physicians entered unknown territory, but also the lawyers. The decision reached by the acting district court in Hersbrück provoked criticism and bewilderment among members of the legal profession. The "grandparents" were selected as "guardians" and a further relative was appointed as a temporary proxy for the brain-dead, pregnant woman. And yet, legally, in Germany a proxy is intended to stand in for *living* adults who are unable to manage their own affairs. The extent to which a specially chosen proxy is capable of representing the "post mortal interests" of a brain-dead, pregnant woman was therefore controversial. The issued death certificate caused further irritation among the lawyers. The registrar in question refused to register the death of the brain-dead, pregnant woman on the grounds that later he would then have to register the birth of a human being *without a mother*, a legal impossibility (Bockenheimer-Lucius and Seidler, 1993, p. 21). Other lawyers criticized this failure to register the death formally subsequent to brain death being established, however, and outlined various scenarios involving, for example, difficulties with inheritance law (Koch, 1993, p. 81).

IV. REPROACHES AND ARGUMENTS

Now let us take a look at the most important arguments against further treatment of the brain-dead, pregnant Marion Ploch put forward by the public and the specialists. First, there was criticism that it was not therapy which was taking place, but an "inhumane" experiment. Second, the physicians faced the reproach that their action was responsible for a renewed and far-reaching breach of public confidence in modern medicine. Third, the concept of brain death was thrown into question.

A. Experiment or Therapy?

Many people criticized the physicians in Erlangen for experimenting with human life irresponsibly. The physicians' appeal for the child's right to live was seen as an attempt to give this human experiment the appearance of humanity. It should be emphasized that the word "experiment" is strongly emotive when used in connection with human beings. The atrocities that occurred during the "Third Reich", and the terrible human experiments which were punished during the Nuremberg Trials (Mitscherlich and Mielke, 1962), burden this term further, at least for the Germans. Many people experience a fundamental sense of discomfort at the thought of human experiments; some even reject the whole idea. It is therefore far from superfluous to emphasize that "experiments on and with human beings are neither totally reprehensible, nor automatically permissible; it always depends on the *reasons* for the experiment, the *means* used, the *conditions* and the *risks* involved" (Eser, 1989, p. 503).

The Erlangen physicians rejected the use of the term "experiment" from the start. They emphasized the importance of saving the child's life; it was never their intention (so said the physicians) to carry out scientific experiments of any kind. The physicians decided to limit their diagnostic interventions to the extent necessary in order to care for the fetus. No samples of blood were taken for experimental or scientific analyses later on, for example (Scheele, 1993 pp. 16ff.). These guidelines were an essential component in the willingness of the nursing staff to care for the brain-dead, pregnant woman. It was a case of "treatment in unknown territory" which was not sought, but only "challenged" by the tragic, accidental death of a pregnant woman (Wuermeling and Scheele, 1992).

In evaluating the behavior of the Erlangen physicians, it is important – both ethically and legally – to distinguish between "human experimentation" and "clinical trials". Whereas medical *treatment* is an attempt to further the patient's individual well-being with standardized medical methods, a clinical *trial* is an attempt to achieve the same goal with *new* procedures (because of a lack of established methods of therapy). Whereas medical treatment and clinical trials are primarily aimed at therapy for the patient, *human experimentation* is primarily interested in the acquisition of scientific knowledge (Eser, 1989, pp.

504ff.; Laufs, 1988, p. 223). A "step into unknown territory" of this nature has to show medical indications of its benefit for the patient, has to be in accordance with medical rules, and must be consented to by the patient, but no physician is obliged to carry it out. If he or she does choose to enter the world of clinical trials, then the "chances of success of, and the dangers involved in" the method he selects should "be relative to the level of affliction" (Laufs, 1988, p. 227). Even if the borderline between clinical trials and human experimentation is not very clear, it is absolutely necessary, particularly for legal permissibility, but also for ethical evaluation, to make a distinction between the two. For example, experiments on human beings may not be carried out without the permission of an ethics committee. Since the Erlangen case did not represent an experiment, it was not deemed necessary to involve the University ethics committee; an ad-hoc-commission was appointed instead. Retrospectively, it was said that in this difficult case the ethics committee should have been asked, if only to prevent public suspicion of manipulation (the commission members were appointed as a result of personal consideration). The fact that the commission did not include a single woman was responsible for most of the outrage, culminating in the sarcastic reproach that "male childbearing envy" had walked abroad in Erlangen (Koch, 1993, p. 80).

B. Breach of Confidence

No other event in Germany over the past few years has made the population so emphatically aware of the significance of ethical decisions within the field of medicine as the case of the "Erlangen baby". The coincidence of *brain death and pregnancy* raised considerably more questions than the medical decision to keep the fetus alive inside the brain-dead, pregnant woman. The *Akademie für Ethik in der Medizin* [Academy for Medical Ethics], an interdisciplinary forum for scientists and health care employees which was formed in 1986 to deal with ethical matters arising within the field of medicine, was bombarded by enquiries during the acute phase of the happenings in Erlangen, although its interdisciplinary nature and the multitude of ethical views represented within it forbade a consensus "Vatican" statement from "the" Academy. Instead, a scientific debate was organized at short notice, in the course of which very different assessments of the situation came to light (Bockenheimer-Lucius and Seidler, 1993). The physicians and nursing staff related the events in question from their points of view. During the ethical reflection that followed, many were of the opinion that the procedure chosen in this case was neither forbidden nor imperative. One point of criticism, however, was that the intensive care efforts in the Erlangen case had led to a breach of public confidence in the medical profession and modern medicine, not least because the decision in Erlangen had the appearance of "physicians granting themselves privileged access to moral decisions affecting persons other than themselves" (Schöne-Seifert, 1993, pp. 20f.). Furthermore, the Erlangen case had caused a breach of confidence in the private and personal nature of motherhood, in the sensibility of the medical profession, in the humanity of medical progress, and in the definition of brain death. By stopping the intensive care efforts, these far-reaching social consequences could have been avoided, especially as the physicians were not morally obliged to let a fetus grow inside the womb of its "mother's body" (Schöne-Seifert, 1993, p. 13). The physicians' choice not to apply the technology available would have sent out a "signal to the public" as far as maintaining trust in modern medicine was concerned (Schöne-Seifert, 1993, p. 23).

The neonatologist V. v. Loewenich countered this reproach regarding a breach of confidence with his comment, that trust in a collective term like "medicine" cannot possess a status as high as that of a *single* human being's bodily freedom from injury, spiritual well-being, or right to live. Physicians' decisions do not affect abstract things, but individuals' fates; the Erlangen case also involved such an *individual ethical* decision (Loewenich, 1993). This brings to light a conflict to which we have already referred in another context, namely the conflict between the concern of medicine for individual patients on the one hand, and the interest of society to control medical progress and its social consequences on the other.

> A satisfactory compromise between these competing interests has yet to be found. There are many reasons to believe that there can be no 'smooth' solution to this conflict, i.e., one that is satisfactory in all respects for all parties. There is a real conflict of goals between individual interest in medical aid at all costs and socio-political interest in controlling the progress of medical technology (Bayertz, Paslack and Schmidt, 1994, p. 467).

It is impossible to grant maximal medical intervention and maximal safety at the same time. The conflict is a structural one.

C. Brain Death

We have already mentioned that at no other time in Germany had there been a public discussion of this intensity about the concept of brain death. *Before* the Erlangen case, the brain death criteria could be regarded as socially accepted, not only within the medical profession, but also by the public. The brain death criteria are the result of norms that have been generated over more than ten years. The problems involved were first mentioned by a group of experts, brought together by the *Bundesärztekammer* [German National Medical Association] in 1979, which published the first version of brain death criteria in 1982. Due to further medical and technological developments, a first addendum was necessary in the mid-1980s (Bundesärztekammer, 1986) and a second followed in the early 1990s (Bundesärztekammer, 1991), both again the work of committees formed by the *Bundesärztekammer* especially for this purpose. From the very beginning, there were individual physicians, theologians, and philosophers who rejected this consensus, and yet at no time did this rejection find extensive public support. This situation did not change until the Erlangen case, when the opinions of a few previously critical voices were now adopted by the outraged public.

The debate surrounding the Erlangen case became very significant for public perception of the concept of brain death in general – beyond the pregnancy problem – and public acceptance of organ transplantation. The same difficult questions that appear in connection with brain death in a pregnant woman ("Is she really completely dead if she can still become a mother?") can also apply to the problem area of organ donation ("How can a man be 'completely dead' if his heart can still beat and his kidneys still function inside another body?"). Until the Erlangen case, an independent legal regulation of organ removal had not existed in Germany, although, after many failed attempts, a very promising bill was finally drafted. A silent social consensus, which in the meantime had really existed, was destroyed by growing mistrust in the brain death concept. The drop in heart, kidney and pancreas transplantations in Germany in 1992 had many causes; *one* reason for the decreased willingness to donate organs was the public's skepticism as a result of the Erlangen case (An, 1993).

At this point it should be emphasized, however, that the debate provoked by the Erlangen case is not about to lead to the *abolishment* of the brain death criterion. Future decisions in Germany (for example, the legality of organ removal) will be as dependent upon brain death criteria as their predecessors. Moreover, not even pronounced critics of brain death are calling for a radical prohibition of all incidences of organ removal or an immediate stop to the entire practice of organ transplantation. What they do want is to reduce the pool of organ donors. In cases of brain death, organ removal should be permitted only when the donor has previously given his expressed permission to this intervention (Grewel, 1992, p. 407); proxy decisions may not substitute for this permission. According to the critics' views, the brain-dead patient is *dying*, beyond hope of recovery and the point of no return, but not yet dead. The removal of heart, lung, or liver would represent a "lethal intervention" and would make an extension of § 216 of German criminal law ("death on demand") necessary (Hoff and Schmitten, 1994, pp. 227ff.).

IV. THE TWO CULTURES OF DEATH

Just a few days before the Erlangen case, Daniel Wikler had spoken at the *Inaugural Congress of the International Association of Bioethics* in Amsterdam. He stated that "the definition of death as death of the brain as a whole is widely regarded as a settled matter." From his point of view, it is "a point of pride to bioethicists, who are vulnerable to the charge that they offer arguments but not solutions," that in a once-controversial issue a wide number of countries could be found to be in agreement, and that the debate on brain death is almost at an end. "Indeed, those nations which have so far resisted the global movement toward the whole brain death criterion risk being seen as retrograde, held back perhaps by widespread misinformation, anti-scientific attitudes, or archaic folkways" (Wikler, 1993, p. 239). Here, the brain death criterion appears to be the product of a context free rationality; its metaphysical and cultural foundations are simply ignored.

And yet, the presentation by Kazumasa Hoshino (1993) at the very same congress on the reticence of the Japanese public toward brain death could have drawn attention to the fact that consensus regarding this definition of death depends upon certain cultural prerequisites. Only a multitude of the most different events and anthropological views could enable us to begin to understand the Japanese reservation – the fear that the supporters of brain death might actually try to "produce" fresh donors of organs for transplantation. We should take into account here that the first heart transplant, carried out in Japan in 1968, raised some unclarified questions concerning the correct procedure, which remain unanswered today and have led to a deep mistrust within much of the population (Hoshino, 1993, pp. 236f.). In addition, the Japanese national sentiment toward the corpse seems to play a decisive role in Japanese reticence toward brain death criteria. For many Japanese, it is important to see the deceased *as dead*, in order to be convinced of his/her death. And yet brain death

> is an invisible death contrary to the cardiac death which is a visibly recognizable death. Moreover, brain death is diagnosed by medical staff using a number of sophisticated medical equipment and machines in a closed intensive care unit (...). Survivors are placed in the position where they must rely solely on the conclusion of the medical staff (Hoshino, 1993, p. 238).

For the Japanese, the concept of brain-death "is a foreign concept and [Japanese are] far from being able to witness the death themselves visually at the bedside of the deceased" (Hoshino, 1993, p. 238).

The greatest difficulty for Europeans probably lies also in *seeing* a dead person as an artificially respirated brain-dead patient whose chest rises and falls, whose body is warm, whose skin is rosy, who perspires, and who is capable of reflex movements controlled by the spinal cord. The situation seems to have been simplified by the dualism of body and soul prevalent in Western culture, as well as the emphasis placed upon rationality when the concept of brain death was introduced. Since Aristotle, we have been used to comprehending the human being as an *animal rationale*, a being that is essentially characterized by its ability to think and make decisions rationally. This interpretation remains, even within traditional Christian thinking. In its report on brain death, the U.S. President's Commission emphasized this embedding of brain death criteria in the history of Western philosophy (President's Commission, 1981).

Western culture is not homogenous, however, but multi-structured and complex. It contains dominant currents but not an omnipotent consensus. It is home to a multitude of (partly divergent, partly convergent) metaphysical, anthropological and ethical views, which lead to varying opinions about the problems surrounding brain death. One example of this is "anthroposophic medicine", advocated by a minority, especially in Germany and Switzerland, and based on the teachings of Rudolf Steiner, the Hungarian-Croatian philosopher (1861-1925). From an anthroposophic point of view, a human being can only be deemed dead when *heartbeat and respiration* have ceased and the spiritual-mental element has "left" the physical element; this does not occur until three days after death (as has been established by "traditional" medical methods) (Steiner, 1987, pp. 105ff.) Since the human being is not really dead until *after* the separation of a special part, which is essential for *living* beings (the *Ätherleib*), from the body has taken place, brain death can only be one stage within this separation process, for in a brain-dead patient the individuality of this person, his/her "Ich" (ego), is still present. From an anthroposophic point of view, a brain-dead patient is still alive. The concentration of "traditional" medicine on brain-activity as proof of "ego-activity" is, for an anthroposophic physician (who always has traditional medical training, but who has extended and influenced his/her knowledge of the human being as a result of anthroposophic views), wrong, and brain death a "complete non-term," since the ego of the human being is still present in other regions of a brain-dead person (cf. Glöckler, 1993, p. 37). Furthermore, the case of irreversible brain failure represents a "severe disease," the start of the dying process (Bavastro, 1994, pp. 123f.). A "brain-dead", pregnant woman, whose heart is still beating and who is artificially respirated, cannot therefore be "dead"; this is "proven" by the course of treatment carried out on her (Bavastro, 1994, p. 110). One year before the case of the Erlangen baby – albeit without any accompanying turbulence in the media – a brain-dead, pregnant woman was treated in the anthroposophic Filderstadt Hospital in Stuttgart until she gave birth to a healthy child. In the reports which were later written by the hospital's physicians and the patient's husband, the individuality of the event was emphasized, as well as the lack of similarity to the Erlangen case (Lamerdin, 1994; Bavastro, 1994, pp. 141-153; Siegel, 1994). This example is nevertheless evidence of the fact that different philosophies do not necessarily in practice have to lead to different actions. The anthroposophic physicians in Stuttgart, guided by their view that the pregnant woman in question was *not yet* dead, arrived at a similar conclusion as did the Erlangen physicians a year later, guided in turn by their view that she was *already* dead. Both advocated further treatment aimed at saving the life of the fetus.

More important for an understanding of the Erlangen case are the fundamental differences existing within one overall culture between different groups – between the official scientific and technological culture on the one hand and the popular everyday culture on the other. The cultures are connected by complex links involving not harmony but friction and tension, and are forever being reinforced by the high speed of development within the cultural realm of science and technology. It usually takes a while for society to assimilate scientific and technological innovations; sometimes it takes an entire generation or longer. This is especially the case when these innovations touch upon deeply rooted elements of human self-understanding. The concept of brain death is obviously one such case. Independent of all the progress made by modern medicine, death still represents one, if not *the* central problem of human existence. One indication of this is the fact that death is one of the few events within a human lifespan that is ritualized, even within modern societies. If we take this seriously, then it should come as no surprise that fundamental innovations, like the use of brain death criteria, must be subject to serious debate. Even *before* the Erlangen case and *before* the irritations and protests that it provoked, the grave moral problems raised by brain death criteria were apparent (cf. Bayertz, 1992). With this in mind, the public's irritation and protests which erupted so vehemently in the Erlangen case seem far less in need of explanation than the quick acceptance of brain death after 1968!

One reason for this acceptance is certainly the *medicalization of death* that has taken place over the past 100 years. Within this period, scientific and technological culture has eclipsed the supremacy of religion in interpreting death, with the field of medicine slowly but surely becoming the authoritative body in matters of death. Among other things, this medicalization of death (Ariès, 1982, pp. 720f.) gives rise to a remarkable dynamism of interpretation. Interpretations of death no longer follow just the placid rhythm of cultural evolution, but are spurred on by the constantly increasing rate of theoretical and technological progress within the field of medicine.

VI. CONCLUSION

A large portion of the public reaction to the Erlangen case was obviously the product of one-sided and shortened reports in the press that reinforced the already widespread picture of the physician as a "technical manipulator", guided more by scientific interest than care for a patient's well-being. In the assessment that followed the case, it was therefore suggested that in the public debate, the uncertainty on the part of the physicians should have been more strongly emphasized, in order to curb the prejudice that they had decided between life and death "in their own absolute power." In so doing, one would have created within the public a consciousness of the problems involved and thus avoided the radical polarization that occurred (Bockenheimer-Lucius and Seidler, 1993, p. 63).

It is necessary that we learn from events like the Erlangen case and draw consequences for the future. And yet we believe that it will not be possible to avoid such cases completely. The irritations it caused are no more the result of mere "clumsiness" on the part of the medical profession than they are an expression of "irrationality" on the part of the public. It is indeed our view that such irritations are, to a certain extent, necessary and unavoidable: they are an expression of the tension between scientific and technological progress on the one hand and moral and cultural tradition on the other. This tension has always accompanied the history of Western science and technology, and there is no reason to assume that it will disappear in the future.

It has been said that the public, within developed industrial societies, is today as far from an adequate understanding of science as the inhabitants of remote villages in the Middle Ages were from an adequate understanding of Thomas Aquinas's theology. This observation, however, does not go far enough. In the Middle Ages, theological innovations did not influence the everyday lives of village farmers, whereas the practical application of scientific innovations in our time revolutionizes our lives time and again, right down to their smallest and most intimate ramifications. The public has not only learned to view this influence as necessary; it now takes it for granted. Yet it also feels challenged, and rejects a world in which everything seems possible, and in which nothing is holy. The achievements of medicine and biology, in particular, are seen by many as an increasing threat to their individual identity *as human beings*.

University of Münster, Münster, Germany
St. Markus-Hospital, Frankfurt/M., Germany

NOTES

* This essay was translated into English by Sarah L. Kirkby

1 It is unclear whether further experiments of this kind have been carried out, since negative proceedings are rarely published.

REFERENCES

An (1992). 'Amtsgericht ordnet "Betreuung" für hirntote Schwangere an,' *Frankfurter Allgemeine Zeitung* 244 (Oct. 12), 12.

An (1993). 'Organverpflanzungen weiter rückläufig,' *Frankfurter Allgemeine Zeitung* 64 (March 17), N 1.

Ariès, P. (1982). *Geschichte des Tode.* Munich: Deutscher Taschenbuch Verlag.

Bavastro, P. (1994). *Anthroposophische Medizin auf der Intensivstation. Historische Hintergründe. Schlaf- Narkose – Hirntod – Organtransplantation. Eine besondere Krankengeschichte*, Persephone. Arbeitsberichte der Medizinischen Sektion am Goetheanum, Vol. 8. Dornach, Schweiz: Verlag am Goetheanum.

Bayertz, K. (1992). 'Techno-Thanathology. Moral consequences of introducing brain criteria for death,' *The Journal of Medicine and Philosophy* 17, 407-417.

Bayertz, K., Paslack, R. and Schmidt, K.W. (1994). 'Summary of "Gene transfer into human somatic cells. State of the technology, medical risks, social and ethical problems": A report,' *Human Gene Therapy* 5, 465-468.

Bockenheimer-Lucius, G. and Seidler, E. (1993). [Editorial], *Ethik in der Medizin* 5, 1-2.

Bockenheimer-Lucius, G. and Seidler, E. (Eds.) (1993). *Hirntod und Schwangerschaft. Dokumentation einer Diskussionsveranstaltung der Akademie für Ethik in der Medizin zum 'Erlanger Fall'*, Medizin in Recht und Ethik, Vol. 28. Stuttgart: Ferdinand Enke.

Bräutigam, H.H., Kruse, K. and Rückert, S. (1992). 'Schneewitchens Kind,' *Die ZEIT*, No. 45 (Oct. 30), 17, 19.

Brody, B. and Engelhardt, Jr., H.T. (eds.) (1987). *Bioethics. Readings and Cases*. Englewood Cliffs, N.J.: Prentice-Hall.

Bundesärztekammer (1986). 'Kriterien des Hirntodes. Entscheidungshilfen zur Feststellung des Hirntodes,' *Deutsches Ärzteblatt* 83, 2940-2946.

Bundesärztekammer (1991). 'Kriterien des Hirntodes. Entscheidungshilfen zur Feststellung des Hirntodes,' *Deutsches Ärzteblatt* 88, 4396-4407.

Eser, A. (1989). 'Humanexperimente/Heilversuch: (3.) Recht.' In:A. Eser et al. (Eds.), *Lexikon Medizin Ethik Recht* (pp. 503-514). Freiburg/ Basel/ Wien: Herder.

Feinberg, J. (1974). 'The rights of animals and unborn generations.' In: W. T. Blackstone (Ed.), *Philosophy and Environmental Crisis* (pp. 43-68). Athens, Georgia: University of Georgia Press.

Fletcher, J. (1988). 'Ethics and genetic control.' In: J.F. Monagle and D.C. Thomasma (Eds.), *Medical Ethics. A Guide for Health Professionals* (pp. 3-11). Rockville, MD: Aspen Publishers.

Glöckler, M. (1993). 'Medizin an der Schwelle.' In: M. Glöckler (ed.), *Medizin an der Schwelle. Erkenntnisringen – Liebe als Heilkraft – Schicksalsgestaltung* (pp. 13-62). Persephone. Arbeitsberichte der Medizinischen Sektion am Goetheanum. Vol. 3, Verlag am Goetheanum. Schwiez: Dornach.

Grewel, H. (1992). 'Gratwanderung der Transplantationsmedizin', *Pastoraltheologie* 81, 391-408.

Hoff, J. and Schmitten, J.i.d. (1994). 'Kritik der "Hirntod"-Konzeption. Plädoyer für ein menschenwürdiges Todeskriterium.' In: J. Hoff and J. in der Schmitten (Eds.). *Wann ist der Mensch tot? Organverpflanzung und Hirntodkriterium* (pp. 153-252). Reinbek: Rowohlt.

Hoshino, K. (1993). 'Legal status of brain death in Japan: Why many Japanese do not accept "brain death" as a definition of death,' *Bioethics* 7, 234-238.

Kerényi, K. (1966). *Die Mythologie der Griechen. Band 1: Die Götter- und Menschheitsgeschichten*, Munich: Deutscher Taschenbuch Verlag.

Koch, H.-G. (1993)., 'Stellungnahme,' in G. Bockernheimer-Lucius and E. Seidler (Eds.), *Hirntod und Schwangerschaft. Dokumentation einer Diskussionsveranstaltung der Akademie fur Ethick in der Medizin zum 'Erlanger Fall'* (pp. 72-83). Medizin in Recht und Ethik Bd. 28.

Lamerdin, M. (1994). 'Sterben und Geborenwerden kreuzen sich. Geburtshilfe im Lichte zweier Welten,' *Die Drei*, 22-28.

Laufs, A. (1988). *Arztrecht*. Schriftenreihe der Neuen Juristischen Wochenschrift, 4th ed., No. 29. Tübingen: C.H. Beck.

Loewenich, V. v. (1993). 'Leserbrief,' *Ethik in der Medizin* 5, 220.

Mappes, T.A. and Zembaty, J.S. (Eds.) (1991). *Biomedical Ethics*, 3rd ed. New York: McGraw-Hill.

Menzel, H. (1976). 'Ziel und Grenzen ärztlichen Handelns im Extrembereich menschlicher Existenz.' In: A. Auer et al. (Eds.), *Zwischen Heilauftrag und Sterbehilfe. Zum Behandlungsabbruch aus ethischer, medizinischer und rechtlicher Sicht* (pp. 53-74). Köln/Berlin/Bonn/München: Carl Heymanns Verlag.

Mitscherlich, A. and Mielke, F. (Eds.) (1962). *Medizin ohne Menschlichkeit. Dokumente des Nürnberger Ärzteprozesses*. Frankfurt/M: Fischer.

Petersen, P. (1994). 'Mütterlicher Hirntod und Schwangerschaft,' *Die Drei*, 477-485.

President's Commission for the Study of Ethical Problems in Medicine and Biomedical and Behavioral Research (1981). *Defining Death. Medical, Legal, and Ethical Issues in the Determination of Death*, Washington, D.C.

Scheele, J. (1993). 'Fallbericht.' In: G. Bockernheimer-Lucius and E. Seidler (Eds.), *Hirntod und Schwangerschaft. Dokumentation einer Diskussionsveranstaltung der Akademie fur Ethick in der Medizin zum 'Erlanger Fall'* (pp. 11-18). Medizin in Recht und Ethik 28..

Schöne-Seifert, B. (1993). 'Der "Erlanger Fall" im Rückblick: eine medizinethische Lektion?', *Ethik in der Medizin* 5, 13-23.

Siegel, K.-E. (1994). *Wir durften nicht aufgeben!*, 2nd ed. Gütersloh: Gütersloher Verlagshaus.

Steiner, R. (1987). *Theosophie. Einführung in übersinnliche Welterkenntnis und Menschenbestimmung*, Gesamtausgabe No. 9, 31st ed. Dornach, Schweiz: Rudolf Steiner Verlag.

Wedemeyer, G. (1992). 'Das darf nie wieder passieren.' *Stern* 49 (Nov. 26), 220-221.

Wikler, D. (1993). 'Brain death: A durable consensus?' *Bioethics* 7, 239-246.
Wuermeling, H.-B. and Scheele, J. (1992). 'Das Kind in der toten Mutter,' *Frankfurter Allgemeine Zeitung* (Oct. 17), 242, 9.

MAURIZIO MORI

BIOETHICS IN ITALY UP TO 2002: AN OVERVIEW

INTRODUCTORY REMARKS AND PRELIMINARY DISTINCTIONS

There are at least two general features of Italian culture that a foreigner should keep in mind in order to understand Italian bioethics. The *first* is that until the late '60s Italy really was a "Roman Catholic country" in the sense that on issues concerning family life and medicine there was a widely "shared morality" roughly corresponding to the Catholic perspective, which was enforced by legislation and built into major social institutions. For instance, divorce was introduced only in 1970, and one article of the 1929 Lateran Pacts between Italy and the Vatican State stated that the whole of Italian family law had to be consistent with the Roman Catholic view on the matter. This situation changed drastically in the course of about 15 years. Beginning in the late '60s, a joint movement involving the judiciary (at different levels), the parliament and civil society succeeded in introducing reforms aimed at adjusting (or updating) social institutions to the new life-styles of Italian society, which was becoming industrial and secularized. One consequence of this reformative process was that some basic laws concerning health care and family departed in significant aspects from the standards of the Roman Catholic tradition.[1] However, apart from some technical adjustments to ease divorce for childless couples (and now a recent law on organ donation), since the early '80s no new law has been approved concerning family life or bioethical issues, and therefore we must conclude that this reformative season ended in the early 1980s.

The *second* general feature of the Italian situation to be kept in mind concerns the close relationship between the "intellectual work" and "political involvement" (or "affiliation") of a scholar. While in other Western countries "academic research" is (or at least appears to be) a peculiarly self-regulating institution, rather unaffected by political influence, in Italy (peculiarly in philosophical and historical matters) extra-academic considerations are often quite weighty. Thus, an "intellectual contribution" is often valued not on the basis of academic criteria (originality, clearness, etc.), but on other criteria, such as possible social or political consequences, etc. Some argue that this peculiar feature

H.T. Engelhardt, Jr. and L.M. Rasmussen (eds.), Bioethics and Moral Content: National Traditions of Health Care Morality, 97–120.

is due to the Italian mind, which is fond of clear-cut polarization. Others explain this feature by means of historical reasons, going back mainly to the opposition between Roman Catholics and Protestants, and subsequent contraposition between "clericals" and "anti-clericals" in the ninetieth century and "communists" and "anti-communists" in the twentieth century. Be that as it may, one should not forget that in Italy the "logic of (political) coalition" is stronger than the "logic of (scientific) argumentation". In bioethics – willy nilly and in spite of lamentations coming from everywhere – the major opposition remains between Roman Catholics and non-Catholics, where this latter category includes secularists, Protestants as well as Jews – the Muslims being almost unheard of, at least so far. A straight consequence of such a polarization is that we should carefully distinguish between *bioethics as a cultural movement* (or *intellectual debate*), devoted to the critical evaluation of received opinions and elaboration of new ideas to be advanced by scholars and people; and *bioethics as an institutional setting* aimed at influencing public opinion or controlling social change in the field of health care and issues concerning living stuff.

These remarks are helpful for understanding the three different stages of Italian bioethics. The first one goes from its very beginning (the late '70s), up to the late '80s or early '90s, and is characterized by a magmatic situation, which was consequential to the intellectual discovery of the new ethical problems examined in bioethics. The second stage goes from the late '80s or early '90s up to the end of the century, and is characterized by a division into schools of thought and an attention to bioethics institutions which had to be influencing public policy –if not public opinion. The third stage is in its early beginning, but there are already some clear signs indicating that a new trend is already taking shape.

In this paper I will outline major features of various stages and try to sort out the main reasons leading to the new situation.

II. THE FIRST STAGE OF ITALIAN BIOETHICS: BIOETHICS AS A CULTURAL MOVEMENT

The first Italian author to use the term "bioetica" was Menico Torchio, a biologist who read Potter's *Bioethics. Bridge to the Future* (1971) and presented such a perspective in some papers written in the mid-'70s

(Torchio, 1973). However, Torchio's works circulated in very limited circles, remaining completely unknown even to scholars until the early '90s, when bioethics had already been cultivated for other reasons. Torchio's views hardly stimulated any debate and are mentioned only for history's sake.

In Italy bioethics began as an intellectual interest and a cultural inquiry in the late '70s in two different scholarly circles: a group of analytical philosophers attracted to the development of English-speaking philosophy by Rawls' celebrated book as well as by the growth of applied ethics; and a group of Catholic scholars (theologians and physicians) who came to know of "bioethics" through the Kennedy Institute (Washington, D.C.) and the Borja Institute (Barcelona, Spain). The birth of Italian bioethics is strongly connected with these two groups, so it is instructive to look at each of them.

Already in the mid-'70s, a few analytical philosophers perceived that the sudden passage from "metaethics" to "normative ethics" and then to "applied ethics" marked a significant shift of interests opening "new directions in ethics."[2] Being eager to examine practical issues (such as abortion, witholding treatment, etc.), which were already hotly discussed in Italy as well as in other European countries, they welcomed the new turn toward "practical philosophy". However, this trend was firmly opposed by a large majority of Italian philosophers, though for different reasons. Most Italian philosophers espouse the so-called "continental approach" to philosophy, and therefore they rejected bioethics simply because – given its American origins – it was seen as a mere by-product of analytical philosophy.[3] But even the far smaller group of Italian philosophers working in the "analytical tradition" were quite hostile to "applied philosophy". Most of these philosophers came from legal philosophy and they argued that any involvement in practical issues was incompatible with the (evaluative) "neutrality" proper to philosophy and implied a violation of *Hume's law* ("no ought from an is"). Not only does bioethics rest on a sort of "logical" mistake, but – Hume's law being the main argument for the thesis of strict separation of morality between law – the new field is also *politically dangerous* because it challenged the separation thesis which justified the (above-mentioned) change in the '70s toward a more liberal legislation. In brief, most analytical philosophers perceived bioethics as a sort of "Trojan horse" introduced into the citadel of a sane secular world-view in order to re-introduce the obsolete idea of an *ethical State* justifying the enforcement of *one* specific morality (the Roman Catholic one).

In Italy the birth of secular bioethics would have been in serious danger if Uberto Scarpelli had not supported the new reflection. Scarpelli was a professor of philosophy of law at the State University of Milan as well as an esteemed analytical philosopher holding a version of legal positivism grounded on an original interpretation of Hume's law. His "orthodoxy" in the analytical tradition was beyond any doubt, and by joining his intellectual prestige with his strong interests in practical issues he succeeded in making of bioethics a philosophically respectable field of inquiry. As a member of the board of the *Rivista di filosofia* (the oldest and most influential Italian philosophical journal), in 1979 Scarpelli presented the project for a special issue devoted to the "right to life", which is possibly the first work produced in Italy inspired by the new interdisciplinary spirit of bioethics.[4] Scarpelli did not publish much scholarly work in bioethics, and his contributions to the field consist mainly in short papers and presentations to conferences. But he introduced to the field an analytical rigor that forced other philosophers to do as well.[5] Scarpelli's teaching was crucial for the birth of Italian bioethics because he contributed to changing the unfavorable attitude manifested by most Italian secular philosophers toward the new subject. Moreover, Scarpelli encouraged the activity of some early groups working in bioethics: he cooperated with the *Centro di Bioetica* established in Genoa in April 1984, which devoted particular attention to "animal rights" issues;[6] he was associated with *Politeia*, a private research center on "applied ethics" established in Milan in 1983, which soon started to work on bioethics; and was a founding member of the Consulta di bioetica in 1989. His association with *Politeia* was particularly relevant because in the late '80s *Politeia* had already organized a few successful conferences devoted to major issues debated in Italy such as the status of the human embryo, organ transplants, definition of death, witholding treatment, etc., resulting a most active and influential group in nascent bioethics as well as in the ongoing debate.[7]

Scarpelli died an untimely death in July 1993, which was a great loss not only for Italian philosophy but also for the whole culture. He was a leading figure in philosophical circles as well as an acute writer commenting on legal and political events. Without his influence, Italian bioethics would certainly be much poorer and possibly would have suffered a much slower development. He framed a basic tenet of current Italian debate by clarifying the concept of "secular bioethics" (*bioetica laica*) as the view in which one argues "as if god wouldn't exist" (*etsi deus non daretur* – using Grotius' famous latin sentence). This view does not entail by itself atheism or agnosticism, and a person can believe in God's existence while holding this view. But one cannot claim that the thesis of God's existence rests on a rational proof to be accepted by everyone. Therefore, bioethical arguments cannot rely on religious premises, and therefore the "logic of (religious) coalition" is subordinated to the "logic of (scientific) argumentation" which recognizes the limits of reason in ethics. None can claim to know absolute moral truth (for Scarpelli, any moral *truth* is logically forbidden by Hume's law), and therefore we have to recognize that there are different and incommensurable moral views, so that *ethical pluralism* is not only an empirical fact but also a *value*. People have a basic right to live according to their fundamental moral beliefs (if others are not harmed), and therefore *tolerance* is the utmost moral value of bioethics, and frank and free debate is the only way to achieve an adequate social consensus. Granted such a conceptual (secular) frame, on specific substantive issues Scarpelli was sometimes quite in agreement with tradition. For instance, he morally condemned abortion, even though he held that such a practice should be legal and regulated carefully. In any case, he was very open to a dialogue leading to possible social consensus and was very far from any sort of enthusiasm for new technical possibilities.

While secular philosophers debated (or quibbled?) over the intellectual "legitimacy" of the new field, bioethics had an enthusiastic reception among some theologians and legal doctors based at the faculty of medicine of the Catholic University in Rome.[8] Since 1951 – founder fr. Agostino Gemelli established the journal *Medicina e morale* – the Catholic University of Milano paid special attention to medical morality, and saw bioethics as a good opportunity to restate the Roman Catholic point of view, revitalizing a field that appeared agonized, having suffered a great defeat with the approval of the abortion law in 1978. The first (1982) issue of *Medicina e morale* was devoted to genetic engineering, and in the editorial of that issue, the editor (Msgr. Elio Sgreccia) remarked that such a topic was rather new and unusual for a journal of medical ethics conceived in traditional terms, but it was justified and welcome because the journal was widening its scope of inquiry, as indicated by the new subtitle: *Rivista trimestrale di Bioetica, Deontologia e Morale Medica* (Trimestral Journal of Bioethics, Deontology and Medical Morality).[9] In 1983-84 Sgreccia taught a new course in *bioethics* at the faculty of medicine, and in 1985 Pope John Paul II officially opened the new *Centro di bioetica*, the first institution of its kind within an Italian university. Since then the group has been very active in promoting and supporting Vatican positions on bioethical issues. The journal firmly opposes any form of "etica laica" as well as "ethical pluralism." The first view is unacceptable because being the very foundation of morality God cannot be bracketed as claimed by holders of the "etica laica". "Ethical pluralism" is criticized because "pluralism" in reality is a self-defeating version of ethical relativism and dangerous skepticism, leading to some totalitarian drift.[10] When human life is at stake (as it is in the case of human embryos), there is no room for alleged doubts or different views, and people must recognize the moral truth on the issue.

Other Catholic groups had an early interest in the new issues emerging in medicine and contributed in some way to the early stage of bioethics, in a wide sense of the term. This qualification is needed because at first these scholars were somehow reluctant to accept at least the name *bioethics* (if not the concept), and approached the subject from a different viewpoint. Sandro Spinsanti, for instance, approached "bio-medical ethics" – as he prefered to call it – through psychology and the social sciences as well as theology (his original field), so that his research ended up at the foundation of a new center in Rome (and a new quarterly, *L'arco di Giano*) devoted to "medical humanities" (in 1999 he abandoned this Center and founded another journal called *Janus*). His perspective is more flexible and open to dialogue than that of the Catholic University center and represents a version of so-called "liberal Catholicism". Another early Catholic group interested in the field was based at the San Raffaele hospital in Milano. In 1983, this group paid attention to issues of philosophy of medicine, and only later came to be involved in bioethical issues. Applying a phenomenological approach to medicine, this group held that there is a sort of intrinsic guidance for medicine and medical ethics. Paolo Cattorini directed the center from the late '80s to 1997, giving to it a kind of visibility and developing a dialogue with other positions.[11] This work is now continued by Roberto Mordacci and Massimo Reichlin.

In a short presentation like this I cannot mention all the contributions to the birth of bioethics, but it is important to emphasize that in early '80s bioethics was a *cultural movement* promoted by a relatively small group of scholars who had two basic problems: a) trying to convince other collegues that bioethical issues were intellectually interesting and culturally respectable, and b) trying to understand exactly what bioethics was about. People perceived that something new was emerging, but they couldn't say exactly what it was. From an intellectual point of view it was an exciting period, because the attention was focused on arguments justifying the different positions. Scholars were trying to understand the different possible moves in the debate and were open to various perspectives. The situation was characterized by a magmatic confusion because, on the one hand, new perspectives and issues were at stake, and on the other, people were ready to accept the challenges and think on them. This attitude for a time was shared by secular scholars as well as by some Roman Catholics, many of whom still hoped for the *aggiornamento* concerning moral matters recommended by the Vatican II council. In this sense, for a time bioethics seemed to be something really new, escaping traditional moves of the "logic of coalition".

However, this time was unfortunately short. The Instruction *Donum Vitae* (1987) was a blow to this intellectual debate, because it altered the cultural atmosphere and set heavy limits on theologians' freedom of research and expression. This trend was reinforced a few years later by the *Instruction on the Function of the Theologian* (1990), which suppressed any form of public dissent within the Italian Catholic church closing any possible openings of Catholics.

The combined influence of these factors (the new policy endorsed by the Catholic church and the ongoing process of institutionalization) brought to a close the first stage of Italian bioethics, a stage characterized by doubts and an openness to new solutions as well as a friendly and sincere dialogue between various participants who met without any previous "school positions" to defend.

III. THE SECOND STAGE OF ITALIAN BIOETHICS: BIOETHICS AS AN INSTITUTIONAL SETTING DEVOTED TO CONTROLLING SOCIAL CHANGE IN BIOMEDICAL MATTERS

In the early '90s, bioethics had gained cultural "respectability", but was still considered a sort of "sophisticated interest" limited to people looking after quite "peculiar and rare" situations distant from normal daily life. At the same time, the primeval situation of magmatic confusion had come to an end, and the overarching influence of different "schools of thought" emerged powerfully – with peculiar strength for the Catholic perspective.

These schools were the following: there is an active minority composed by some *analytical* scholars involved mainly in academic work, defending a liberal secular perspective; there is a large fraction of scholars following the *continental approach*: using the conceptual framework of philosophers such as Martin Heidegger, Hans Gadamer or Emmanuel Levinas, some defend liberal views, but most of them hold a very traditional view of bioethics issues. Finally, there is another fraction defending a strictly Vatican view, using a more thomistic frame. In general the Vatican perspective can easily be in agreement with positions coming from *continental approaches* because both are against technical "manipulations" and condemn what they call "scientism", i.e. the view that science should not be subordinated to (sanctity of life) ethics or to "humanism". In this sense, bioethicists of the continental school are always paying attention to Catholic thought. This explains the general influence of Catholic thinking upon Italian bioethics and why the influence of the analytic school remains quite limited.

In this context the publication of *Veritatis Splendor* (1993) and even more of *Evangelium Vitae* (1995) had a significant role in the process of institutionalization. As is well known, *Evangelium Vitae* affirms that our time is characterized by the radical opposition between two irreconcilable world-views or moral paradigms, the so-called "culture of life" (supported by Catholics and all the people of good will) and the "culture of death" (supported by all the others). This perspective provided an authoritative cultural background for the ongoing institutionalization, reinforcing the tendency to polarization.

The process of institutionalization which occupied most of the '90s issued prolific results for the Catholic perspective. Even though bioethics as a cultural movement started within secular culture, where the new field attracted some positive interest among educated people, it was completely disregarded at an institutional level by secular politicians and bureaucrats.[12] Catholic scholars, on the other hand, had a tremendous impact on institutions at different levels: several private research centers were established and Catholics also got control of some pivotal state institutions. As early as 1983, during a general reform of university studies, Catholics succeeded in including the newborn discipline "bioethics" within the group of *legal medicine* (ruled by a large majority of Catholic professors), so that in 1990, Msgr. Elio Sgreccia became the first tenured professor of bioethics appointed in Italy, and Paolo Cattorini got an associate professorship in 1993 at the University of Florence (and later moved to the University of Varese). The general result is that in the first part of the '90s, Catholics had a complete monopoly on the teaching of bioethics in the universities.

Moreover, Catholics had an almost complete control of the several governmental commissions appointed from the '80s up to the mid-'90s, starting the first one, the so-called Santosuosso Commission (from the name of judge Fernando Santosuosso, who chaired it), instituted in 1984 to elaborate a possible regulation for assisted reproduction. The "Santosuosso bill" suggested a strong limitation of *in vitro* fertilization, and considered "Artificial Insemination by Donor" (AID) as a kind of "surrogate-adoption", so that a couple could apply for it only after the application for an adoption was unsuccessful. Even though this proposal came from a Catholic oriented commission, since it only discouraged AID – but did not forbid it – it may have appeared too "liberal" to some hidden rulers, so it was abandoned.[13]

Other "ad hoc commissions" on various topics (such as AIDS epidemics, end of life issues, etc.) have been formed over more than a decade and all of them ruled by a large majority of Catholics. Even Italian representatives at the international organizations were designated accordingly. Even more attention was devoted by Catholics to the National Committee for Bioethics (*Comitato nazionale per la bioetica*), which was appointed in March 1990 by the Christian Democrat Prime Minister, Mr. Giulio Andreotti, and chaired by Adriano Bompiani, a professor of gynecology at the Catholic University in Rome. The history of the Committee would require more space, and here I can only say that it had four major stages corresponding to the four different chairmen. Bompiani chaired for about two years (having then to leave because he became a cabinet minister) a Committee formed by more then 30 Catholics out of the 40 members, which produced a number of reports, most of them about issues that in Italy are almost non-controversial, such as genetic therapy and organ donation or issues concerning childhood.[14] Bompiani was replaced in 1992 by professor Adriano Ossicini (another Catholic physician involved in psychology and less influenced by the Vatican views) who chaired a more pluralistic Committee since the two vice-presidents were secular scholars and the number of Catholic members was about 30 out of 40. However, only a few reports were published so the influence of this short period (a bit more than one year) was minimal. The Committee was renewed at the end of 1994 by the resigning right-wing cabinet, which appointed so many Catholic members that three secular scholars immediately resigned, and the Committee was baptized as "the bishops' committee" (*il comitato dei vescovi*"). Apart from the lively controversies which ensued, this Committee, chaired by professor Francesco D'Agostino, a philosopher of law holding positions of strict Roman Catholicism, endured for the whole term, being therefore (implicitly) confirmed by the left-wing cabinet – a fact which showed that on bioethical issues there still holds a sort of *political* consensus. The Committee was very productive and issued about 40 reports on several topics, but the most important one was on the "Identity and status of the human embryo" (27 June 1996), stating that a human embryo is "one of us" and ought to be treated accordingly.[15]

For about a decade, Catholics had almost full control of institutions devoted to bioethics. This explains why at the public level the only voice which was heard came (and often still comes) from the Catholic arena or is (roughly) consistent with such a view. In the secular area no institutional attention was devoted to the growing bioethical reflection and in some cases bioethics was still seen with some suspicion.

Responses to the new need for bioethical reflection came from some academics and citizens, who worked to found some private bioethical institutions. In 1985 *Politeia* established a special branch devoted to bioethics, and in 1989 Renato Boeri, a well-known Italian neurologist, founded the *Consulta di Bioetica*, another voluntary association devoted to promote "secular bioethics" (in Scarpelli's sense). *Politeia* organized some successful congresses on crucial topics as well as regular seminars that tried to convey an interdisciplinary and pluralistic style of debating. It also supported the new reflection, publishing several papers in its journal, *Notizie di Politeia*, that for a few years was the only voice for secular bioethics. The *Consulta* has had a prominent role in the first stages of the euthanasia debate prompted by the decriminalization of the practice in the Netherlands in the early '90s. Catholics tried to stop any open discussion on the issue, making it a sort of taboo in the name of the absolute immorality of any intentional killing. The *Consulta* succeeded in breaking such an effort and keeping the discussion open. Moreover, the *Consulta* launched a version of the *Living will* – called *Carta dell' autodeterminazione* – which received a good reception among the public and was supported by a number of the members of Parliament, who in February 1999 presented a bill to make it legal.[16] Finally, since 1993 the *Consulta* published *Bioetica. Rivista Interdisciplinare*, which is still the only bioethical journal informed by ethical pluralism, where scholars of different opinions (Catholic and secular) can debate and confront their views. Together with some academics, attention was paid to obtaining university positions even for secular scholars, and by the end of the '90s this goal was reached. Now there are several bioethicists doing good scholarly work in a secular perspective.

This hard work resulted in some public success, and both *Politeia* and *Consulta* are esteemed and well-known institutions on the Italian scene. But their action is mostly limited to a minority of educated people and has hardly any impact on state or governmental settings. At this level, Catholics still have full and strict control of the situation. This occurs either from a sort of traditional inertia or because secular politicians and bureaucrats tend to leave things as they are as far as possible in order to avoid possible controversies with Catholics. Two pieces of evidence confirm this attitude.

The first is provided by the 1999 National Committee of Bioethics, which was appointed by Mr. Massimo D'Alema, a secular politicians ruling a center-leftist government. This fourth Committee was chaired by Giovanni Berlinguer, a professor of hygiene at the University of Rome and one of those secular scholars who didn't accept the appointment in the former Committee: the new Committee could have been a good opportunity to establish a solid state institutional basis for secular bioethics. But, apart from some positive efforts to establish new relationships with other social institutions,[17] the Committee avoided a re-examination of former reports and failed to become the reference point for an authoritative non-Catholic perspective.

The second piece of evidence is given by reactions to Veronesi's stands on bioethical issues. Professor Umberto Veronesi is a famous oncologist who was Minister of Health from April 26, 2000 up to the end of May 2001 in a center-leftist government. Being a minister, he was asked about the problem of Permanent Vegetative State (PVS) patients, when the Appeal Court of Milan denied withdrawing of artificial feeding. He said that we cannot continue to treat PVS patients as "normal patients" and that a better solution to such a tragic situation should be found .[18] Commenting on another sentence on non-voluntary euthanasia issued in July 2000, Veronesi said that in his long career he was never asked to perform euthanasia, but he acknowledged that terminal suffering is a serious problem to be faced, showing a moderate openness to euthanasia. He supported also the opportunity of the wider use of opium for therapeutic reasons and changed the law accordingly; he received in

Italy the European directive concerning the use of the "day-after pill" ("emergency contraception"), saying that the reception was not only a due act, but also that the new service was for women's reproductive health. Finally, in September 2000 he nominated an *Ad hoc* Commission to report on stem cells research chaired by Nobel Laureate Renato Dulbecco and formed by a large majority of secular scholars, and just before leaving office, Veronesi presented the Oleari report on withdrawing artificial feeding from PVS patients.[19]

"Never again one like Veronesi, the worse minister of health Italy ever had!" was a comment of a Catholic journal when he left his office. This comment manifests how angry Catholics were at his actions, which on the other hand were approved by most Italians (opinion polls revealed that a large majority agreed with Veronesi's view). What is most surprising, however, is that Veronesi was not supported by his fellows: other secular politicians did not enter into such issues, keeping themselves out of such controversies. This shows the lack of commitment of secular politicians for bioethical struggles and explains why Catholics still have strict control of most state bioethical institutions.

There is a sense in which this situation is quite odd and somewhat incomprehensible, since in Italy public opinion is largely dissonant with Catholic teachings. This was shown by empirical research commissioned by Italian bishops in 1994, which revealed that only a small minority of Italians agree with Catholic teachings on bioethics. The dean of the Italian moral philosophers, Pietro Prini, says that there is a "submerged schism" going on in the church, and even cardinal Camillo Ruini, president of the Italian bishops, at the end of 2000 admitted that Catholics are already a minority in the country.[20] Nevertheless, Italian secular politicians had been hesitant or unwilling to engrain secular views into state bioethical institutions.

The result of this situation is that while Italians' opinion and conduct are increasingly secular, most bioethical institutions (university research centers, the National Bioethics Committee, etc.) are controlled by Catholics and convey conservative positions. This discrepancy is at the basis of Italian bioethics' third stage, which seems to be at its onset. The exact shape of this new stage is not defined yet, but there are already some signs indicating its direction. Those aspects emerge from different issues, but are more prominent in the debate on assisted reproduction and more clear with the appointment of the latest (the fifth) National Committee for Bioethics (July 12, 2002).

IV. THE THIRD STAGE OF ITALIAN BIOETHICS. ATTEMPTS TO CONTROL BIOETHICAL MATTERS THROUGH INSTITUTIONS

Debates on assisted reproduction have been (and still are) crucial in Italian bioethics, to the extent that in many quarters "bioethics" is identified with the issue. It has raised several controversies since 1984, when AID was banned by the NHS by a decree of the Minister of Health. Since then it has been practiced only in private fertility clinics, which are totally unregulated. Even from a technical and hygienic viewpoint, no state control was performed until 2001, when minister Veronesi established a Commission to monitor the number and activities of fertility clinics.[21] This long-lasting situation explains some "queer cases" which received public attention and explains why Italy is spoken of as a sort of "reproductive Far West", i.e., a land in which everyone is entitled to do what she likes. Since the early '80s, many bills (about 50) to regulate or forbid the practice have been presented to the Parliament, but none have been considered. However, controversies over assisted reproduction and human embryos have from time to time come to the fore. Apart from some scandals, the issue received wide attention from the public when the National Committee for Bioethics presented its report on the identity of the human embryo in July 1996. A few weeks later, news of the destruction of about 3,300 embryos in the U.K. got the front page for several days and about a hundred women were willing to "adopt" these embryos in order to prevent their destruction.[22] Moreover, on the 1st of February 1997 (just before the "life day" celebrated by the Catholics), four renewed intellectuals (including the chairman of the National Committee, professor D'Agostino) supported a new bill proposing a change of art. 1 of the Italian civil code, which would transfer the acquisition of "legal capacity" from birth to "conception". This bill is considered the founding stone of the so-called "party of the embryo."[23]

Within this general context, the impression produced by the birth of the sheep Dolly at the end of February 1997 was so strong and effective that it convinced a number of parties that the time was ripe for new legislation on assisted reproduction. Ms. Marida Bolognesi was appointed to chair a parliamentary commission to prepare a "unified bill", which was presented in early 1998.[24] In its frame the bill was rather conservative, because it admitted assisted reproduction only as a remedy to infertility, and applicants had to prove their infertility (considered a burden, if not a stigma). However, it had some "liberal" openings since it allowed AID even to non-married couples and was vague enough concerning embryo protection to allow some possibilities for cryoconservation. This bill was a "political mediation" among secular views and some "liberal Catholic" perspectives, and should have gained the majority of the Parliament. However, the results of discussion in the lower chamber in the first months of 1999 were appalling. Even though the bill was proposed by the ruling center-leftist government, leaving the MPs free to vote according to personal conscience, it was clear from the beginning that Catholics and other conservatives would have been strongly against the bill. After some crucial amendments passed, Ms. Bolognesi left the leadership of the bill, which progressively became quite different from that prepared by the commission. The bill was finally approved by the lower chamber on May 26, 1999: apart from very heavy penalties for any violation, it included the following features: an opening general clause declaring that an embryo's rights are to be protected by law; a general proscription of AID and of embryo conservation and even a provision allowing "pre-adoption" of embryos currently stored in Italian fertility clinics.

When the bill arrived in the Senate, in the Fall, the strategy of the ruling center-leftist group was to present many amendments, in order to send the bill back to the lower chamber. All these attempts were defeated by the majority. Even an amendment to redress some heavy penalties (an AID was punished with prison like a murder) was rejected by a large majority. In mid-March 2000 cardinal Ruini spoke in favor of the bill, expressing his hope for a prompt approval. For technical reasons discussion and votation of the bill were postponed to early June, and prospects were in favor of an approval. However, on June 7, 2000 from 9.30 to 11.00 a.m. the Senate approved two amendments: the first erasing the "rights of the embryo", and the other allowing AID. This occurred because a large number of right-wing Senators had not arrived on time. The official justification was that they had been trapped in Rome's traffic jam or couldn't find a taxi. As a matter of fact the bill had to go back to the lower chamber and did not pass.

Given the unbelieveability of the traffic jam excuse, the Senators' behavior needs to be explained: why did right-wing Senators, who had strenuously defended the bill, not show up to vote it? On the matter there are several conjectures. One is the following: considering that the absent Senators came mainly from Catholic parties joining the right wing coalition, they did not show up because (as the bill came from the center-left ruling coalition) the merit of the new law would have been ascribed to the Catholic party joining the ruling coalition, which would have earned the Church's gratitude. Right wing Catholic senators did not show up in order to prevent the left-wing Catholic party from gaining the Church's gratitude from the new law.

Such strategic behavior was productive, because in the Spring 2001 political election the Church endorsed those parties which had peculiar attention to protection of human life and promotion of (traditional) family. As a matter of fact the right-wing coalition won the election and now a new cultural climate seems to influence bioethical debate. In his speech for Sunday the "life day" (Sunday March 3rd 2002), the pope explicitly approved the initiative of the Italian Pro-Life Movement leading to the presentation again of the bill for changing article 1 of the civil code. Political and social conditions are now significantly different from what they were six years ago, and the proposal might be successful. On March 27, the bill on assisted reproduction approved by the lower chamber in the last legislature started to be discussed again, and on June 18 it passed with a 268 for, 144 against and 10 abstaining. Once again, the "conceptus" is endowed with rights, AID is banned, the embryo's creation is strictly restricted and no spare embryo is permitted, and a further decree will decide for existing abandoned spare embryos.[25] Different polls give different responses concerning Italians' opinions on the matter, but what is most astonishing is that never before have appeals to "natural law" and "respect for natural procreation" been offered to justify a legislation.

The bill is already scheduled for vote in the Senate in the Fall. Any prediction is hazardous, but it is likely that by the end of 2002, Italy will have a new restrictive law on assisted reproduction. It is too early to predict what will be the real consequences of this new possible law: at a social level it will favor what has been called "reproductive tourism", i.e. the practice of people going abroad to get the service. From a legal point view it represents a step back for the Italian system, which since the '70s has favored individual freedom in family matters. Now this perspective has come to a tidy stop. From a political point of view there are parties that are ready to start the process of having a referendum to abrogate the law, which would be a violation of people's basic rights on reproductive freedom.

It is not possible to predict what will occur, but the new law on assisted reproduction is a clear effect of Catholic control of bioethical institutions in the '90s. Attitudes of most Italians on bioethical matters appear to be more secularized and "liberal" than is assumed by this law. Debates in the Parliament and the speed of its *iter* show the willingness of the ruling coalition to use institutional means to control social processes concerning bioethical issues. This is rather worrying: granted that bioethical institutions are controlled by Catholics, there a serious risk that Italy will undergo a stage leading to a very conservative legislation. After three decades of liberal legislation on family and other bioethical matters, the pendulum's swing seems to be changing. This is occurring not to satisfy people's new need for the stability of familiar customs, but because Catholics and other conservatives use institutional settings, hoping to redress or direct the social *milieu* according to their views. For this reason some have already spoken of a sort of "renewed Counterreformation" or a "new Restoration".

Further evidence of this new trend is the composition of the new National Committee for Bioethics: chaired once again by Francesco D'Agostino, it is formed by 56 members, of which about 40 are Catholics, with the remaining split between secularists and Jews (the Committee includes no Protestants or Muslims). Interesting also is the appointment of the Italian Pro-life Movement President and a number of scholars from the Catholic university to a sort of "task force" for the defense of the "culture of life".

V. POSSIBLE EXPLANATIONS OF THE ITALIAN SITUATION CONCERNING BIOETHICS

In this short historical overview of Italian bioethics I distinguished three different stages: the first characterized by efforts to gain intellectual respectability; the second devoted to creation of institutions devoted to promote bioethical thinking, which was dominated by Catholic bioethics; and the incoming third, in which bioethical institutions are used to justify conservative perspectives and legislation. Institutions have the function of *legitimizing* new ideas, which usually die out after some time if left without such cultural support. In Italy there is a risk that there is a dissonance between intellectual reflection and institutional directives, because most cultural institutions are controlled by Catholics.

At this point we are left with an historical problem: how could it happen that secular politicians, who in the '70s supported and successfully accomplished liberal legislation on abortion and other family issues, a decade later did not understand the social significance of bioethics and bioethical institutions and left to Catholics the development of the field?

The answer cannot be simple, because several factors are interwined. According to Scarpelli this happened simply because secular culture was "inattentive" to bioethics (see Scarpelli's paper, 1991). Demetrio Neri holds that the "historical reluctance of secular culture to invest intellectual energies" in ethics was more important (see Neri, 1994). Both theses are correct in so far as we consider the earlier period of the cultural debate. As I mentioned, at first bioethics was seen from the Communist parties with a sort of hostility, being considered a form of "*bourgeois* ethics", if not Yankee imperialism. But at a later period these remarks are not enough. Bioethics was not on the agenda of the secular leftist parties and other secular institutions for much deeper reasons connected with the nature of Italian culture in general. A large portion of secular Italian culture is influenced by "Continental philosophy" with its aversion to technology and scientific thinking in general. This attitude prevented secular culture from understanding that bioethics stems from the ongoing "biomedical revolution". Instead of being conceived as the vanguard of a larger movement, assisted reproduction was seen as a kind of hybrid to be limited. Consider the fact that the Bolognesi bill started as a consequence of Dolly's birth. The panic generated by the first cloning of a mammal brought about all over the world, in Italy gave the impulse for a new legislation on assisted reproduction. The frame of the Bolognesi bill tries to discourage as much as possible access to the practice, even if after such a declaration of principle the clauses were rather loose. The new bill, approved by the Chamber in June, 2002, brings this trend to its logical conclusion, admitting assisted reproduction in its minimal form. Catholics have been and are working hard in this process, but they can succeed in their work because their views concerning limits to science and technique is rather agreed upon even in the secular arena. Evidence for this can be found in debates on other issues that I could not comment on, i.e., those about Genetically Modified Organisms and research on stem cells.[26] This anti-scientific thinking is deeply rooted in Italian culture: as a result Italian biomedical research is dying, and pro-scientific perspectives are not strong enough to reach political levels. Of course no one despises science or scientific research, which formally is praised by everyone, but it is a qualified approval: scientific research should respect the limits of ethics, which are more or less tradition (or the Catholic view). In this sense science is seen with some suspicion, in Italy. This is a long-term reason for the lack of attention to bioethics in an "analytical style", a term to be understood not in a strict linguistic sense but as indicating an approach keen on exactness and precision. In this sense in Italy "analytic philosophy" is a general term used to indicate a philosophy respectful of "scientific methodology". But this philosophy is not engrained in the framework of Italian culture, which is more inclined to "history and arts". In this way metaphors are the major arguments and gamete donation is conceived as a sort of "technological adultery" instead of as an aid to the reproductive process provided to someone who asks for it.

This "long-term reason" is at the basis of the "lack of attention" paid by secular culture to bioethics. But there are other sorts of reasons. One is a "short-term" reason depending on the fact that in early '90s – after the end of the Soviet Union in 1989 and some scandals for political corruption – Italy underwent a sort of "political revolution" leading to two major consequences: the electoral system was reformed in favor of a version of bipolar coalition, and most historical parties either transformed themselves or simply disappeared. This latter solution occurred to the so-called "liberal secular parties," to whom the social reform of the '70s is to be ascribed. Therefore, the liberal secular perspective was left without any political voice. On the other hand both the Communist party and the Christian Democracy (the two historically opposite leading parties) disappeared and split. In particular Christian Democracy gave birth to several different parties which are crucial in both coalitions. In the left-wing one they are revered and respected as an essential part of the coalition, while in the right-wing one they are even more influential, claiming the leadership in matters of life and family: even if this coalition is called the "Liberties' Pole", freedom is understood in merely economic terms – trying to dismantle the welfare state. In the '70s Christian Democracy was the relative majority party, but it had to look for secular allies to support a position. On the other hand, now Catholic parties are dispersed in both coalitions and can control the policy on bioethical issues. For this reason secular politicians avoid controversies and the situation is favorable to Catholics.

This "short term reason" can cooperate with three other "middle term" reasons. The first of these is about the kind of issues to be faced: having failed to understand that there is a "biomedical revolution", some new interventions (such as assisted reproduction) are seen as excesses to be limited. In the '70s issues such as divorce, abortion, etc. had a long history and involved a large number of people, so that a liberal legislation could be presented as measures of "social prophylaxis" needed to prevent greater social evils. They were justified as "remedies" to an otherwise unbearable situation of widespread illegality, and not as challenges to traditional (Catholic) morality. On the contrary, nowadays most bioethical debates are focused on assisted reproduction, which appeared to be the crucial topic. But assisted reproduction involves only a minority of the population and sometimes the new regulations appear, not as a "practical necessity" to help "good people in trouble", but a sort of "license" allowing eccentric people to satisfy desires in clear contrast to traditional morality. From this viewpoint, bioethics is considered uninteresting from a political viewpoint, and therefore is not on the agenda of secular and liberal parties.

The remaining two reasons are about the cultural *milieu* and run in opposite directions. The first concerns the situation within Catholicism. In the '70s the so-called "dissent within the Catholic church" was very active, and influenced many people and politicians, convincing them to support reforming processes. This sort of "liberal Catholicism" had a crucial role because it softened Catholic opposition and suggested an "intermediate" position, so important in political bargaining. Many theologians campaigned for divorce and even for abortion, while now there is no dissent. Catholics are compact, and dissent is never public.

The other reason concerns the situation within secular culture: many secularists are convinced that after Vatican II Catholicism has changed significantly, now accepting the basic tenets of a liberal and democratic society. In this sense, it is still assumed that citizens' basic rights are not in danger. Catholic representatives have to declare their oppositions to some new practices, but they would never have dared to use the force of the law to impose their view to all citizens. Their public declarations were (and still are) interpreted as merely "tactical", but the light was the usual: as an old proverb says, "a barking dog never bites." In this sense the strategy was to concede the principles and get substance (this may be an explanation of the Bolognesi bill).

All these reasons had some role in the great disregard shown by secular culture for bioethics. We do not know yet what will be the consequence of the new legislation on assisted reproduction. It may be that a referendum to abrogate the new law will be called, and nobody can foresee whether it will be successful or not, and what the consequences will be. Only two points can be asserted with some confidence: Italian attitudes to bioethical issues are as secularized and liberal as in most industrialized countries; and Catholics never change: they are unable to accept ethical pluralism and are always ready to use the force of law to impose their moral views on other people.

University of Turin
Turin, Italy

NOTES

[1] A *legal* start to this process was prompted by a 1968 decision of the Constitutional Court stating that the law forbidding a wife's adulterous act (and only a wife's, not a husband's) and punishing it as a criminal offence (with up to two years of prison) was unconstitutional, being against the basic equality of people. In 1970 the divorce-act was approved by the Parliament and in 1974 a majority of 63% confirmed the new law in a widely attended popular referendum. In 1975 a new general reform of family law was approved, raising a strong Catholic opposition for its allegedly individualistic character (for these criticisms, see L. Mengoni's illuminating paper, 1979). In 1978 a general reform of health care was accomplished and a National Health Service modeled on the British system was instituted, guaranteeing free public assistance to every citizen. In the meantime, the legal ban on contraception was abolished, and within the NHS a woman could ask her physician for prescriptions to receive free contraception. On May 22, 1978 a quite liberal abortion law was approved by the Parliament, and confirmed three years later (1981) by a 68% majority in another hotly debated popular referendum. For this earlier stage of Italian health care, also see my 1984 and 1987.

[2] This is the title of a successful book edited by J.P. De Marco and R.M. Fox in 1986. Italian scholars knew of such a shift in English-speaking philosophy, and discussed it on various occasions. For a general presentation of these issues see my 1980.

[3] A frequent objection was that bioethics was totally useless as any "applied ethics". Ethics being by definition "practical" and "applied", the term "applied ethics" is meaningless, and therefore it makes no sense to invest resources in the field. Moreover, one should not forget that up to 1989 (the fall of the Berlin wall), Marxism was the most important philosophical perspective in Italy, and accordingly ethics did not deserve much attention. For a thoughtful statement of this view, see Colajanni (1987).

[4] Scarpelli's proposal was debated and accepted by the board of the journal, and publication of the issue was programmed for early 1981. Unfortunately, the financial bankruptcy of the publisher delayed its publication, and the issue was available only in June 1984, even though the official date is 1983. The publisher never distributed it, in some cases even to regular subscribers, and therefore, unfortunately, this early work was without larger impact.

[5] Scarpelli's papers are now collected in a volume: *Bioetica laica*, edited by M. Mori, Baldini and Castoldi, Milano, 1998. For a critical examination of this book, see issue *Bioetica. Rivista interdisciplinare* VII (1999), no. 2. For an earlier critical discussion of Scarpelli's views, cf. the special issue of *Biblioteca della Libertà* XXII (1987), n. 99 devoted to his early seminal paper. For a general overview of his contribution to bioethics, cf. my paper (1997).

[6] See the proceeding of a seminal conference held in Genoa in May 1986, edited by S. Castignone and L. Battaglia (1987).

[7] Apart from regular seminaries in bioethics, since 1985 *Politeia* has published *Notizie di Politeia*, which for some time was the only journal devoted to "applied philosophy" available in Italy. Proceedings of many conferences organized over the years have been published under the following titles: *Un'etica pubblica per la società aperta*, Bibliotechne, Milano, 1987; *La bioetica: questioni morali e politiche per il futuro dell'uomo*, Bibliotechne, Milano, 1991, *Quale statuto per l'embrione umano: problemi e prospettive*, Bibliotechne, Milano, 1992.

[8] According to this group, bioethics began at the Nuremberg Trials (1946-1947) and had its first systematic presentation in Pius XII's speeches to doctors. In the '70s, bioethics had an American influence, assuming a utilitarian and individualistic orientation, but in the '80s it came back to Europe where it got its original "personalistic orientation."

[9] Following a time of deep crisis in the '60s, *Medicina e Morale* is now a bi-monthly publication with over 1200 pages a year, including many documents from the church teachings and various governments.

[10] This view is presented in Sgreccia (1996, 1998). In November 1996 Sgreccia received a letter from Pope John Paul II (1996) praising him and the Center for its activities.

[11] For a comprehensive presentation of this view, see the collected volume *Introduzione allo studio della bioetica*, Europa Scienze Umane Editrice, Milano, 1996. Cattorini also promoted a dialogue with secular groups which is now published in the volume edited by Cattorini, D'Orazio and Pocar (1999). For more recent contributions, see Reichlin (2002).

[12] Many examples will be listed below, but the following fact illustrates in a paradigmatic way the lack of attention I am referring to: in its early beginning, *Politeia* had a good connection with the Italian Socialist Party, and in 1986 presented to the Socialist prime minister, Mr. Bettino Craxi, a project for creating a National Ethics Committee analogous to the French *Comité d'Ethique*, appointed in 1983 by the Socialist president François Mitterand. This proposal was unheard and the new Italian National Committee for Bioethics had to await a Christian Democrat prime minister in 1990.

[13] For a critical review of the Santosuosso bill, see Mori (1988), especially ch. 5.

[14] For a general overview of the work done in this first stage, see the report of Comitato Nazionale per la Bioetica (1992). For a critical overview of different reports, see Boeri (1994). For further evaluations of the subsequent activities of the new Committee, see Defanti (1995). For an evaluation of the last two Committees, see Pocar (1999; 2002).

[15] However, in the official report no sentence like this can be found, even though this slogan was spoken by the president of the Committee in a television interview, and immediately reported in the press. For a critical evaluation of this report, see issue no. 3 of *Bioetica. Rivista interdisciplinare*, IV (1996), which contains a paper by C. Flamigni which started a lively correspondence published in the subsequent issues of the journal. For further discussion of this report, see the papers published in *Rivista di teologia morale* XXVIII (1996), no. 112; and in *Iride. Filosofia e discussione pubblica* IX (1996), no. 19.

[16] For the text of this bill, see *Bioetica. Rivista interdisciplinare* VI (1998), no. 2, 313-324. Concerning the euthanasia debate, for earlier controversies, see the special issue edited by E. D'Orazio, *Notizie di Politeia* VII (1991), no. 22. For a later statement, see various issues of *Bioetica. Rivista interdisciplinare*, and more specifically the papers of Defanti and of Neri criticizing a report of the National Committee for Bioethics on the topic (*Bioetica. Rivista interdisciplinare* V (1997), no. 1.).

[17] In this view the National Committee supported an agreement with the ministry of education for bioethics teaching in high school and dialogued with local ethics committees in order to prepare a report concerning a proposal of ethics committees' reform. However, such a proposal has had no impact on the Ethics committees system, at least so far. Moreover, a report on ethical issues raised by research on stem cells was complete by May 2000, but it was published only in late October, after the British government in August accepted the proposals of the Donaldson Report. What is strange is that a large majority of the Italian National Committee held conclusions similar to Donaldson's, but this Report had hardly any impact on the Italian debate.

[18] For the text of the Appeals Court decision, cfr. *Bioetica. Rivista interdisciplinare*, VIII (2000), no. 1. Veronesi's speech was delivered at a Conference organized to present the issue of *Bioetica* devoted to such a decision (June 4, 2000).

[19] The appointment of the Dulbecco Commission was followed by much controversy, generated by Catholics, who were worried about a permissive Report. As a matter of fact on December 28, 2000, the Report was published with a dissent statement by 7 Catholic members out of 25 and recommendations which are similar to those advanced by Donaldson's Report in the UK and by the Italian National Committee. For a presentation of the debate, cf. Neri (2001), who was an active member of both the National Committee and the Dulbecco Commission. For the Oleari Report and some comments see *Bioetica. Rivista interdisciplinare*, VIII (2000), no. 2.

[20] The report for the values of Italians, cfr. Cesareo, Vincenzo, et al., *La religiosità in Italia* (1995). For a short comment concerning bioethics, cf. my paper (1995). Further confirmation of this fact is given by the "silent revolution" which occurred in the '90s concerning informed consent. For an interesting story of the issue, cf. Santosuosso (2001).

[21] It was not until 2001 that a Commission chaired by professor Carlo Flamigni was appointed by minister Veronesi to monitor the number of fertility clinics existing in Italy. They are 384, of which only 323 are actually active. Some of them only perform simple insemination (124), while 190 perform IVF with embryo transfer, 153 the ICSI and 65 FIVET. 73 practice embryo freezing; 25 oocyte freezing.

[22] It may be interesting to note, in passing, that this proposal was warmly approved by cardinal E. Tonini (quite popular in Italy and often on various television programs) and criticized by bishop E. Sgreccia, who held that – apart from other practical problems – such an "adoption" was not acceptable because it implied a moral recognition of a sort of "surrogacy," which is never permitted.

[23] For the text of this bill and a favorable comment by Casini, see his 1996.

[24] The original bill proposed by the Commission can be found in *Bioetica. Rivista interdisciplinare* VI (1998), no. 1, pp. 124-134. Various "Manifestos" promoted in early 1998 on the issue are collected in *Bioetica. Rivista interdisciplinare* VI (1998), no. 2, 324-336. For a critical analysis of some aspects of that proposal, see the editorial of *Bioetica. Rivista interdisciplinare* VII (1999), no. 2; and for the final text approved by the lower chamber in 1999, see *Bioetica. Rivista interdisciplinare* VII (1999), no. 3, 531-536.

[25] For the text of the bill, see *Bioetica. Rivista interdisciplinare*, X (2002), no. 3

[26] In Italy on February 13, 2001, over 1500 scientists came to Rome to protest in the streets against a decree of the Ministry of Agriculture forbidding the use of GMO outside laboratories. For some comments on the event, see the paper by C.A. Viano (2001) and the issue of the *Rivista di filosofia* (2002, n. 2) (edited by C.A. Viano) devoted to relations between science and society.

REFERENCES

Biblioteca della Libertà, XXII (1987), n. 99.

Bioetica. Rivista interdisciplinare, VII (1999), no. 2.

Boeri, R. (1994). 'Primo bilancio dell'attività svolta dal Comitato Nazionale per la Bioetica.' *Bioetica. Rivista interdisciplinare* III (1), 109-121.

Casini, C. (1996). 'Presentation of the bill.' *Bioetica. Rivista interdisciplinare*, IV (2), 334-350.

Castignone, S. and Battaglia, L. (Eds.) (1987). *I diritti degli animali*. Genova: KL Publishers.

Cattorini, P., D'Orazio, E. and Pocar, V. (Eds.) (1999). *Bioetiche in dialogo. Le nozioni di dignità della vita umana e della autonomia individuale*. Milan: Zadig Publishers.

Cesareo, V. *et al.* (1995). *La religiosità in Italia*. Milan: A. Mondadori Publishers.

Colajanni, N. (1987). 'Socialismo senza statalismo.' In: Politea (Ed.), *Un'etica pubblica per la società aperta*, (pp. 70-73). Milan: Bibliotechne Publishers.

Comitato Nazionale per la Bioetica (1992). *Rapporto al presidente del consiglio sui primi due anni di attività del Comitato Nazionale per la Bioetica 13 luglio 1990 – 18 luglio 1992*. Rome: Presidenza del Consiglio dei ministri.

Defanti, C. (1995). 'Secondo bilancio dell'attività svolta dal Comitato Nazionale per la Bioetica (Presidenza Ossicini, 1993-1994).' *Bioetica. Rivista interdisciplinare* IV (2), 249-55.

De Marco, J.P. and Fox, R.M. (1986). *New Directions in Ethics*. New York: Routledge & Kegan Paul.

John Paul II (1996). *L'osservatore romano* (Nov. 10).

Mengoni, L. (1979). 'La famiglia nell'ordinamento giuridico italiano.' In:. *La Coscienza Contemporanea Tra "Pubblico" e "Privato": La Famiglia Crocevia della Tensione* (pp. 267-288). Milan: Vita e Pensiero.

Mori, M. (1980). 'Recenti sviluppi nella filosofia pratica di lingua inglese.' *Rivista di Filosofia* LXXI, pp. 139-156.

Mori, M. (1984). 'Abortion and nationalized health care.' *The Hastings Center Report* 14 (November-December), 23-24.

Mori, M. (1987). 'Italy: Pluralism takes root.' *The Hastings Center Report* 17 (June), 34-36.

Mori, M. (1988). *La Fecondazione Artificiale: Questioni Morali nell'Esperienza Giuridica*. Milan: Giuffrè.

Mori, M. (1996). 'Il recente aumento di interesse per la bioetica e il cambiamento dell'ethos in Italia.' *Bioetica. Rivista interdisciplinare* IV (1), 111-116.

Mori, M. (1997). 'Il contributo di Uberto Scarpelli alla bioetica.' In: *Scritti per Uberto Scarpelli* Letizia Gianformaggio e Mario Jori (Eds.) (pp. 653-703). Milan: Giuffrè Editore.

Neri, D. (1994). 'Nuove vie per la bioetica italiana? Una critica di tre idee di bioetica.' *Bioetica. Rivista interdisciplinare* II (2), 323.

Neri, D. (1998). 'Quale futuro per i Comitati etici?' *Bioetica. Rivista interdisciplinare* VI (3), 447-461.

Neri, D. (2001). *La bioetica in laboratorio. Cellule staminali, clonazione e salute umana*, Rome-Bari: Laterza.

Pocar, V. (1999). 'Terzo bilancio dell'attività svolta dal Comitato Nazionale per la Bioetica (Presidenza D'Agostino, 1994-1998).' *Bioetica. Rivista interdisciplinare* VII (3), 505-508.

Pocar, V. (2000). "Perché i cattolici italiani sono contro la Carta dell'autodeterminazione? Risposta ad alcune critiche", *Bioetica. Rivista interdisciplinare* VIII (2), 319-329.

Pocar, V. (2002). "Quarto bilancio dell'attività svolta dal Comitato Nazionale per la Bioetica (Presidenza Berlinguer, 1999-2001).' *Bioetica. Rivista interdisciplinare* X (3).

Reichlin, M. (2002). *L'etica e la buona morte*. Turin : Comunità Publishers.

Santosuosso, A. (2001). *Corpo e libertà. Una storia tra diritto e scienza* Milano: Raffaello Cortina. Milano.

Scarpelli, U. (1983). 'Il dirito alla vita' *Rivista di filosofia* LXXIV, 25-27.

Scarpelli, U. (1991). 'I compiti dell'etica laica nella cultura italiana di oggi.' *Notizie di Politeia* VII (23), 4.

Scarpelli, U. (1998). *Bioetica laica*. Milan: Baldini e Castoldi.

Sgreccia (1996; 1998). *Bioetica. Manuale per medici e biologi*, 3rd ed. Milan: Vita e Pensiero.

Torchio, M. (1973). 'Rapporti uomo-natura secondo le principali metafisiche orientali, loro implicazioni bioetiche ed ecologiche.' *Natura* 2, 101-132.

Viano, C.A. (2001). 'La protesta degli scienziati', *Rivista di filosofia* XLII 2, 201-217.

FABRICE JOTTERAND

DEVELOPMENT AND IDENTITY OF SWISS BIOETHICS

> Every ethical system ... is ultimately a synthesis of intuitive and rational assertions, the proportions of each varying from culture to culture.
>
> Kazumasa Hoshino

I. INTRODUCTION

The discourse surrounding bioethical issues is characterized by its fundamentally contentious nature, which in turn reflects the divisions in Western contemporary moral culture. One source of discord lies in the content of morality and in the specific conditions necessary for the possibility of a generally justifiable moral discourse intelligible to all. The Enlightenment project, especially as it developed under Kant, sought to create such a context and attempted to justify a common moral language by rational arguments and analysis. It proved unable to provide the intellectual and rational tools for a single moral discourse able to justify the social structure of the West. As a result the fragmentation of Western moral identity reveals eclectic "rationalities" rather than an agreement about the content of the good life. New ways to confront the realities of moral existence have emerged, typically defined by a disbelief in traditional sources of morality (particular communities, religion, etc.) and by an appeal to procedural conventions (Engelhardt, 1996).

In the absence of shared philosophical assumptions about morality, the current inclination is toward a *politicization* of (bio)ethical norms, especially in European countries that attempt to (re)discover or (re)create a uniquely European identity concerning bioethical matters. (It would be interesting to explore whether or not this is in part a deliberate attempt to respond to American bioethics.) This effort to establish a moral identity is apparent in the development and institutionalization of bioethics. Most significantly, in 1996, the Council of Europe adopted the final draft of *The Convention for the Protection of Human Rights and Dignity of the Human Being*, the aim of which is to generate what Hans-Martin Sass

H.T. Engelhardt, Jr. and L.M. Rasmussen (eds.), Bioethics and Moral Content: National Traditions of Health Care Morality, 121–142.

calls a "common European market of values and valuables" (Sass, 2001, p. 215).

More recently, Research Commissioner Philippe Busquin, speaking at a meeting of the European Parliament's temporary committee on human genetics and representatives of civil society, underscored the need for a common effort among countries of the European Union to elaborate consensual rules on biotechnology and called for a *pluralist* debate on bioethics and biotechnology (European Parliament, 2001). The result is far from a uniform European bioethical moral vision. Thus, in the European context, on the one hand, there is a move in the direction of a globalization of values, as is the case in the development of a European bioethics. On the other hand, however, this harmonization is confronted by the fact that not every European state has created, so far, a *full national system* addressing the control of bioethical issues and biomedical research. Some countries, such as Switzerland, are still in the process of developing their own "bioethical" identity. For some, the vestiges of post-Enlightenment Europe still represent a compelling source enabling people of various cultural and religious backgrounds to construe a moral identity for European (bio)ethics.

In this essay I address the inevitable tension between traditional values and the emergence of the phenomenon called bioethics. Bioethics is an attempt to create a common moral framework that will examine and assess contemporary medical practice and new biotechnologies.[1] This common moral framework is, however, constituted out of different moral understandings that render difficult the possibility of moral discourse that can be heard and recognized or justified by all parties. I will illustrate this through examining bioethics in Switzerland. I first describe how Swiss bioethics developed and then comment on the arduous task that confronts this new field in Switzerland (i.e., the task of finding common moral ground in a culture that not only rejects traditional moral understandings but also in which professional ethics is questioned). What I demonstrate is that, even in a country with plural cultural identities such as Switzerland, the tendencies toward globalization do not provide the conditions for a common bioethics.

II. SOME SOCIO-CULTURAL PARTICULARITIES OF SWITZERLAND

Any attempt to understand the evolution of bioethics in the Swiss context must take into account particular socio-cultural considerations. In particular the linguistic and religious diversity of its inhabitants is an important aspect in any understanding of the identity of Switzerland. From a linguistic perspective, three main groups constitute the Swiss population: (Swiss)-German (63.3%), (Swiss)-French (19.2%), and (Swiss)-Italian (7.6%). The rest of the population is either part of the fourth national group, that is, Romansch (less than 1%–0.6%) or part of various other linguistic groups (8.9%) (Office Fédéral de la Statistique, 1997b). These numbers, however, do not show the real cultural diversity of Switzerland. Analysis of the permanent resident population by nationality shows that 19.8% (more or less 1.45 million people of a population of 7.28 million) are in fact foreigners. This 19.8% is broken down as follows: 5.1% are from Asia, 3.5% from North America, 2.6% from Africa, and 0.2% from Australia/Oceania. The rest of the foreign population is from other European countries (Swiss Federal Statistical Office, 2001). On a religious level, the two primary denominations share almost the same percentage of *nominal* believers.[2] In 1990, Roman Catholics represented 46% of the population and Protestants 40% (Office Fédéral de la Statistique, 1997a).

Although Switzerland has remained one of the most stable democracies in the world despite its socio-cultural diversity, the above statistics show, to a certain extent, the eclectic composition of the social fabric of Swiss identity. This plurality becomes more obvious when we examine how each ethnic (and religious) group compares to others in its moral and political orientations. For instance, a 1977 vote on the question of abortion-on-demand in the first trimester of pregnancy revealed that Protestant Swiss-French cantons (states) favored its liberalization whereas cantons with a majority of Catholic Swiss-Germans rejected the new proposal (Schoene-Seifert, et al., 1995, p. 1585).[3] Furthermore, there seems to be a tendency for each ethnic group to look to its "linguistic representative", that is, to the countries in Europe that share its linguistic identity. In relation to the evolution of bioethics, the Swiss-German scholars tend to observe the developments in Germany (and to some extent The United States[4]), the Swiss French France and Quebec[5], and the Swiss Italians Italy.[6]

Interestingly, Alberto Bondolfi (Professor of Medical Ethics at the University of Zurich) remarked, in an interview at the University of Zurich, that the German influence on Swiss-German universities is not only due to "linguistic" influences but also to the fact that many professors in positions key to the development of bioethics are Germans. (Professor Johannes Fischer of the University of Zurich and Professor Stella Reiter-Theil of the University of Basel are two good examples) (Bondolfi, 2001). To a certain extent, the same "linguistic attraction" holds for the Swiss-French universities in relation to France, although Quebec seems to have a recognizable influence. Jean-François Malherbe (University of Sherbrooke) and Hubert Doucet (University of Montreal) are two scholars who often travel to Switzerland to lecture on medical ethics at the University of Lausanne and University of Geneva. The bridge between the canton of Ticino (the Swiss-Italian part of Switzerland) and Italy is mostly due to Alberto Bondolfi's numerous publications in Italian.

The extent to which Germany (and the United States), France and Quebec, and Italy influence and shape the context of bioethics in Switzerland is difficult to assess. Each tradition affects, in a specific way, how bioethics is construed in the Swiss context. One of the main differences can be found in the "juridical culture" each country represents. Jean-François Malherbe notes that Anglo-Saxon bioethics and French-speaking bioethics are tied to specific legal systems. On the one hand, the Anglo-Saxon tradition is determined by a system of "common law" which is conceived according to an *inductive method.* In this procedure the ethical and the legal are intertwined in the attempt to resolve "medical suits" (Malherbe, 1996, p. 120). A good example of this type of ethico-legal imbroglio is the Kevorkian affair. In 1993, after Dr. J. Kevorkian assisted fifteen patients to commit suicide, the Michigan legislature passed legislation establishing that assisted suicide would be considered a felony requiring a sentence of up to four years in prison. In reaction, the American Civil Liberties Union of Michigan (ACLU) challenged the decision by bringing a lawsuit arguing that the new law was unconstitutional. This case epitomizes how ethical and legal concerns interact in the attempt to resolve the moral controversies. On the other hand, the French tradition (or Roman Law) is *deductive*, that is, law and ethics remain separate and aim at the protection of the ethical values of citizens. It also controls the right application of the law through tribunals (Malherbe, 1996, p. 120).

To sum up the main difference between these two traditions of law, Malherbe concludes that "in the 'Roman Law' system, ethics and law are articulated through the mediation of the legislative process. But, in the 'Common Law' system much more defined by jurisprudence, tribunals are less dependent upon the decisions of the central power" (Malherbe, 1996, p. 120). As a consequence, in the "Common Law" tradition, bioethics operates mostly under the control of lawyers and physician whereas in the "Roman Law" system theologians and philosophers occupy more of the scene (Malherbe, 1996, p. 120).

The "legal culture" of Switzerland reflects the tradition of the "Roman law". We may wonder, however, whether this situation will prevail in bioethics. It is true that European countries seem to have a different approach to handling ethical issues in comparison with the North American context (emphasis on rights). The difference between these two models resides essentially in the fact that the U.S. legal system creates new laws as Courts respond to particular cases (abortion being a good example) whereas in Europe, and as a matter of fact in Switzerland, the legal system remains very general in so far as ethical issues are concerned. Moral questions are interpreted in the light of the law as a whole rather than simply understood with reference to a specific law that deals with a particular bioethical issue. However, there has been a trend to politicize bioethical issues in Europe, as exemplified not only by *The Convention of Human Rights and Biomedicine* at the European level, but also by the creation of governmental commissions at the national level.

III. THE DEVELOPMENT OF BIOETHICS IN SWITZERLAND

In what follows, I examine two distinct periods. The first constitutes what I have called "the pre-bioethics period" (from the foundation of the Swiss Academy of Medical Sciences in 1943 to the creation of the Swiss Society of Biomedical Ethics in 1988). During this period bioethical issues were analyzed almost exclusively by physicians within the context of the medical profession. The latter part of this period is characterized by a crisis of medicine's relation to the public due to controversies about bioethical issues (abortion, euthanasia, new assisted reproduction technologies, genetic engineering, etc.). The second period is connected to the creation of the Swiss Society of Biomedical Ethics and compasses recent developments in bioethics in Switzerland, particularly the emergence of an "institutionalization" (although limited) of bioethics and a reform of the teaching of medicine in Swiss medical schools.

A. The Pre-Bioethics Period: Medical Ethics and the Swiss Academy of Medical Sciences (1943-1988)

Besides the complex socio-cultural identity of Switzerland, there is another important aspect that deserves our attention in relation to the development of bioethics. Compared to the United States and other European countries, bioethics developed somewhat late. I do not examine at length the specific reasons for this state of affairs, but it is worth mentioning a few factors: the absence of a civil rights movement that would defend patients' rights; a strong tradition of medical paternalism; and general access to medical care and therefore the absence of a debate concerning the allocation of resources. Finally, medicine has had professional organizations that have sustained a tradition of professional self-regulation (Schoene-Seifert, et al., 1995, p. 1579; Sass, 1992, pp. 211-212). The last peculiarity, that is, the role of professional organizations, deserves particular attention because professional organizations played an important role in the formulation of the first bioethical guidelines and recommendations for the Swiss medical profession. Furthermore, this circumstance reflects an awareness of the need for moral examination that prepared the way for a more extensive development of medical ethics in the subsequent period.

In the second half of the 20th century, the Swiss Academy of Medical Sciences (SAMS) regulated medicine in Switzerland. It did so not only in order to promote the development of medical research (Thevoz, 1992, p. 42) and the professional training of future generations of physicians (SAMS, 2001b) but also in order to deal with some of the ethical conundra of the time. The Academy was founded in 1943 by the deans of five medical and two veterinary faculties as well as the Swiss Medical Association (Foederatio Medicorum Helveticorum – FMH). The period of its creation coincides with the "Nazi era" which is, according to Jean-Marie Thévoz, precisely one of the reasons for the Academy's establishment: it was undertaken in order to remain detached from Nazi "medicine" (Thévoz, 1992, p. 42).

The Academy issued its first guidelines in 1969, which concerned the diagnosis and definition of death. In the early part of 1970s other recommendations were published, specifically concerning abortion and the care of newborns and the dying. It is important to note that bioethical issues were not handed over to ethicists (whether theologians or philosophers) as is the case today. Specifically, the task of medical ethics was accomplished by physicians within the medical community for members of the medical profession. The first outsiders to collaborate with the Academy were two theologians. One, a Jesuit, Father Albert Ziegler, was the chaplain at the University of Zurich with a particular interest in medical ethics. The second, Professor Hermann Ringeling, was a Protestant theologian and a professor at the University of Bern who likewise was concerned with issues of medicine and ethics. These two figures helped the Academy to address and formulate its initial medical-ethical guidelines.

Subsequently, confronted with increasing bioethical issues and in order to clarify ethical questions, the Academy appointed, in 1979, a Central Ethics Committee (CEC). Its primary aim was (and remains) the protection of patients and society through the establishment of working-groups (constituted of members from the medical profession, the nursing profession, the legal profession, and ethics) whose task was (and is) to discuss the problems raised by the practice of medicine in the contemporary context and anticipate new challenges so to elaborate guidelines,[7] recommendations or position papers.[8]

Today, experts from various fields and with diverse interests are members of the Academy. Their principal task is to reflect on the future developments of medical practice and the potential problems it may encounter. This involves discerning the real potential of medicine as well as the impact it may have on life, health and society. The central charge of the Academy may be summarized under three rubrics – as formulated by the Academy:

1. Training – Research:

(a) promotion of the professional training of the coming generation of physicians, especially in clinical research;

(b) support of the high quality of research in biomedical and clinical research;

(c) acquisition of knowledge from basic research and from practical clinical research, taking into account in particular the needs of the basic providers.

2. Bioethics – Social Accountability

(a) identification of new ethical questions arising from top biomedical research and from the development of new technologies, and the drawing up of ethical and procedural instructions;

(b) clarification of continual ethical questions relating to medical developments and their impact on society;

(c) development of information for the public about the contentious aspects of medical developments and their consequences for society.

3. Future Perspectives:

(a) the reflection on the future of medicine;

(b) the identification of perspectives for the future development of medical science and the assessment of the impact of such developments on the provision of health care to the population (SAMW, 2001a; SAMW, 2001b).

In the introductory comments of this section, I pointed out that the slow development of bioethics in Switzerland was partially due to a strong tradition of self-regulation within medicine. As a matter of fact, the first non-physician to be a member of the Central Ethical Commission of the Swiss Academy of Medical Sciences was Catholic theologian Alberto Bondolfi, who was nominated in 1988 (1988-2000). Furthermore, as the three commissions demonstrate (Central Ethics Committee, The Committee on Scientific Integrity in Medicine and Biomedicine, and The Ethics Committee for Animal Studies), ethics is a preoccupation of the Academy but still remains within the walls of medical institutions and under control of physicians. In other words, medical ethics was formulated *by* physicians (with few exceptions), *for* physicians.

B. The Advent of Bioethics: The Foundation of the Swiss Society of Biomedical Ethics (1989-)

The creation of an institution outside the medical community able to reflect on moral issues related to the practice of medicine in a clinical setting or to medical research occurred within the parameters of two events. The first was a social questioning of the almost "untouchable" status of the medical establishment. Public opinion (especially of groups or associations such as pro-life organizations) demanded more accountability regarding certain medical practices. Second, this period witnessed a rapid enhancement in genetic research: in 1989 the first intervention on the human genetic make-up occurred and a year later the first attempt of gene therapy took place. A few years earlier (1985), the initial steps toward the idea of the mapping of the human genome and the sequencing of its genes were promoted by biologist Robert Sinsheimer. These scientific advances raised questions and worries in the public mind. In Switzerland, this took the form of a public initiative for the protection of life and the environment with regards to genetic manipulations ("Initiative populaire pour la protection de la vie et de l'environnement contre les manipulations génétiques"), which addressed issues concerning the ethical implications of genetic manipulation (Confédération Suisse, 1992). As a result, a new article (formerly Article 24 novies which is now Article 119) was added to the Constitution, stating that "the genetic endowment of a person cannot be analyzed, registered, or revealed without that person's consent or else on the basis of legal prescription" (Confédération Suisse, 2001; Sass, 1995, pp. 250-251). The need for ethical guidelines was also a concern of the Swiss Academy of Medical Sciences which issued medical-ethical guidelines with regards to genetic research and gene therapy (Swiss Academy of Medical Sciences, 1993, 1998). This particular context of biotechnological progress and its potential applications, according to the bioethicist Rehmann-Sutter, provided the grounds for further bioethical reflections in genetic research and interventions (Rehmann-Sutter, 1999, pp. 15-16).

In response to this "social protest" some scholars reached the conclusion that "themes and problems in medical ethics [should not] be (mis)understood as the 'hunting privilege' of fundamentalist groups."[9] In response to this concern, two scholars, Bernard Courvoisier, former president of the Swiss Academy of Medical Sciences from 1985 to 1990, and Protestant theologian Eric Fuchs, professor of ethics at the University of Geneva, created in 1989 the Swiss Society of Biomedical Ethics (Schweizerische Gesellschaft für Biomedizinische Ethik SGBE – Société Suisse d'Ethique Biomédicale SSEB) in order to address bioethical issues, especially medicine and biotechnology.

With the founding of the society it was necessary to develop an identity with a strong academic base. The academic context of Swiss universities, however, proved to have insufficient structures to sustain a rich philosophical endeavor concerning ethical issues. This meant that the discipline of ethics was not *per se* recognized as a field of investigation worthy of full consideration. The only chairs in ethics existed within theology faculties, with the exception of the University of Fribourg (a university with strong Catholic roots) that had a chair in philosophical ethics – in the Neo-Thomist tradition. Some of the reasons for the lack of an "ethical culture" outside theology are historical. The Swiss government used to think of Swiss culture as fundamentally Christian in its moral outlook (the preamble of the Swiss Constitution begins with the following words: "In the name of God Almighty!"). Consequently, due to the bi-confessional character of Switzerland and as a way to reflect the Christian values of the country, Catholic and/or Protestant Churches specifically addressed ethical issues. Hence, numerous theologians – whether Catholic or Protestant – participated in the development of the SSEB. Nevertheless, as Bondolfi (first president of the SSEB from 1990 to 1996) remarks, there was no "logic of proselytism or confessional indoctrination" in the sense of the promulgation of a particular moral teaching derived from Christian principles, either Protestant or Catholic. The absence of institutions either in philosophy or in medicine with a particular interest in bioethical issues can explain this state of affairs (Bondolfi, 1999, p. 19).

Due to numerous socio-cultural changes that have occurred in Swiss culture, theologians currently do not have preponderance in the examination of ethical issues. Also, due to the subsequent secularization of Swiss society, the dichotomy between Protestants and Catholics is no longer clear. Denominational affiliation does not necessarily mean conformity with the ecclesial authority. Furthermore, as a Post-Enlightenment society, Switzerland accepts moral pluralism so that the government reflects the plurality of *Weltanschauungen*.

The second pillar on which the SSEB wanted to rely was the provision of a framework for an open discussion reflecting the wide range of views in Switzerland, which had become a democratic and pluralistic society. In particular, the SSEB intended to create a place for reflection that would not be defined by a particular ideological, political, and religious perspective, while at the same time considering each main ethnic group represented in Switzerland (SSEB, 2001). The society clearly stipulates that it aims at the promotion of interdisciplinary research and teaching in the field of biomedical ethics. It seeks also to encourage the dialogue between people and groups of different training and convictions (SSEB, 1999, p. 6).[10] Currently the SSEB gathers people from different backgrounds (physicians, nurses, theologians, philosophers, biologists, lawyers, etc.). It exercises its "influence" through two specific channels: first, it publishes the journal *Bioethica Forum* which aims at dispensing bioethical reflection. The second is the organization, every two years, of seminars in medical ethics to educate those engaged in professional activities involving bioethics. As such the SSEB compensates for the current absence of specific teaching in medical schools (Bondolfi, 1999, p. 19).

C. Toward an Institutionalization of Bioethics

Because of its socio-economical influence, medicine in society is one of the Academy's concerns. To begin with, medical progress is obvious and legitimate, so that expectations about the great potential benefits of research create political support for research. On the other hand, according to a report on the future of Swiss medicine (ASSM, 2000 and ASSM, 2001), the medical profession faces a cluster of challenges including improving the relationship of medicine and patients/society, containing the cost of health care, improving society's level of scientific knowledge, assessing biotechnological progress and coming to terms with societal mores, etc. In particular, the health care system, as currently organized, does not seem to meet the expectations of Swiss society. Despite efforts by public collectivities, health care insurance, and political powers to find broad based solutions, it has become necessary to rethink what medicine entails (ASSM, 2000, p. 4).

The report articulates a crucial point in relation to the development of bioethics: the education of medical students appears one-sided because of its nearly exclusive emphasis on "objective knowledge" – curative medicine – as opposed to the development of the physician as person with his or her personality ("Le développement de la personalité et du sens de l'orientation – par opposition au savoir objectif – sont sous-estimés dans les études.") (ASSM, 2001, p. 36). In other words, the committee that issued the report identified a key aspect for the enhancement of medical practice: not only does medicine require the acquisition of better scientific data based on natural sciences, but it also must take into account knowledge obtained by the humanities and social sciences (ASSM, 2001, p. 37).

The first steps toward that goal were taken by what is called the Commission Fleiner II. Between 1997 and October 1998, this expert commission, headed by Professor Th. Fleiner, issued a draft for a preliminary project on basic medical training (LPMéd basic training) between 1997 and October 1998. This recommendation, which came in the form of proposed legislation, combined with a previously proposed legislation on postgraduate and specialized post-academic training in the medical professions (LPMéd of 1996), was presented to the Federal Council and to the Parliament for approval in 2001. The new LPMéd should come into force in 2003.

LPMéd constitutes a reform of medical training in Switzerland with the main objective "to maintain and promote quality health care by warranting the best possible education for academically trained medical professionals..." (Swiss Department of Home Affairs, 1999). The reform has two foci: first, reforming the *approach* of medical education. Following the motto "Problemorientierten Unterricht" (problem-based learning), education will not be isolated within the various medical disciplines, i.e., cardiology, urology, endocrinology, etc. Instead, specific problems will be addressed by involving all relevant fields of specialization. The second focus of reform involves the *content* of medical education. In addition to the traditional curriculum, new fields of investigation will be added, such as preventive medicine, the sociology of medicine, and, most importantly for our purposes, medical ethics/bioethics.

Currently, and before the LPMéd becomes regulative, only the University of Geneva requires medical students to have education in bioethics. As the continuation of a project that used to be directed by the Fondation Louis Jeantet in medicine, since 1995 the Unité de Recherche et d'Enseignement en Bioéthique has offered instruction in bioethics through Alex Mauron, the first individual with full professorship teaching bioethics in a medical schools in Switzerland.[11] The chair has as its charge not just teaching bioethics to medical students but also teaching and doing research in clinical ethics.[12]

Finally, at a federal level the willingness to reflect on moral issues in medicine and biotechnology has been translated into the creation of two national commissions. The first, formed in 1998, is a commission concerned with research on genetic engineering in non human areas (Commission fédérale d'éthique pour le génie génétique dans le domaine non-humain). It focuses on examining and evaluating from an ethical perspective the evolution and applications of these new biotechnologies. The second commission (Commission nationale d'éthique pour la médecine humaine), appointed by the government in 2001, is comprised of 21 members (including ethicists, medical professionals, biologists, lawyers, and members of the social sciences) whose task it is to work in an interdisciplinary manner, reflect on the development of the medical sciences and medicine, and subsequently identify ethical, social and legal questions entailed by medicine as whole.

IV. MORAL IDENTITY AND MORAL PLURALISM

The above analysis of the development of bioethics in Switzerland reveals the inability of traditional mores and social institutions to provide and sustain the moral identity of bioethics within the context of postmodernity. Secularization combined with the rejection of a range of traditional values has transformed the moral landscape of Switzerland – within and without bioethical reflection. The result has been the salience of a number of disparate moral understandings. Thus the question: In a pluralistic context, do people of different cultural, social, and political affinities have enough commonality to create and sustain a shared morality? The limited core of mutual moral commitments seems to suggest that the moral culture of particular practices (e.g., medicine) takes place outside of specific moral traditions. Hence the creation and development of a field that tries to bring together different visions of life and moral and social understandings under one heuristic term: bioethics.[13]

The field of bioethics, both in Switzerland and in Europe, has the arduous task of establishing the conditions for a pluralistic debate on moral issues. The difficulty lies in the co-existence of competing ideologies in the face of the need to make concrete decisions. There is as well an inevitable tension between allowing a pluralism of ideas to exist and the globalization of (bio)ethical values.[14] Pluralism has permeated moral reflection as is expressed in seemingly interminable disagreements (MacIntyre, 1984, pp. 6ff.). Yet, the current trend is to settle moral controversies in a legal language of rights, which tends to universalize its authority beyond cultural and social diversities. It follows that the politicizing of morality emerges as the only option social-democratic societies of the West can produce.

John Rawls's work on liberalism epitomizes this political move. He attempts to remove the discussion from endless debates by appealing to political values, which are, in his view, morally neutral. He distinguishes between two kinds of doctrines: the ones that cannot be used in public discourse and those that, although incompatible, remain reasonable. Thus he argues that a modern democracy entails not simply "a pluralism of comprehensive religious, philosophical, and moral doctrines" but also "a pluralism of incompatible yet reasonable comprehensive doctrines" (Rawls, 1993, p. xvi; see also 1997, p. 766). Since the doctrines of the former kind (religious, philosophical, and moral doctrines) represent a source of disagreement they cannot constitute a basis for social collaboration or moral agreement. On the other hand, the latter kind (incompatible but reasonable) constitutes what he calls the ground for a "public reason" which strives not to criticize or attack any comprehensive doctrine (religious or nonreligious), except when a doctrine is incompatible with the "essentials of public reason and a democratic polity" (Rawls, 1997, p. 766).

In Rawls' work, the idea of a "public reason" is closely related to the concept of justice in the sense that "public reason" reflects a political conception of justice outside moral doctrines. Although he recognizes that the concept of justice is a moral concept, he points out that justice is a moral conception for *political*, *social*, and *economic* institutions (Rawls, 1993, p. 11). Hence, justice within the context of political liberalism does not refer to morality *per se*, but to a *reasonable* understanding of justice that attempts to provide the basic structure of society without any reference or commitment to any other doctrine (Rawls, 1993, pp. 11-13).

Ultimately, Rawls suggests replacing "comprehensive doctrines of truth and right" by "an idea of the politically reasonable addressed to citizens as citizens" (Rawls, 1997, p. 766). In order to achieve the goal, he introduces the concept of *justice as fairness*. It constitutes the core of a fair political system of cooperation in which each citizen, as a free and equal individual, participates in civic life according to three requirements: (1) *a list of certain basic rights, liberties, and opportunities*; (2) *the assignment of special priority to those rights, liberties, and opportunities*; and (3) *measures ensuring for all citizens adequate all-purpose means to make effective use of their freedoms* (Rawls, 1997, p. 774). Justice, then, is limited to the realm of the political (i.e., public reason) and is understood as the implementation of established rights and liberties so that each individual can justify his or her use of freedom. It also implies that any reference to secular philosophical doctrines (what he calls first philosophy) or religious arguments cannot provide public arguments not only because they are susceptible to disagreements but because they are at odds with the ideal of discourse in a constitutional social democracy.

This is a crucial point that deserves careful attention with regards to morality and social order. By recasting the notion of justice in terms of reasonableness, Rawls separates the realm of the political from the concept of the good (morality), thus grounding the social order exclusively on hypothetical consent and a new theory of the good independent of a common substantive understanding of the good for society. Indeed, Rawls justifies his claim by arguing that political values are not moral doctrines and consequently they can and must constitute the ground for public reason:

> Political values are not moral doctrines, however available or accessible these may be to our reason and common sense of reflection. Moral doctrines are on a level with religion and first philosophy. By contrast, liberal political principles and values, although intrinsically moral values, are specified by liberal political conceptions of justice and fall under the category of the political (Rawls, 1997, pp. 775-776).

Rawls' assumption here is that political values are morally neutral and therefore their public use is justified as a means for consensus in a well-ordered society.

A second point to stress is that the principles and ideals derived from his political conception of justice as reasonableness do not assume any particular common end or goal. Rather, Rawls promotes a liberal society in which each individual creates his or her own conception of what is reasonable and fair. This is negotiated in the social arena through a self-interested transaction bound by a social democratic political consensus. Political power is gained by those – the "dominant and controlling citizens" – who succeed in reaching agreement out of "irreconcilable yet reasonable comprehensive doctrines" and therefore are able to impose certain doctrines on minorities (Rawls, 1997, p. 807).

The consequence of this "political move" is the emptying of morality of its content on behalf of socio-political interests. Morality is transformed into a set of procedures that attempts to justify what is socially suitable for the sake of social order.

V. CONCLUDING REMARKS

The tendency to move from ethical norms to legal concerns is an ineluctable trend in medical ethics whether in Switzerland (see Ummel,

1995, p. 87) or in Europe generally. Indeed, regulations and laws certainly have their validity and usefulness. They do not, however, suffice to sustain the moral identity of the medical profession for reasons addressed in the preceding section. Thus, in order to provide a content-full morality, two approaches appear possible. On the one hand, one might want to confine moral reflection exclusively to the realm of particular communities, affirming that the content of moral discourse and moral actions are limited to and defined by the individuals (belonging to a particular moral community) who, let's say, practice medicine. In other words, the outcome of the decision making process is almost exclusively the result of the practitioner's own moral commitments. On the other hand, it could be argued that right reasoning and the willingness to put aside particular irreconcilable moral commitments could provide the ground for ethical principles and moral actions. What would be needed is to find consensus on various issues, which in turn would constitute a morality in itself.

Both perspectives, however, seem problematic. In the first case, it would mean that the practice of medicine and certain ethical issues related to it can be understood only within particular communities independently of the ends and goals of medicine. But if medicine can be practiced by people of different philosophical, religious, and social backgrounds, there must be at its core some fundamental principles regulating its practice. Being a physician involves not simply the acquisition of technical skills for curing the sick; it is a social and communal endeavour in which one agrees to respect certain professional rules. In the latter case, if moral reasoning is muted into a political consensus (as is the case in a Rawlsian world), there is the danger of emptying morality of its content and also its deep and rigorous analysis. Hence, it is my contention that, in a pluralistic society such as ours, moral issues should be part of a political debate in which various ethical perspectives must be heard – even though agreement might not occur. More importantly, a (re)consideration of the ends and goals of medicine can provide a constructive analysis concerning bioethical issues. As the morbid condition of the field of the philosophy of medicine suggests, there is little interest in the philosophical analysis of the nature of medical practice. An effort to revisit the philosophy of medicine seems necessary in the light of the current condition of bioethical reflection (i.e., the politicization of bioethics) because such a study could inform us about the nature of medicine. In the light of such a study, the political, economical, and social aspects of medicine could be considered in terms of a philosophically enriched understanding of final analysis of bioethical issues.

The legal, economic, and political aspects of bioethical problems are legitimate but not exclusive concerns. Bioethical reflection should encompass all the relevant factors that shape a moral identity in a pluralistic framework. As Denis Durand de Bousingen and Arthur Rogers remark in their work *Une bioéthique pour l'Europe*, cultural, political and philosophical traditions diverge quite dramatically among European nations. There are, nevertheless, some points of convergence and consensus among European ethical committees from which a European bioethics can be established.[15] Hence, a national bioethics (Swiss bioethics, for instance), cannot and must not be reduced to generalizations concerning European principles but rather it must reflect its own national cultural, political and social identity. Only then can it participate in a larger and more meaningful discussion with other approaches.

* * *

I would like to thank Professor Alberto Bondolfi and Professor Denis Mueller who allowed me to interview them at the University of Zurich and at University of Lausanne (June 2001). I would like to thank also Professor H. Tristram Engelhardt, Jr. and Ana Smith Iltis for their comments on previous drafts of this essay.

Rice University
Houston, Texas, U.S.A.

NOTES

1 For a critical assessment of the idea of a neutral and secular moral framework see Engelhardt, *The Foundations of Bioethics* (1996).

2 What I mean by *nominal* is the denominational affiliation of Swiss citizens to a state church whether Protestant or Catholic. This affiliation does not signify necessarily a religious commitment but it is a way for the state to collect taxes in order to meet the financial needs of parishes belonging to the state churches.

3 More recently, however, there seems to be a change in how confessional belonging – whether Catholic or Protestant – affects people's decision in moral issues. The official churches will take specific stands on particular ethical problems but generally the tendency is towards autonomous decisions regardless of the individual's own denominational background.

4 For example, Hans-Martin Sass, director of the Zentrum für Medizinishe Ethik at Ruhr-Universität in Bochum is also Senior Research Scholar at the Kennedy Institute of Ethics, Georgetown University in Washington D.C. At the Kennedy Institute, he supervises the European Program in Professional Ethics in which the expertise of the institute provides a substantial resource for the development of programs, courses, and symposia in Germany and subsequently in other European countries.

5 One might think that due to Quebec's geo-political situation, American philosophy and ideology might be influential. Hubert Doucet, one of the leading scholars in bioethics in Quebec, however, epitomizes the hindrances to adopting uncritically American bioethics. He notes that "comme Nord-Américan francophone, j'ai toujours été fasciné par le dynamisme de la pensée américaine dans son face-à-face avec les problèmes de la vie réelle, en même temps que par les limites profondes qui caractérisent ce pragmatisme. Ma pensée éthique est nourrie de lectures américaines, mais garde ses distances à l'égard de l'approche qui s'est imposée aux Etats-Unis" (Doucet, 1996, p. 11).["as a French-speaking North American, I always have been fascinated by the dynamism of American thought in facing real life issues, but also by the profound limits that characterizes this pragmatism. My ethical thought is nourished by American readings, but keeps its distance from the approach that forced itself in United States," translation mine.]

6 For an overview of the traditions of bioethics in Germany, France and Italy see Dell'Oro & Viafora (1996). For the German-speaking world see Alberto Bondolfi, "Orientations and Tendencies of Bioethics in the German-Speaking World," pp. 199-227 in Dell'Oro & Viafora (1996), see also Hans-Martin Sass "Bioethics in German-Speaking Western European Countries: Austria, Germany, and Switzerland" (Sass, 1992, pp. 211-231) and by the same author "Bioethics in German-Speaking Western European Countries: Austria, Germany, and Switzerland" (Sass, 1994, pp. 247-268); for the French-speaking world see Jean-François Malherbe, Orientations and Tendencies in the French-speaking World," pp. 119-154 in Dell'Oro & Viafora (1996); and for an outline of Italian Bioethics see Adriano Bompiani, "The Outlines of Italian Bioethics," pp. 229-286 in Dell'Oro & Viafora (1996).

7 The guidelines issued by the Central Ethical Committee do not have a legal force but they are considered as having a considerable moral force. Here are some of the latest issues covered by these guidelines:

(1) Medical-ethical guidelines for genetic investigations in humans (1993)
(2) Medical-ethical guidelines for the medical care of dying persons and the severely brain-damaged patients (1995)
(3) Medical-ethical guidelines for organ transplantation (1995)
(4) Medical-ethical guidelines on the definition and determination of death with a view to organ transplantations (1996)
(5) Medical-ethical guidelines for the transplantation of human fetal tissue (1998)
(6) Medical guidelines for somatic gene therapy in humans (1998)
(7) Medical ethical guidelines on borderline questions in intensive-care medicine (1999)

Other guidelines (e.g., medical-ethical guidelines for assisted reproduction technologies (1990), and medical-ethical guidelines for xenotransplantation (2000), etc.), are also available in French or German. For further details on the content of these recommendations see SAMW (2001c).

8 Recently, the Academy extended the scope of its regulative task. In order to deal with the question of scientific integrity in scientific research (false data, plagiarism, etc.) the Academy

appointed, in 1999, another committee (The Committee on Scientific Integrity in Medicine and Biomedicine – CIS) specifically charged to oversee and ensure appropriate scientific behavior. It also commissioned an Ethics Committee for Animal Studies as a regulative agency overseeing the use of animals in biomedical research. For more details see SAMS: Ethics (SAMS, 2001a).

9 Bondolfi, (1999, p. 19, translation mine): "Beide [Courvoisier and Fuchs] waren schnell darin übereingekommen, dass Themen und Probleme der Medizin-ethik nicht als 'Jagdreservat' für fundementalistische Gruppierungen (miss-)verstanden werden dürfen."

10 Article 2 stipulates: "La SSEB a pour buts: a) de promouvoir la recherche et l'enseignement interdisciplinaires dans le domaine de l'éthique biomédicale; b) de promouvoir l'ouverture et le dialogue entre personnes et groupes de formation et de convictions différentes..." ["The SSEB has as its goals: a) to promote interdisciplinary research and teaching in the field of biomedical ethics; b) to promote the openness and the dialogue between people and groups of different education and conviction...," (translation mine).]

11 A second position has been created at the University of Basel where Professor Stella Reiter-Theil is Anne Frank-Stiftungsprofessur at the medical school. She also supervises an interdisciplinary institute for bioethics (Institut für Angewandte Ethik und Medizinethik). For further detail on the institute see <www.unibas.ch\aeme>.

12 In relation to clinical ethics, the profession of clinical ethicist is currently not as well defined in Switzerland as it is in North America. Currently, there exists only one full-time position in Switzerland held by Carlo Foppa, ethicist at the CHUV (Centre Hospitalier Universitaire Vaudois) in Lausanne. For an account of his experience as ethicist in a clinical setting see Foppa (2000).

13 This terminology is used by Engelhardt. He writes: "A new word [bioethics] often allows us to name elements of reality in a way that conveys new control over our cultural environment. ...In fact, it is often the imprecision, the lack of clarity, that allows us to name and bring together at one time many areas of interest. An apt word can assemble a rich set of images and meanings and thus help us to see relations between elements of reality that were previously separated in our vision and thought of only as disparate. ...This has been the case with 'bioethics.'...The word 'bioethics' [has done] brilliant service in bringing together a wide cluster of important cultural concerns. The term is profoundly heuristic" (Engelhardt, in Potter, 1988, pp. vii, ix).

14 Interestingly the idea of a global bioethics has come to be challenged not only within Western culture (see for instance the drafting of the *Basic Ethical Principles in European Bioethics and Biolaw* (1998) which establish the ethical foundation of European bioethics as opposed to the "Georgetown mantra"; see also Sass (2001) for developments on the some particularities of European bioethics) but likewise in Asian culture (for a particular Asian perspective see the volume on Filipino bioethics edited by Angeles Tan Alora and Josephine M. Lumatao (2001), which demonstrates how economical, social, and political factors condition bioethical reflection.

15 See particularly Chapter VIII "Voyage en éthicie: un aperçu de l'organisation de l'éthique biomédicale en Europe" in which the authors notes that although each countries has diverse cultural, political, and philosophical traditions there are many converging points: [L]es points de convergences et de consensus restent nombreux parmi les comités européens, au-delà de leurs différences d'approche et de fonctionnement...Toutes ces grandes tendances se retrouvent ainsi dans la plupart des pays et se déclinent au gré des traditions et des structures politiques ou législatives propres à chaque Etat; c'est sans doute d'ailleurs la variété des

réflexions et la multiplicité des formes de pensée qui, au bout du compte, constituent la force et la specificité de ce que l'on peut appeler 'la bioéthique européenne'..."(1995, pp. 195-196). ["The points of convergence and consensus remain numerous among European committees, beyond their differences in approach and functioning...All these tendencies are thus found in most countries although their exact forms vary according to the traditions and the political or legislative structures of each particular state; it is, for that matter, certainly the variety of reflections and the multiplicity of thought forms that, in finality, constitute the strength and the specificity of what we might call 'European bioethics", translation mine).]

REFERENCES

Académie Suisse des Sciences Médicales (2000). Nouvelle orientation de la médecine: Rapport intermédiaire de la 1ère Séance de réflexion, 25/26 août 2000, Bienne.

Académie Suisse des Sciences Médicales (2001). Nouvelle orientation de la médecine: Rapport intermédiaire de la 2ème Séance de réflexion, 19/20 janvier 2001, Bienne.

Amstad, H. (1999). 'Medizinethik: Who's who?' *VSAO Journal*, 8. Available on-line: <http://www.vsao.ch/journal/8_99/amstad.html>

Bondolfi, A. (2001). Personal interview, University of Zurich, June.

Bondolfi, A. (1999). 'Zur Lage der Medizinethik in der Schweiz. 10 Jahre SBGE.' *Bioethica Forum* 29, 17-20.

Bondolfi, A. (1996). 'Orientations and tendencies of bioethics in German-speaking world.' In: Dell'Oro, R. & C. Viafora (Eds). *History of Bioethics: International Perspectives.* San Francisco: International Scholars Publications.

Confédération Suisse (2001). *Constitution fédérale de la Confédération suisse.* Available on-line: http://www.admin.ch/ch/f/rs/101/

Confédération Suisse, Initiative populaire fédérale (1992). 'Initiative populaire fédérale pour la protection de la vie et de l'environnement contre les manipulations génétiques (initiative pour la protection génétique).' Available on-line: <http://www.admin.ch/ch/f/pore/vi/vi240t.html>

European Parliament (2001). 'Busquin calls for pluralist debate on biotechnology.' Cordis RTD-News/© European Communities.

Dell'Oro, R. & C. Viafora (Eds) (1996). *History of Bioethics: International Perspectives.* San Francisco: International Scholars Publications.

Diezi, J. (1995). 'La commission d'éthique de la recherche clinique: A la recherche de l'éthique.' *Cahiers Médico-sociaux, 39*, 91-93.

Doucet, H. (1996). *Au pays de la bioéthique. L'éthique biomédicale aux Etats-Unis* . Labor et Fides, Geneva.

Durand de Bousingen, D. and Rogers, A. (1995). *Une bioéthique pour l'Europe.* Les éditions du Conseil de l'Europe.

Engelhardt, H.T., Jr. (1996). *The Foundations of Bioethics*, 2nd ed. Oxford: Oxford University Press.

European Union, Biomed II Project Partners (F. Abel, M. Bothobol-Baum, P. Kemp et al.) (1999 and 2000). In: J.D. Rendsorff and P. Kemp (Eds.), 'Basic Ethical Principles in European Bioethics and Biolaw,' Institut Borja de Bioetika, Center for Ethics and Law, Barcelona (2 volumes).

Foppa, C. (2000). 'Entre les livres et les patients: l'éthicien. A propos d'une expérience d'éthicien en milieu hospitalier.' *Médecine & Hygiène* 58, 1201-1206.

Hoshino, K. (Ed.) (1995). *Japanese and Western bioethics: Studies in moral diversity.* Dordrecht: Kluwer Academic Publishers.

MacIntyre, A. (1984). *After Virtue*, 2nd ed. Notre Dame: University of Notre Dame Press.

MacIntyre, A. (1988). *Whose Justice? Which Rationality?* Notre Dame: University of Notre Dame Press.

Malherbe, J.-F. (1996). 'Orientations and Tendencies of Bioethics in the French-Speaking World,' pp. 119-154. In Roberto Dell'Oro and Corrado Viafora (eds.) *History of Bioethics: International Perspectives.* International Scholars Publications. San Francisco.

Mueller, Denis (2001). Personal interview, University of Lausanne, June.

Office Fédéral de la Statistique (1997a). 'Le paysage religieux helvétique: des tendances nouvelles.' Berne: Office Fédéral de la Statistique. Available on-line: <http://www.statistik.admin.ch/news/archiv97/fp97063.htm>

Office Fédéral de la Statistique (1997b). 'Les frontières linguistiques en Suisse sont pratiquement stables.' Berne: Office de la Statistique. Available on-line: http://www.statistik.admin.ch/news/archiv97/fp97104.htm

Potter, Van R. (1988). *Global Bioethics.* East Lansing: Michigan State University Press.

Rawls, J. (1993). *Political Liberalism.* New York: Columbia University Press.

Rawls, J. (1997). 'The idea of public reason revisited.' *The University of Chicago Law Review* 64, 765-807.

Rehmann-Sutter, C. (1999). 'Zur Aufgabe der Schweizerischen Gesellschaft für biomedizinische Ethik.' *Bioethica Forum* 29, 15-17.

Reich, W.T. (1995). 'The word "bioethics": The struggle over its earliest meanings.' *Kennedy Institute of Ethics Journal, 5*, 19-34.

Sass, H.-M. (1992). 'Bioethics in German-Speaking Western European Countries: Austria, Germany, and Switzerland.' In: B. Andrew Lustig, Baruch A. Brody, H. Tristram Engelhardt, Jr., & Laurence B. McCullough (Eds.), *Bioethics Yearbook Vol. 2: Regional Developments in Bioethics-1989-1991*, pp. 211-231.. Dordrecht, Netherlands: Kluwer Academic.

Sass, H.-M. (1995). 'Bioethics in German-Speaking Western European Countries (Austria, Germany, and Switzerland): 1991-1993.' In: B. Andrew Lustig, Baruch A. Brody, H. Tristram, Jr., & Laurence B. McCullough. *Bioethics Yearbook Vol. 4: Regional Developmenst in Bioethics-1992-1993*, pp. 247-268.. Dordrecht, Netherlands: Kluwer Academic.

Sass, H.-M. (2001). 'Introduction: European bioethics on a rocky road.' *The Journal of Medicine and Philosophy* 26(3), 215-224.

Schoene-Seifert, B. (1995). 'History of medical ethics: Europe.' In: Warren T. Reich (Ed.) *Encyclopedia of Bioethics.* New York: Macmillan Pub. Co.

Société suisse d'éthique biomédicale (2001). '*Présentation*.' Available on-line: <http://bioethics.ch/presentation.htm>

Societé suisse d'éthique biomédicale (1999). 'Status de la SSEB.' *Bioethica Forum* 29 (November).

Swiss Academy of Medical Sciences (2001a). *Ethics.* Available on-line: <http://www.samw.ch/content/e_Ethik.htm>

Swiss Academy of Medical Sciences (2001b). *SAMS at a glance.* Available on-line: <http://www.samw.ch/content/e_Samw.htm>

Swiss Academy of Medical Sciences (2001c). *Medical-ethical Guidelines*. Available on-line: <http://www.samw.ch/content/e_Richt.htm>

Swiss Academy of Medical Sciences (1998). *Medical-ethical guidelines for somatic gene therapy in humans*. Available on-line: <http://www.samw.ch/>

Swiss Academy of Medical Sciences (1993). *Medical-ethical guidelines for genetic investigations in humans*. Available on-line: <http://www.samw.ch/>

Swiss Department of Home Affairs (1999). 'The Medical Professions.' *EDI/FDI-themen-e-Die Medizinalberufe*. Available on-line: <http://www.edi.admin.ch/e/themen/medizin.htm>

Swiss Federal Statistical Office (2001). 'Population: Permanent resident population by nationality.' Neuchâtel: Swiss Federal Statistical Office. Available on-line: <http://www.statistik.admin.ch/stat_ch/ber01/eufr01.htm>

Tan Alora, A. & Lumitao, J. M. (Eds.). (2001). *Beyond a Western Bioethics: Voices from the Developing World.* Washington: Georgetown University Press.

Thévoz, J.M. (1992). 'Research and Hospital Ethics Committees in Switzerland.' *HEC Forum* 4(1), 41-47.

Ummel, M. (1995). 'Les commissions d'éthique en Suisse. Développements factuels et questions critiques.' *Cahiers Médico-sociaux, 39*, 81-90.

PART III

DEATH, CULTURE, AND MORAL DIFFERENCE

MICHAEL D. FETTERS AND MARION DANIS

DEATH WITH DIGNITY: CARDIOPULMONARY RESUSCITATION IN THE UNITED STATES AND JAPAN

I. INTRODUCTION

Bioethicists continue to debate whether there are fundamental universal moral precepts that apply to all cultures or whether morality is relative and defined by cultural norms. Tom Beauchamp, for example, argues for universal moral precepts (Beauchamp, 1997), while others such as H. Tristram Engelhardt and Kevin Wildes point out the inevitability of post-modern pluralism (Engelhardt, 1996; Engelhardt and Wildes, 1994). As the longstanding leader of the Japan Association of Bioethics and advocate of bioethics in Japan, Kazumasa Hoshino has cast considerable doubt on universal moral precepts in his explication of the inadequacy of Western bioethical precepts for Japanese bioethics (Hoshino, 1997a). In the context of this current debate, we examine the use of cardiopulmonary resuscitation (CPR) in the United States (US) and Japan and how it reflects differing cultural beliefs about death with dignity. We begin with a brief description of the development and dissemination of CPR. We present data grounded in the reports of US and Japanese physicians about their own experiences and approaches to CPR. We describe how decisions are made to provide CPR, and the goals and preferred outcomes when CPR is provided in the US and Japan.

Not long ago medicine had little more to offer than sympathy and compassion for the dying and their families. However, the development and rapid dissemination of a variety of technological interventions in the last several decades have given medicine the capacity to postpone death for individuals afflicted with illnesses that only a short time ago invariably caused imminent death (Rothman, 1997). These successes have given medicine a great deal of credibility and enhanced the rapid dissemination of and desire for technological treatments. One of the most noticeable applications of life-sustaining technology is the use of resuscitation techniques after cardiopulmonary arrest. CPR includes basic life support in the form of assistance with breathing and chest compressions, and advanced cardiac life support techniques, which involve additional administration of electrical shock (defibrillation) and

H.T. Engelhardt, Jr. and L.M. Rasmussen (eds.), Bioethics and Moral Content: National Traditions of Health Care Morality, 145–163.

medication treatments. These procedures were developed based on a scientific understanding of physiology and pharmacology (American Heart Association, 1997-99).

With the adoption of the technique of external cardiac compression, it became possible to prolong patients' lives, and initially, both in the US and Japan, it became a virtue to do so. For example, the phrase, "*Ichibyou demo nagaku*" (even if just for a minute), is a phrase that captures this symbolic change that occurred in Japan and reflects the physician's duty to save the patient's life. Fueled by the technological imperative (Koenig, 1988; Rothman, 1997), ventilator support and the general techniques of CPR rapidly spread throughout the US and Japan. This intervention offered the hope of rescue to the patient who had fallen victim to sudden cardiopulmonary arrest. As the technological equipment necessary to conduct advanced cardiac life support interventions became available in the US and Japan, attempted resuscitation quickly became the standard of care for hospitalized patients who experienced a cardiac arrest, regardless of the illness. Automatic use of CPR in the event of cardiopulmonary arrest became the default approach.

CPR can save the life of a patient who has suffered acute cardiac or pulmonary arrest, though the patient's chance of making a full recovery drops precipitously if effective circulation and ventilation is not established within minutes. US physicians often discontinue resuscitation after 15 to 30 minutes because the likelihood of survival diminishes and the probability of neurological damage increases with the duration of resuscitation. In reality, the vast majority of resuscitation attempts fail. The overall survival from CPR is around 10-15% (Schultz et al., 1996).

As information about the use of life-sustaining treatment gained publicity in the US through such nationally renowned court cases as Karen Ann Quinlan and Nancy Cruzan, a public reaction calling for limitation of treatment ensued. The Patient Self-Determination Act was passed to promote the use of advance directives, in the context of public opinion that was skeptical of aggressive, end-of-life treatments that were infrequently effective, or might leave the patient in a persistent vegetative state, or other debilitated, technology-dependent state (Omnibus Budget Reconciliation Act of 1990). Public pressure mounted to require patient involvement in decisions about whether to use resuscitation, and is exemplified in a President's Commission report entitled, "Deciding to forgo life-sustaining treatment" (President's Commission for the Study of

Ethical Problems in Medicine and Biomedical and Behavioral Research, 1983).

No sooner had resuscitation become an almost universal intervention used on dying, hospitalized patients in the US, than it was restricted by public interest in quality of life and death with dignity. The tangible development and use of advance directives (Omnibus Budget Reconciliation Act of 1990; Emanuel et al., 1991; Emanuel and Emanuel, 1989; Orentlicher, 1990), and professional efforts from ethicists and many physicians, pressured clinicians to limit resuscitation efforts to cases where the patient desired the intervention or there was a reasonable chance of effectiveness (Blackhall, 1987; Tomlinson and Brody, 1988).[1] Recognition that resuscitation should not be employed in every case led to the development and common use of Do-Not-Resuscitate (DNR) orders in the US (Blackhall, 1987; Tomlinson and Brody, 1988). US physicians became less aggressive about providing resuscitation and DNR orders became common. In a recent study of 42 US hospitals, 60% of deaths in intensive care units were preceded by DNR order (Jayes et al., 1993; Jayes et al., 1996).

In Japan, there is no legislation like the PSDA and there is no legal status of living wills or other advance directives (Masuda et al., 2001). However, citizen groups have begun to form, to draw attention to patient rights to participate in medical decision making (Shibazaki, 1991). Moreover, there is growing interest in advance directives. For example, a group called the Japan Society for Dying with Dignity has formed to pressure lawmakers to legalize living wills. Though these efforts have not been successful to date, the group has developed a substantial membership (Japan Society for Dying with Dignity, 1998). Court cases to date have not demarcated clear lines of support for patient rights, and preserve family and physician influence (Kimura, 1998). Despite these many changes, the family takes a central role in end-of-life decisions (Hattori et al., 1991; Hoshino, 1997a; Kimura, 1998; Fetters, 1998; Long, 1999).

In the following, we draw upon data collected during our investigation designed to understand patients' and physicians' preferences for decision making about end-of-life issues (Danis et al., 1996; Fetters and Danis, 2000; Hanson et al., 1996). Interviews for the US arm of this research began in October 1990 and continued until July 1993 at a teaching hospital in North Carolina. During this time, 158 physicians were enrolled. Japanese data collection was initially conducted from June to

August 1992 in a variety of university hospitals, geriatric hospitals, and a private clinic. Follow-up research was continued during subsequent visits to Japan in 1995 and 1998. During these time periods, a total of 40 Japanese physicians participated. During the 1995 and 1998 visits, we conducted member checking with original participants, a process used in qualitative research traditions for ascertaining the validity and reliability of the project results (Creswell, 1998). Further details about the interview instrument and methods are reported elsewhere (Fetters and Danis, 2000). We have also conducted a number of informal interviews with members of the lay public and hospital workers. Moreover, both authors have been participant observers of end-of-life care as medical students, residents, fellows, and attendings, Fetters as a family physician and Danis as a medical intensivist and former intensive care unit director.

II. APPROACHES TO CARDIOPULMONARY RESUSCITATION IN THE UNITED STATES AND JAPAN

Detailed description of the advanced cardiac life support interventions are beyond our purposes, but suffice it to say that the technical aspects of care are provided based upon scientific principles of physiology and pharmacology and are similar in both the US and Japan. Still, there are minor environmental differences in the US and Japanese approaches. For example, most US hospitals have organized code teams that include a designated code team leader and an anesthesiologist or anesthetist. This code team is often called by a special beeper, or notified of an arrest by voice paging system using special terminology such as "code blue". In Japan, nursing staff contact the attending physician or an accessible physician when a patient arrests, and it is generally expected that this physician will orchestrate the resuscitation effort. Moreover, anesthesia specialists for airway support are available 24 hours a day only in the largest hospitals, which makes management of the airway an additional primary duty for physicians conducting a resuscitation event in Japan. Moreover, there is greater room for physician discretion about whether and how long to conduct a resuscitation effort in Japan since advance directives are highly uncommon, and because direct, concrete discussions about patient and family preferences appear to occur less commonly.

In both countries the hospital staff make an effort to notify the family as soon as possible after arrest. Sometimes this occurs at the outset of the arrest, and at other times it may not occur until the resuscitation attempt is completed and the outcome is clear. These biomedical aspects of and approach to resuscitation are very similar. However, when the patient does not respond to CPR, the Japanese response differs from the usual course in the US.

A. Termination of resuscitation and timing of death in the US

In the US, according to the protocol of the American Heart Association, the resuscitation team leader will assess the patient's response to resuscitation and potential for meaningful recovery (American Heart Association, 1997-99). Once there is agreement that further resuscitation efforts have a negligible probability of effecting the patient's recovery, resuscitation efforts are ceased. This usually occurs in fifteen to thirty minutes, though the resuscitation may be shorter if it is obvious that resuscitation is pointless, and may be longer if the patient was exceptionally healthy or the arrest was completely unexpected. The code team leader has the responsibility of declaring the patient dead. Standard protocol calls for the resuscitation leader or other representative, usually someone who participated in the resuscitation effort, to talk to the next-of-kin and review the reason for the patient's arrest and the general course of the resuscitation effort. This is also often used as an opportunity to ask for an autopsy, or organ donation for transplantation[2]. After preparation of the body, the family is called in to the room and given time to grieve with the patient for as long as several hours. In most cases, the length of time spent is at the family's discretion, though not uncommonly, there are pressures to expedite removal of the deceased patient in order to prepare the room for another patient. In this way, death in the hospital is viewed primarily as a physiological event with the time of death determined by the physician orchestrating the resuscitation effort.

In very unusual circumstances, physicians in the US will continue life-sustaining treatments in order for the family to be at the bedside at the time of the patient's death. In most cases, treatment involves the continuation of life-sustaining treatments such as fluid resuscitation, ventilator support, medications (so-called "pressors") to maintain blood pressure and heart rhythm, or antibiotics. More commonly, US physicians reported continuation of treatment because the *patient* had a compelling need to participate in or contribute to a social event that had special meaning for the patient. For example, these US physicians indicated circumstances when they had continued life-sustaining treatments to keep their patients alive long enough to see such things as high school graduations or other social events. One US internist stated,

> ... I would be reluctant to do most of these [life-sustaining treatments] but would do some of them if there was a good rationale [given by the patient, such as], "My son is in Europe and I have bad pneumonia. He can't get here until ten days from now. It is important for me to see him, even if the pneumonia needs a respirator." "Okay, lets see if we can tide you through to accomplish that." I would be reluctant but would look very carefully at all these situations.

A US pulmonologist echoed the importance of considering the goals and social circumstances of the patient. In his discussion of a cancer case he reported,

> If I thought he had some reason for living and wanted to live, I would again let him make that decision and he would have to decide at what level he wanted to make that cutoff. So his heart stops beating for a non-cancer-related reason. Would I advise it? See, we don't know what his prognosis is for this cancer. You know he may want to finish his book, see his daughter graduate from college or something. I think we just have to talk about the nature of his disease and let him make that call. I guess I am a very non-directive doctor.

In summary, a minority of US physicians discussed their willingness to continue or employ life-sustaining treatments for *family* reasons, but in the majority of cases when it was discussed, the impetus for employing life-sustaining treatments had to come from the *patient*. Even then, it would usually include mechanical ventilation, antibiotics, or perhaps pressors to maintain blood pressure – interventions that are less labor intensive than physically providing chest compressions or ventilating by hand with an ambu bag.

B. Termination of resuscitation and timing of death in Japan

In Japan, after a patient does not respond to efforts in a time frame in which patient survival is possible, there are two primary patterns. In some cases, these efforts are discontinued as is the custom in the US. This usually occurs when there has been some advanced discussion about limitations of treatment and family preferences not to conduct heroic measures. In other cases, the resuscitation effort sometimes continues for several more hours. The purpose of resuscitation is not to promote patient survival, but rather to prolong the time of death in order for the family to come to the bedside to witness the last moments of the patient's life. One Japanese physician referred to this effort as a "ceremony" (*gishiki*). When the patient is intubated, it is uncommon to connect the patient to a ventilator when the goal is the arrival of the family. Japanese physicians are reluctant to withdraw ventilator support once it has been initiated. Hence, this "ceremonial code", a prolonged resuscitation effort to prolong the time of death until the arrival of the family, is a highly labor intensive, physical process and further highlights the dramatic nature of prolonged CPR in Japan.

The actual length of time of the additional family-focused resuscitation effort typically varies from one to two hours, though efforts not infrequently continue for several hours, and some physicians stated they had continued resuscitation for as long as 24 hours. The medical team's commitment to resuscitation designed to allow the family time to come to the patient's bedside is reflected by the case of one family member who was living in the US at the time when her father arrested in Japan. The medical team inquired by telephone whether she would like treatment to continue until she was able to make arrangements to return to Japan in order to see her father prior to his "death". The level of intensity of CPR varies by doctor and ward. Some physicians will continue a full resuscitation while others conduct only the absolute basics of chest compressions and ventilation with the ambu bag. As a rule, CPR is most aggressively pursued in the emergency room. For patients who are accident victims for whom death is completely unexpected, emergency room doctors tend to be much more aggressive about continuing CPR. However, on the wards, the doctors will often alert the family that the patient is approaching a serious condition. They will ask the family if they want the patient to have resuscitation measures until the family can get there, or if they prefer to let the patient die without any intervention. Family preferences are variable. Some wish for CPR to be continued until they can come, while others prefer to let the patient die without any intervention.

Major influences on the decision between terminating treatment and continuing "resuscitation" are the family's desires or physical ability to come to the bedside for the final moments of the patient's life. Sometimes family members arrive within minutes of notification of the patient's impending death. In other circumstances, it may take considerable effort to reach the family by telephone, and in some cases, they may require several hours to come to the hospital. If the family is comfortable with discontinuing CPR, the effort is discontinued. If the family requests CPR to be continued until their arrival, the attending physician usually honors their request. When the family indicates such a desire to be there prior to "death", the CPR ceremony typically involves at least the basic resuscitation procedures of chest compressions and ventilating the patient with an ambu bag.

The endpoint for the resuscitation ceremony is the arrival of family members. When the family has assembled, they are invited into the room to witness the resuscitation effort, namely the cardiac compressions and ventilation with the ambu bag. The medical team directs the family to watch the waveforms from the compressions on a cardiac monitor. The attending physician then directs cessation of chest compressions and ventilation. The treatment team and family watch the cardiac monitor together. This usually reveals a flat line or displays agonal rhythms. Though not always in a precise order, the physician then looks for a light reflex (*taikou hansha*) and listens to the heart and lungs. After this short activity, the examining physician turns to the family and states "*Go rinju desu*", that is, "The patient is dead".

One Japanese physician's discussion about his approach to the use of life-sustaining treatments illustrates his own experiences of resuscitation efforts for the family:

> MF: In general, under what circumstances would you advise life-sustaining treatment?
>
> Doctor: I think it's difficult to define life-support treatments.
>
> MF: Really?
>
> Doctor: It depends on the degree of support. For example, depending on if it's resuscitation, heart massage [i.e., chest compressions], intubation, or whether or not to attach a respirator, I think that the way you would answer would be different. Even if you do nothing for the actual problem, with any type of sickness, it depends on whether the family has come yet or is in the hospital; we wouldn't pronounce a person's death until the family came. Most of the time we wait for the patient's family to arrive and after they've come we pronounce the patient's death. For example, if a person had terminal cancer and we

determined that he didn't even have a week left, we would intubate the patient. If that's considered life-support treatment, then we do it. Next, if it's a question of attaching a respirator, I don't think that we would go that far. So I think depending on the level, the answer is slightly different. It depends on the judgment made at that time. It's that way even with heart massage. For example, if nobody had come yet and it looks like they'll arrive shortly, but the patient goes into arrest and has apnea, no matter how terminal the cancer is I think we would do it.

MF: Have you had any cases like that?

Doctor: I have. In the evenings, regardless if it's my own patient, there are cases when the patient arrests after the family has gone home. In these situations, without even considering a long-term life support system, I would treat them for the short term.

MF: How long do you continue?

Doctor: Even then about an hour.

MF: How many times have you done this?

Doctor: In my experience up until now there have been at least 20 or so cases, even where I thought that with support there was no chance of resuscitation. Especially in Japan where it is said that death is something you should see. We value this idea. It isn't a matter of going after one has died, rather, it is very important be there at the time of death. This is what I was thinking about.

From the above description it is clear that when conducting CPR the technical strategies are very similar, but the goals and preferred outcomes differ in significant ways in the US and Japan. To understand these differences more clearly with an eye toward death with dignity, we now address two questions: 1) How do US and Japanese physicians decide whether to do CPR?; and 2) What are the goals and preferred outcomes when US and Japanese physicians perform CPR?

C. How US and Japanese physicians decide whether to do CPR

Based on the law and ethical articulations of informed consent, US hospitals have an obligation to educate patients about their right to complete an advance directive specifying their wishes for care at a future time when they may no longer be able to make decisions (Omnibus

Budget Reconciliation Act of 1990). Physicians are routinely encouraged and, in principle, required to learn whether the patient has completed an advance directive, to discuss with patients their preferences for resuscitation in the event of catastrophe, and to refrain from heroic measures when requested. Very specific guidelines have been developed to determine who can and cannot make decisions for incapacitated patients (Buchanan and Brock, 1990). When the patient is incapacitated, the family or other surrogate is asked to provide input about what the *patient's* wishes would be if he/she were able to participate in decision making. The DNR order is commonly used to implement requests not to have treatment. While it would be naive to believe that this is an accurate representation of real-world practice all the time, it reflects the ideals to which physicians aspire in the US. These mechanisms have been developed expressly to enhance the opportunity for the patient to exercise autonomy. Death with dignity in the US is construed to mean the patient has participated, or at least the patient's surrogate or physician has acted in ways that are believed to best represent what the incapacitated patient's preferences would have been if he/she were able to participate.

In contrast, there is no legislation like the PSDA in Japan, there is no legal recognition of advance directives, and discussions about whether to provide CPR, when the discussions happen at all, usually are held between the physician and the family (Kimura, 1998). There are *not* clear guidelines about who does and doesn't qualify as substitute decision makers for the patient. As articulated by Hoshino, these professional matters are often held to be the province of physicians, and patients may resent physician insistence on patient participation in decision making (Hoshino, 1992; Hoshino, 1995; Hoshino, 1997a). Physicians who seek family or patient preferences may be construed as incompetent and thus not trustworthy.

D. Goals and preferred outcomes when US and Japanese physicians perform CPR

In both the US and Japan, the primary goal of performing CPR is to restore the patient to their prior state of health. A second goal is to avoid complications of the resuscitation, e.g., cracked ribs or laryngeal trauma from resuscitation.[3] A third common, but not necessarily ubiquitous goal that is similar in the US and Japan is to avoid bad outcomes in which the patient regains cardiopulmonary function, but has significant neurological disability, such as permanent coma, as a consequence of prolonged hypoxia. Specifically, resuscitating a previously competent patient, thereby allowing him/her to survive indefinitely in a markedly compromised state of health and dependent on life-support technology, is generally thought to be worse than allowing the patient to died. Thus in mainstream US practice and culture, a good outcome is the prompt cessation of the resuscitation effort after the critical window of about fifteen minutes of CPR, in order to avoid successful return of cardiopulmonary function complicated by devastating neurological injury. Herein, the goals of resuscitation in the US become less consistently held. Some physicians, patients, families, and organizations that strongly believe in miracles and/or the sanctity of life believe that keeping the patient alive in any state is always a better outcome than allowing the patient to die. The heterogeneity of opinion about this issue is, in our experience, a relatively common cause of tension and a reason for ethics consultation. This conflict appears to occur on occasion in Japan as well, but to our knowledge happens less frequently than in the US.

E. Family involvement at the deathbed in the US and Japan

US families often go to great lengths to be at a loved one's bedside. Stories abound of family members who completely put their lives on hold in order to spend the final moments of a loved one's life with him or her, even if the dying person is unconscious. Clearly, the family's presence at the deathbed helps define a death with dignity in both cultures. There are many religious beliefs and customs regarding the role of the family at the deathbed, though discussion of these diverse practices is beyond the purposes of this work. Not infrequently, US physicians will either employ or delay withdrawal of life sustaining treatments such as mechanical ventilations, antibiotics, or pressors to postpone death until after arrival of the family. It is noteworthy, however, that active CPR to delay the pronouncement of death until the arrival of the family in the US is not the norm, and at minimum conflicts with mainstream US perceptions of death with dignity. While we would not venture to claim that it never happens in the US, we do assert that it is unusual, and moreover that the practice is not unusual in Japan.

A common, but not necessarily ubiquitous goal in Japan is to have the family come to the bedside in order to witness the chest compressions, electrical monitoring, and hand-ventilations if the family so desires, and to pronounce the patient's death in the presence of the family. That is, CPR is continued for the family and not with the intent of the physiological recovery of the patient. Consequently, ancillary goals are not to intubate the patient, as this might precipitate a long course of ventilator dependency in a debilitated state. This would clearly be a bad outcome, as most Japanese physicians and organized medicine in Japan do not recognize the withdrawal of support as ethical practice. The Japanese physician's discussion above illustrates the reluctance of Japanese physicians to connect a ventilator. Moreover, overly aggressive treatment could paradoxically result in the return of cardiopulmonary function. Thus, the goal is to continue the resuscitation effort but avoid the return of cardiopulmonary function if there is a risk of neurological sequelae. Even if the resuscitation effort lasts several hours, even if the effort is only a "ceremony", even if the patient sustains cracked ribs or other trauma, use of CPR for the patient to symbolically spend the final moments of life together with his/her family is preferred. One accepted definition of a dignified death is continued resuscitation until the arrival of the family members, who then witness the discontinuation of resuscitation and the loss of a viable cardiac rhythm.

The motivation and rationale for prolonged resuscitation efforts at the end-of-life, that is, the ceremonial code, in Japan can be found by examining the cultural context. First, from participating Japanese physicians' perspectives, CPR at the end-of-life helps the patient avoid a lonely death without the family. When questioned about this "ceremony" at the end-of-life, and whether he would want such measures for himself given his knowledge of the necessary invasive procedures and the potential for cracked ribs and other trauma, one Japanese physician responded that he would want CPR continued so his family members could come. He said, "I would want my family there. Without the family there, death seems very lonely."

Second and perhaps more importantly, family members are traditionally expected to be at the bedside at the time of the patient's death. This tradition probably has its roots in the concept of filial piety (*oyakokou*), and is reflected by the phrase, *shini me ni au*, literally "to meet the eyes of death." This phrase is symbolic of the Japanese sense of a family member's duty to be at the patient's bedside at the time of death. The phrase *shini me ni atta*, literally, "I met the eyes of death," is used by Japanese people to convey that they were at the family member's bedside as their loved one took their last breath. The phrase, *shini me ni aenakatta*, literally, "I was unable to meet the eyes of death," refers to being unable to be at the loved one's bedside at the time of death and conveys a sense of remorse. Family members who are unable to be at their loved one's bedside at the time of death may agonize for the rest of their life and it may be a substantial source of guilt. The relative social importance of *shini me ni au* is reflected by social criteria for not going to the pronouncement of death. Actors or performers who have an obligation to a large audience are expected to complete their performance even if this precludes them from meeting the eyes of death. Only the obligation to such a large audience is considered sufficient to justify not meeting the eyes of death.

Third, many Japanese people, consciously or unconsciously, believe that ancestors (*sosen*) can influence the current world. Moreover, a belief that the spirit (*tamashii*) remains in the patient's body for a while after physiological death is commonly held. While some believe that displeased ancestors can harm them, this appears to be the exception (Smith, 1974). Investigation of ancestral rites suggests that there is a significant gap between physiological and social death, such that the deceased continues to exert considerable influence on the family after physiological death (Smith, 1974; Smith, 1989; LaFleur, 1992).

Fourth, failure to be at the bedside at the time of death may be a source of embarrassment or even scorn from neighbors or peers (*henna me ni mirareru*). One physician summarized his thoughts about how the patient dies in this way: "Once the patient dies, it is over because the patient is dead, but the family has to live with how the patient died for the rest of their life." Based on all these pressures, the importance of being at the bedside for the pronouncement and showing respect by being at the patient's deathbed cannot be overemphasized.

III. REFLECTIONS ON CEREMONIAL CODES AND DEATH WITH DIGNITY

From a standard Western ethics account, the Japanese ceremonial code is arguably an inappropriate use of financial and human resources, and disrespectful to the dying individual. First, from a purely physiological perspective, continuation of CPR in the face of no expected hope for return of function or survival is futile. Second, according to mainstream sensibilities, use of CPR interventions with no expectation of recovery and passive avoidance of cardiopulmonary function is an almost unquestionable compromise of patient dignity. During the course of CPR, the patient's body is subject to invasive procedures and physical trauma. The fragile elderly are particularly susceptible to fractured ribs during CPR, especially when it is conducted over a prolonged period of time. Thus, from a North American perspective, continued resuscitation in the face of inevitable death is not only futile, but also a clear compromise of the patient's right to death with dignity.

In the above interpretation, the ceremonial code, as practiced in Japan, is a culturally justified moral practice that enhances death with dignity. This description of the ceremonial code should not be interpreted as the exclusive view on death with dignity in Japan. There is much interest in re-thinking end-of-life issues in Japan. It should be understood that the above description may oversimplify the status of medical decision making in Japan. There is increasing interest in participation in end-of-life decisions by some patients in Japan (Shibazaki, 1991). Japanese physicians in our research who reported giving patients opportunities to participate in decision making sometimes experienced patients who chose to do so. Other patients chose not to do so, either deferring to their family members or never expressing a clear opinion. Moreover, the term *informed consent* (*infoomudo consento*) has taken root in Japanese medicine. In addition to scholarly discussions (Hattori et al., 1991; Hoshino, 1997b; Leflar, 1996), it is discussed publicly on television and in popular newspapers and magazines (Chang, 1992; Murakami, 1993), and alluded to in Japanese movies (Itami, 1993). Suffice it to say that some individuals in Japan want to and do participate in the decision making process in ways that are consistent with patient autonomy as articulated in Western bioethics. However, such occurrences appear to be exceptions to the rule. Rather, empirical data and scholarly discourse suggest that family members are currently more likely to participate as a substitute decision maker for a competent patient than an incompetent patient (Hattori et al., 1991; Hoshino, 1997a; Kimura, 1998; Elwyn et al., 1998; Long, 1999). In contrast to the US, Japanese medical practice does not routinely incorporate patient autonomy and informed consent. There is undeniable interest in these terms and concepts, though it is unclear that autonomy as understood and practiced in the US will take the same form in Japan (Akabayashi et al., 1999).

Emerging social movements such as the advent and gradual growth of hospice in Japan, as well as a small but significant interest in living wills, also suggest that Japanese notions about death with dignity are evolving. As in other countries, the hospice movement in Japan seeks the provision of palliation and comfort care minus end-of-life heroics (Chihara and Long, 2000). The association of death with Buddhist priests has been a significant cultural barrier to their participation in the hospice movement. The Japanese Society for Death with Dignity was established in 1976 and has unsuccessfully sought legal recognition of a living will in Japan (Masuda et al., 2001). More recently, the group has aggressively expanded its membership, and recent investigation suggests that exponential growth of its membership may indeed make it a social movement to be reckoned with (Japan Society for Dying with Dignity, 1998). There is emerging evidence from family reports after the death of patients who had completed a living will that many physicians are respecting patients' wishes for a death with dignity defined by an emphasis on palliation and comfort as opposed to intervention (Masuda et al., 2001). Finally, Professor Kazumasa Hoshino brought together scholars in 1994 for a Tokyo bioethics congress and published the proceedings in Japanese as the book *The Dignity of Death* (Hoshino, Tsuchida and Akabayashi, 1995).

While these social movements have touched only a minority of Japanese people, this activity does reflect the dynamism of culture in Japan and the questions that are being raised about the role of end-of-life treatments and their impact on human dignity. It might be argued that the ceremonial code is a cultural relic and that Japanese bioethics is lagging behind the inevitable changes that have occurred in the US (Beauchamp, 1997). But these ceremonies, regardless of how enduring they are, attest to the cultural diversity that underlies and influences one's interpretations of morality.

US attitudes about the role of technology and end-of-life care are similarly in flux (Rothman, 1997). The role of the family in medical decision making in Western bioethics and the need to attend to family interests along with individual interests generated considerable recent debate in the US (Hardwig, 1990; Nelson, 1992; Nelson and Nelson, 1993; Nelson and Nelson, 1995; Kuczewski, 1996; Reust and Mattingly, 1996; Fan, 1997, Fetters, 1998, Levine and Zuckerman, 1999). It is natural that Japanese and US notions about proper medical care at the end-of-life will evolve and influence one another, but unlikely that they will ever be completely the same.

IV. CONCLUSION

These comparisons of decisions about whether to use CPR and of the goals and preferred outcomes of end-of-life treatments in the US and Japan illustrate that there are differing interpretations about the value of technology at the end-of-life that are morally defensible given different cultural vantage points. The Japanese practice of CPR for the sake of the family in Japan illustrates the degree to which cultural values and customs about death with dignity influence medical practice. From a US perspective, a ceremonial code seems a violation of the right to be free from unnecessary medical intervention, yet contextual features of this practice in Japan suggest another interpretation that has significant meaning for the patient and family as well. While CPR in the absence of any hope for physiological recovery might be viewed as a cruel compromise of human dignity according to standards in Western ethics, it is culturally sanctioned and according to some accounts, the preferable way to die in Japan. Taken together, these points illustrate that a dignified death is culturally defined, and interpretations of morality must include some understanding of the cultural context. Assertions about the ethical aspects of medical care at the end-of-life must account for cultural notions of death with dignity.

University of Michigan Health System, Ann Arbor, Michigan, USA
Department of Clinical Bioethics, National Institutes of Health, Bethesda, Maryland, USA

NOTES

[1] Clearly physicians continue to have a great deal of discretion about whether to resuscitate patients. Though respect at the time of death for patient wishes expressed in a written advance directive is rising, evidence collected during the SUPPORT study revealed that advance directives infrequently influenced the use of end-of-life treatments (Lynn and Teno, 1998).

[2] Many medical centers now delegate the request for organ transplantation to an organ procurement team with no direct relationship to the treatment team.

[3] There are many other possible goals that physicians, patients, or families might have in both countries, i.e., to keep the patient alive as long as possible to prepare for organ donation, to minimize the use of resources and costs in order to provide cost-effective care, to maximize the duration of financial gain through charges by outside payers, to provide opportunities for learners to practice skills necessary to resuscitate patients, etc. Recent literature has exposed the "slow code" in the US as an unethical goal of resuscitation (Gazelle, 1998). Slow codes are the practice of intentionally delaying resuscitation efforts, or simply staging a resuscitation effort for medico-legal reasons or to appease the family. These practices are considered a violation of patient autonomy, an imprudent use of resources, and deceitful. Slow codes are an example of behaviors conducted in physicians' best interests. A discussion of the morality of these various goals is beyond the purposes of this paper, though we do argue that these are not typical, primary goals and hence not central to the current thesis.

REFERENCES

Akabayashi, A., Fetters, M.D. and Elwyn, T.S. (1999). 'Family consent, communication, and advanced directives for cancer Disclosure: A Japanese case and discussion. *Journal of Medical Ethics* 25, 296-301.

American Heart Association (1997-99). *Advanced Cardiac Life Support*. Dallas: American Heart Association.

Beauchamp, T.L. (1997). 'Comparative studies: Japan and America.' In: K. Hoshino (Ed.), *Japanese and Western Bioethics: Studies in Moral Diversity* (pp. 25-47). Dordrecht: Kluwer Academic Publishers.

Blackhall, L. (1987). 'Must we always use CPR?' *The New England Journal of Medicine* 317, 1281-1285.

Buchanan, A.E. and Brock, D.W. (1990). *Deciding for Others: The Ethics of Surrogate Decision Making*. Cambridge: Cambridge University Press.

Chang, Y. (1992). 'Cancer patients speak out.' *The Japan Times*, p. 17.

Chihara, S. and Long, S. (2000). 'Difficult choices: Policy and meaning in Japanese hospice practice.' In: S.O. Long (Ed.), *Caring for the Elderly in Japan and the United States: Practices and Policies*. New York: Routledge.

Creswell, J.A. (1998). 'Standards of quality and verification, qualitative inquiry and research design.' In: *Qualitative Inquiry and Research Design: Choosing Among Five Traditions* (pp. 193-218). Thousand Oaks, CA: Sage Publications, Inc.

Danis, M., et al. (1996). 'A prospective study of patient preferences, life-sustaining treatment and hospital cost.' *Critical Care Medicine* 24, 1811-1817.

Elwyn, T.S., Fetters, M.D., Gorenflo, D.W. and Tsuda, T. (1998). 'Cancer disclosure in Japan: Historical comparisons, current practices.' *Social Science and Medicine* 46(9), 1151-1163.

Emanuel, L., Barry, M., Stoeckle, J., Ettelson, L. and Emanuel, E. (1991). 'Advance directives for medical care: A case for greater use.' *New England Journal of Medicine* 324, 889-895.

Emanuel, L. and Emanuel, E. (1989). 'The medical directive: A comprehensive advance care document.' *Journal of the American Medical Association* 261, 3288-3293.

Engelhardt, H. T., Jr. (1996). *The Foundations of Bioethics*, 2nd ed. New York: Oxford University Press.

Engelhardt, H. T., Jr. and Wildes, K. W. (1994). 'The four principles of health care ethics and post-modernity: Why a libertarian interpretation is unavoidable.' In: R. Gillon and A. Loyd (Eds.), *Principles of Health Care Ethics* (pp. 135-147). London: John Wylie and Sons.

Fan, R. (1997). 'Self-determination vs. family-determination: Two incommensurable principles of autonomy.' *Bioethics* 11, 309-322.

Fetters, M. D. (1998). 'The family in medical decision making: Japanese perspectives.' *Journal of Clinical Ethics* 9(2), 132-146.

Fetters, M. D. and Danis, M. (2000). 'We live too short and die too long--On Japanese and U.S. physicians' caregiving practices and approaches to withholding life sustaining treatments.' In: S.O. Long (Ed.), *Caring for the Elderly in Japan and the US: Practices and Policies*. New York: Routledge.

Gazelle, G. (1998). 'The slow code--should anyone rush to its defense?' *New England Journal of Medicine* 338(7), 467-469.

Hanson, L., Danis, M., Garrett, J. and Mutran, E. (1996). 'Who decides? Physician specialty and use of life-sustaining treatments.' *Archives of Internal Medicine* 156, 785-789.

Hardwig, J. (1990). 'What about the family?' *Hastings Center Report* 10, 5-10.

Hattori, H., Salzberg, S. M., Kiang, W. P., Fujimiya, T., Tejima, Y. and Furuno, J. (1991). 'The patient's right to information in Japan. Legal rules and doctor's opinions.' *Social Sciences Medicine* 32(9), 1007-1016.

Hoshino, K. (1992). 'Informed consent to medical decision-making.' In: B. A. Lustig (ed.), *Bioethics Yearbook* (pp. 379-381), Vol. II. Dordrecht: Kluwer Academic Publishers.

Hoshino, K. (1995). 'Autonomous decision making and Japanese tradition.' *Cambridge Quarterly of Healthcare Ethics* 4, 71-74.

Hoshino, K. (1997a). 'Bioethics in the light of Japanese sentiments.' In: K. Hoshino (Ed.), *Japanese and Western Bioethics: Studies in Moral Diversity* (pp. 13-23), Dordrecht: Kluwer Academic Publishers.

Hoshino, K.:1(997b). *Infoomudo Konsento: Nihon Ni Najimu Mutsu No Teigen* (*Informed Consent: Six Proposals that Fit Japan*). Tokyo: Maruzen.

Hoshino, K., Tsuchida, T. and Akabayashi, A. (Eds.) (1995). *The Dignity of Death* (*Shi No Songen*). Kyoto: Shibunkaku.

Itami, J. (1993). *Daibyounin (The Really Sick Patient)* [Movie]. Tokyo: Itami Films, Inc.

Japan Society for Dying with Dignity (1998). *Japan Society for Dying with Dignity Newsletter* 91, 18.

Jayes, R., Zimmerman, J., Wagner, D. and Knaus, W. (1993). 'Do-not resuscitate orders in intensive care units: Current practices and recent changes.' *Journal of American Medical Association* 270 (18), 2213-2217.

Jayes, R., Zimmerman, J., Wagner, D. and Knaus, W. (1996). 'Variations in the use of do-not resuscitate orders in ICU's: Findings from a national study.' *Chest* 110(5), 1332-1339.

Kimura, R. (1998). 'Death, dying, and advance directives in Japan: Sociocultural and legal points of view.' In: H. Sass, R. Veatch, and R. Kimura (Eds.), *Advance Directives and Surrogate Decision Making in Health Care: United States, Germany, and Japan* (pp. 187 208). Baltimore: Johns Hopkins University Press.

Koenig, B. (1988.) 'The technological imperative in medical practice: The social creation of a "routine" treatment.' In: M. Lock and D. R. Gordon (eds.), *Biomedicine Examined.* Dordrecht: Kluwer Academic Publishers.

Kuczewski, M. (1996). 'Reconvening the family: The process of consent in medical decision making.' *Hastings Center Report* 26, 30-37.

LaFleur, W. R. (1992.) 'Social death, social birth.' In: *Liquid Life: Abortion and Buddhism in Japan* (Chapter 3). Princeton: Princeton University Press.

Leflar, R.B. (1996). 'Informed consent and patients' rights in Japan.' *Houston Law Review* 33(1), 1-112.

Levine, C. and Zuckerman, C. (1999)., 'The trouble with families: Toward an ethic of accommodation.' *Annals of Internal Medicine* 130(2), 148-152.

Long, S.O. (1999). 'Family surrogacy and cancer disclosure: Physician-family negotiation of an ethical dilemma in Japan.' *Journal of Palliative Care* 15(3), 31-42.

Lynn, J. and Teno, J. (1998). 'A care provider perspective on advance directives and surrogate decision making for incompetent adults in the United States.' In: H.-M. Sass, R. M. Veatch, and R. Kimura (Eds.), *Advance Directives and Surrogate Decision Making in Health Care: United States, Germany, and Japan* (pp. 3-33). Baltimore: Johns Hopkins University Press.

Masuda, Y., Fetters, M. D., Shimokata, H., Muto, E., Mogi, N., Iguchi, A. and Uemura, K. (2001). 'Outcomes of written living wills in Japan: A survey of the deceased's families.' *Bioethics Forum* 17(1), 41-52.

Murakami, A. (1993). 'Level with terminal patients, let them plan, surgeon urges,' *The Japan Times* (Nov. 21), 3.

Nelson, J. (1992.) 'Taking families seriously.' *Hastings Center Report* 22, 6-12.

Nelson, J.L. and Nelson, H.L. (1993.) 'Guided by intimates.' *Hastings Center Report* 23, 14-15.

Nelson, H.L. and Nelson, J.L. (1995.) *The Patient in the Family: An Ethics of Medicine and Families.* New York: Routledge.

Omnibus Budget Reconciliation Act of 1990 (1990). Vol. Pub. L. No. 101-0508, 4206, 4751.

Orentlicher, D. (1990.) 'From the office of general counsel: Advance Medical Directives.' *Journal of the American Medical Association* 263, 2365-2367.

President's Commission for the Study of Ethical Problems in Medicine and Biomedical and Behavioral Research (1983). *Deciding to Forgo Life-Sustaining Treatment.* Washington, D.C.: Government Printing Office.

Reust, C.E. and Mattingly, S. (1996). 'Family involvement in medical decision-making.' *Family Medicine* 28, 39-45.

Rothman, D. (1997.) *Beginnings Count: The Technological Imperative in American Health Care.* New York: Oxford University Press.

Schultz, S., Cullinane, D., Pasquale, M., Magnant, C. and Evans, S. (1996). 'Predicting in-hospital mortality during cardiopulmonary resuscitation.' *Resuscitation* 33 (1), 13-17.

Shibazaki, T. (1991). 'Group wants doctors to inform patients more fully.' *Japan Times International Edition* (July 15-21), 7.

Smith, Robert J. (1974). *Ancestor Worship in Contemporary Japan.* Stanford, CA: Stanford University Press.

Smith, Robert J. (1989). 'Something old, something new: Tradition and culture in the study of Japan.' *The Journal of Asian Studies* 48 (4), 175-723.

Tomlinson, T. and Brody, H. (1988). 'Ethics and communication in do-not-resuscitate orders.' *The New England Journal of Medicine* 318(1), 43-46.

HO MUN CHAN

EUTHANASIA, INDIVIDUAL CHOICE AND THE FAMILY: A HONG KONG PERSPECTIVE[1]

I. INTRODUCTION

In many Western countries, questions regarding how to treat a terminal patient with decency and dignity have become fairly controversial, and this issue has been of rising concern in Hong Kong as well as other Chinese communities. Many terminal patients are severely disabled by their illness, falling into a coma and being deprived of the capacity of self-determination. Confronting such a predicament is a moral dilemma for the medical profession, the patient himself (if he still possesses sufficient capacity for determination) and the patient's family. Together they must decide whether the patient's life should be prolonged, which may cause the patient to experience persistent suffering, or help the patient to end a life which is not worth living. One might wish we were able to invoke some universal moral principles to help solve this matter. However, on many occasions, the application of such moral principles may lead us to contrary resolutions. For example, if we hold both the intrinsic value of life and the patient's interest to be our moral guiding principles, we may be led nowhere. In the case of treating a terminally ill patient, treasuring the intrinsic value of life may compel us to prolong the patient's life at any cost, but the concern for the patient's interest may persuade us to terminate the painful life so as to advance that interest.

Unsettled moral principles cause hot debates in society where members view matters in different ways. It is not uncommon that the medical profession and the terminal patient's family in countries like the United States would bring the matter to the court and the appellate court for adjudication. It may be comforting to note that no such legal proceedings are known in Hong Kong, nor have the matters surrounding terminal patients' lives stirred up much noise in daily discourse. We may explain this relatively quiet position in various ways. First, the Hong Kong health care system in the old days was more paternalistic in character. The medical profession was perceived to be of great authority while the general public was vastly less informed. Prolonging a patient's life is a medical decision to be made by the medical profession. Second, the

H.T. Engelhardt, Jr. and L.M. Rasmussen (eds.), Bioethics and Moral Content: National Traditions of Health Care Morality, 165–190.

medical system in those days, when resources were largely aggregated for saving life, did not enjoy much liberty or capacity to prolong the terminal patient's life. This is no longer the case; Hong Kong society has developed a great deal over the past one or two decades in terms of resources, advancement of medical technology, and people's consciousness of rights. The public has become more concerned with quality of life, while at the same time enjoying a longer life expectancy. However, life expectancy and the quality of life may not always be consistent. Different people view their importance differently. Such differences exist among the public and surely among the medical profession. The care for the terminally ill is gradually becoming a controversial issue in Hong Kong.

This article is an attempt to explore thoroughly the matters surrounding terminal patients. I approach the matter from the perspectives of philosophy (ethics), medicine and public policy, and hold the view that in certain circumstances, the medical profession should cease the medically futile treatment of a terminal patient in light of the fact that such a treatment simply prolongs life, without necessarily adding any quality. This paper spells out what those circumstances are, and distinguishes the essence of such cessation of treatment from that of euthanasia, and argues that although forgoing treatment is morally permissible for the terminal patient, euthanasia should be made illegal. Having established this position, the paper moves to an examination of the justification of the decision to withdraw or withhold medical treatment for the terminally ill. In the liberal model, such a decision is justified in terms of the self-determination and the best interests of the patient, whereas in the model of familialism, which is a popular model in Eastern societies, e.g., Japan, Mainland China, and Hong Kong, the justification is coined in terms of the autonomy and the interests of the family. As a reconciliation of these two rival models, I propose a moderate version of familialism. Based on a comparison of this version of familialism with Engelhardt's idea of autonomy as a side-constraint, I argue that the former is more suitable for resolving the moral conflicts arising from the decision making process for the terminally ill in Eastern societies like Hong Kong. Finally, the paper concludes with an overview of current practices in Hong Kong regarding euthanasia, forgoing treatment, and the role of family in medical decision making. The overview shows that the practices indeed manifest a moderate form of famililism.

II. EUTHANASIA

The New Shorter Oxford English Dictionary defines 'euthanasia' as 'gentle and easy death'. The literary meaning of euthanasia seemingly denotes the patient's dying process. Hospice service also means the effort to help patients die with ease. What is the exact dividing line between 'euthanasia' and 'hospice service'? Euthanasia should mean more than its literary meaning. It should mean not just allowing patients to die with ease, but purposefully activating certain measures and procedures to cause the patient's death with an intention to relieve the patient from intractable suffering. For those advocating euthanasia, it is better to have death than prolonged life with intractable suffering (Foot, 1980).

From the vantage point of the patient, euthanasia could be classified as voluntary, non-voluntary and involuntary. Voluntary euthanasia means that euthanasia is effected with the patient's consent or request. Non-voluntary euthanasia is effected when the patient is without the capacity for self-determination. Involuntary euthanasia is effected when the patient objects to it. Euthanasia could be further classified as active and passive. Active euthanasia is effected by taking measures (such as injecting a lethal substance) to hasten death, while passive euthanasia is effected by ceasing life-sustaining measures or other treatment.

It is apparent that involuntary euthanasia is contrary to the principle of self-determination and is totally intolerable. Dismissing involuntary euthanasia would surely be unproblematic and will thus not be discussed here. We will therefore consider the following types of euthanasia:

(1) voluntary active euthanasia
(2) voluntary passive euthanasia
(3) non-voluntary active euthanasia
(4) non-voluntary passive euthanasia.

III. ACTIVE AND PASSIVE EUTHANASIA

In a very influential piece, James Rachels suggested that there is no distinction between active and passive euthanasia from the moral point of view (Rachels, 1979). He made a powerful analogy: Imagine that person A drowned a baby in a bathtub. A's conduct should be denounced as immoral. If, on the other hand, A is just standing with his arms crossed when seeing the baby drowning in the bath tub, A's conduct is different but still immoral. Rachels thought that both actively pursuing measures to terminate life and passively ceasing treatment of a terminal patient cause the death of the patient. Rachels' proposition is not meant to justify euthanasia but rather to indicate that active euthanasia and passive euthanasia are not essentially different from the vantage point of morality. What is different may be the varying degree of responsibility incurred.

Many consider passive euthanasia to be more acceptable than active euthanasia, as the medical profession is not required in this case to do anything actively to cause the patient's death. They do nothing and they bear no responsibility. However, if a doctor administers active euthanasia, he or she is doing something deliberately to bring about the patient's death. He or she is accordingly morally responsible, and may even be criminally liable.

Rachels thought that the above reasoning was flawed. Reconsider A's second position: if A does not have the capacity to save the baby from drowning, he cannot be blamed; however, if he ceases to do what he is able to, he cannot be regarded as doing nothing, but he does omit to save the baby. By the same token, if the medical profession has the capacity to prolong the patient's life but does not do so, it should be made morally responsible. Rachels went even further by saying that if euthanasia is morally acceptable, active euthanasia is preferable, as it provides an effective and efficient way for the patient to end intractable suffering. If euthanasia is morally wrong, passive euthanasia should also be condemned in spite of its passiveness.

Some insist that there is still a cardinal distinction between active and passive euthanasia. Passive euthanasia allows the patient to wait for a chance of recovery, while active euthanasia would entirely rule out such chances no matter how dim they are (Beauchamp, 1978). Rachels regarded such reasoning as fallible. Try again to envisage A's second position: There may still be a possibility that the baby may by itself crawl out of the bathtub even if such possibility is very dim. It cannot properly be held that keeping your arms crossed with a view to waiting for some dim possibility to materialize is not morally wrong. Therefore, in essence there is no difference between active and passive euthanasia. So we either have to accept both or deny both. I choose to deny both active and passive euthanasia and will provide my justification in the following discussion.

IV. NON-VOLUNTARY EUTHANASIA

We may not be indifferent to witnessing animals suffering indeterminately, and may prefer that they be subject to humane destruction. Yet human beings are different from animals as life experience, good or bad, is of intrinsic value. We are not allowed to reason that the mere fact that a person is suffering or without any quality of life should justify us in terminating his life (Foot, 1980). When the patient is no longer of sufficient capacity to indicate his view of life, who else is authorized or empowered to conclude that his or her life is not worth living? None of us are. It follows that non-voluntary euthanasia is unacceptable. John Harris (1996) disagreed with this view. He held that what is worthy of respect is 'persons', not life. According to Harris, a 'person' is an agent who is capable of "valuing its existence". Taking away the life of a 'person' who wants to live means depriving her of something that she values, and so it is morally wrong to do so. However, a 'person' who does not want to live cannot be wronged in this way because by having the wish to die granted, say through voluntary euthanasia, does not mean taking away something she treasures.

Harris' point is unfounded. Some may suggest that those with mental disadvantages could not live meaningful lives. Even if such a view is true, it does not follow that we are allowed to terminate their lives justifiably. Even though cats and dogs never generate any meaning for themselves, we are not empowered to destroy them at will. To end someone's life on the premise that that 'someone' is unable to live a meaningful life is discriminatory and unjustified. Even if a person in a coma could not generate meaning for himself, it does not follow that he is no longer a 'person' and that taking away his life would not be morally wrong.

We can have different conceptions for the same concept (Dworkin, 1993). Respect for life is not merely respect for the meaning of life. It is also respect for different people's varying conceptions of the meaning of life. We should not assume that there is a single conception as to what kind of life is meaningful. In an open and pluralistic society, we could not impose our conception of meaning of life on our neighbor. To terminate a patient's life against his will is not to respect his or her conception of the meaning of that life.

V. VOLUNTARY PASSIVE EUTHANASIA: A MISLEADING CONCEPT

After arguing that non-voluntary euthanasia is morally unacceptable, the next question to address is whether there is any difference between voluntary active euthanasia and voluntary passive euthanasia from the moral point of view. We do have an immediate answer to that, as so-called "voluntary passive euthanasia" could not be properly be regarded as euthanasia. When a patient requests the medical professional to cease the operation of life-sustaining measures or to cease treatment, he is exercising his right to refuse medical treatment after his consideration of the value of such treatment. To allow the patient to conduct his business in that manner is to respect his right to self-determination. Such cases of refusal of medical treatment are common. For instance, many patients would consider carefully the risks and consequences of a potential operation before they are able to determine whether or not to go ahead with it. A patient may refuse to undergo any operation after such consideration, even though he may be sure his refusal would abridge his life expectancy. In the light of this, when a terminal patient chooses to receive no further treatment, we cannot properly say that he chooses to die or that he prefers death to living. What he is pursuing is simply *living well*. Dying is the final stage of one's life. Living well implies being able to go through different stages of one's life, including the final stage, in one's own way. So a patient should be allowed to choose living through the last journey in his own way. This is not necessarily contrary to our respect for life, as people have different conceptions of respect (Dworkin, 1993, p. 216). Even if the terminal patient regards his request for cessation of treatment as a request for euthanasia, we cannot say that the medical professional who follows the request is practicing euthanasia. The medical professional is simply respecting the patient's choice of dying in his own way. It is not an act of killing or terminating the life of a patient but an act of enabling a patient to *live* through the last stage of his life in his own way.

VI. VOLUNTARY ACTIVE EUTHANASIA AND THE DUTIES OF THE MEDICAL PROFESSIONAL

Now, if a patient is so keen to have his own death, does he have the right to ask assistance from medical professionals to terminate his life? Are the medical professionals duty-bound to assist? From the vantage point of respect for life, the answer must be negative. In the event that a person begs us to kill him, we appreciate that as his will but we cannot concede. This proposition may attract some rejections by analogies. For instance, some people would hold the view that it is exceptional and acceptable for us to kill someone who is unbearably miserable in suffering. Furthermore, isn't it an exception to the respect for life when we cannot avoid killing, out of self-defense, someone who attacks us? Isn't it noble and inevitable for the country to send troops to kill the enemy when there is clear and present danger for national security? The answer to these two questions may well be in the positive but that could not be extended to justify euthanasia.

It is evident that endangering someone's life and country is immoral. Therefore any measure taken to curb such unjustified danger, including killing, is acceptable. However, in the case of a terminal illness, the patient does nothing morally wrong and therefore killing him in self-defense and/or national defense would not be justified (Beauchamp, 1978). On the other hand, even the patient's will would not constitute a justification for euthanasia. The principle of self-determination has its own boundaries and should not be the only guiding moral principle on every occasion (Callahan, 1992). For example, we will not let an individual who suffers from depression commit suicide even if he requests us to let him do so.

Those favoring voluntary active euthanasia may hold that ending the life of a terminal patient is more constructive than letting such a life to go on (Beauchamps, 1978, Callahan, 1992). But such a position has passed judgement on the meaning of the life of a terminal patient, because the advocate of voluntary active euthanasia assumes that the life of a terminal patient is very different from that of others, so it allows for exceptional treatment. Even if the patient himself agrees with the judgement, the medical professional may have reason not to make such a judgement. Euthanasia is incompatible with the mission of the medical profession that is entrusted to cure the sick, to help the sick in the course of recovery and to eliminate the magnitude of suffering. The medical profession has no obligation to make value judgements on the life of the patient. Even if the medical professional is of the view that the patient's life is worthless, he should never terminate the patient's life, nor should he procure and assist the patient in terminating his life (American Medical Association, Code of Medical Ethics, 1994; Callahan, 1992; Pellegrino, 1994).

Furthermore, the legalization of euthanasia would also cause some adverse social consequences. When terminating one's life becomes an expeditious alternative to curing it, the medical profession will inevitably suffer from low morale, and the unending effort to explore possible cures for human health might be discouraged. As a result, a patient may have a hastened death even though there is some chance of recovery (Sommerville, 1993, Ch. 6). Rendering euthanasia legal may abrogate the trust placed in the medical profession by the patient who may have grounds to suspect that euthanasia is committed in order to save time and resources (Pellegrino, 1994). As the population ages, those who are chronically ill may not receive proper treatment due to the limit of resources. They may regard themselves as the burden of society and prefer euthanasia as the dignified way out (Pellegrino, 1994).

Finally, in spite of the fact that some view euthanasia as only applicable in those terminal patients with intractable suffering, what amounts to 'terminal' and 'intractable suffering' is to be determined subjectively. It indicates that euthanasia may be improperly applied to those patients who are not indeed terminal (Callahan, 1992). We thus uphold our view that euthanasia should not be administered to any patient.

VII. EXTRAORDINARY TREATMENT AND PALLIATIVE TREATMENT

We may have no justification for advocating for euthanasia, but it is undisputed that many treatments for terminal patients may accelerate their pain and suffering. How are we able to help them live better? Generally speaking, we may administer two kinds of treatments (Kuhse, 1991; Steinbock, 1979): opiates or sedative drugs. Both are controversial as both may abridge the patient's remaining life expectancy.

Extraordinary treatment used to mean the treatment that is more expensive, risky and that involves high technology. "Extraordinary treatment" in the present day means, more precisely, a treatment procuring benefit disproportionate to the cost. So an extraordinary treatment may even be an inexpensive, low-risk and low-technology treatment, such as administering antibiotics or physiotherapy, if in comparison with the cost incurred the treatment itself produces very little significant effect for curing, or reducing the pain or discomfort of a patient. For example, in the case of a patient in a coma who contracted pneumonia, administering antibiotics would be of trivial assistance. Similarly, as to a patient with progressively worsening cancer, radiotherapy may not even bring negligible improvement, but rather, extensive pain and suffering. In such circumstances, some argue that ceasing to use extraordinary treatment on the patient does not amount to euthanasia, as such cessation is to avert unnecessary treatment, reducing the accompanying pain and suffering (Steinbock, 1979; Kuhse, 1991). However, the question of whether a shortened life with less suffering is preferable to a prolonged life with greater suffering is still controversial. The medical profession is not necessarily in a better position to judge this than others. It follows that the medical profession should not be too ready to cease those extraordinary treatments without consulting the patient and his family members.

Administering higher than normal doses of opiates and sedative drugs could also accelerate the patient's death even though it is admitted that the terminal patient may need such drugs to ease his intractable pain. Those in support of administering such opiate and sedative drugs argue that the objective thereof is to soothe the patient, not kill him, and the accelerated death is the accompanying side effect. Others would argue that when the medical professionals who cease or discontinue the extraordinary treatments or administer heavy opiate or sedative drugs could reasonably foresee that there is definite possibility of accelerating the patient's death, they should somehow be liable for the patient's life irrespective of their primary motive.

I believe that medical professionals who take the above measures to soothe a patient's suffering should not be held liable for the patient's ultimate death, even though the above measures incur risk of accelerated death. We could hardly assert that these medical professionals are practicing euthanasia, as the above measures would not lead to immediate death. As an analogy, we cannot say that people try to commit suicide when they participate in all kinds of risky activities, like smoking, drug use and high-risk sports. Rather, such risky activities may well represent their reasoned decision after calculating the gratification brought about and the risk that accompanies it.

After arguing that ceasing extraordinary treatment and administering high doses of opiate and sedative drugs would help soothe those patients with intractable suffering in spite of the fact that high risk of accelerated death is reasonably foreseeable, what remains unsettled is how we are to define intractable suffering, high risk of accelerated death and the like. It is recommended that the medical profession formulate its code of practice to guide its decision on all these matters after proper public discussion and consultation. The advantage of having such a code of practice is that it averts unnecessary controversy and shields medical professionals from accusations that they are practicing euthanasia when they are not.

VIII. THE DYING PROCESS AND FUTILITY OF MEDICINE

No living person could experience death as death comes only when life evaporates. As Wittgenstein rightly said, "death is not an event in life" (Wittgenstein, 1961, p 72). Many people are often not afraid of death, but rather fear the dying process, especially the accompanying suffering and the possibility of a death without dignity. Dying is inevitable. Therefore, it is important that death should keep faith with the way we want to have lived (Dworkin, 1993, p. 199).

When medical science was not as advanced as it is today, the medical profession tended to take the cessation of a heartbeat as the indicator of death, since this would very soon lead to brain death. However, contemporary medical science can maintain respiration and blood flow even after the heart has stopped functioning, thus avoiding the death of the brain. Today the cessation of the heartbeat is no longer the only indicator of death (Kearon, 1995, p. 27). Rather, the medical profession and our society accept brain death as the indicator of death. The advancement of medical science inserts more intermediate stages between life and death, and therefore medical professionals are more capable of saving a patient from the brink of death (Schneiderman & Jecker, 1995, p. 4). But on many occasions doctors can only prolong the dying process, not necessarily save the patient in any real sense. They are then only administering extraordinary treatment that is indeed futile treatment. Is such futile treatment consistent with the goals of medicine?

When treatment is effective, the medical profession has the duty to use it. When treatment could not cause full recovery, it is still the duty of the medical profession to assist the patient as much as possible, and to soothe his pain and suffering. However, we have to concede that death is inevitable and even the most advanced medical science could not stop that. The fact is that dying is an irreversible process and there are limits to medical science (Caplan, 1995, p. 56; Callahan, 1988). The cessation of futile treatment is not the causation of death, and is accordingly not euthanasia. Incurable illness is the true cause. Hipprocrates in 'The Arts' even held out that medical professionals are able to refuse to pursue any treatment when such treatment is deemed to be futile (Schneiderman & Jecker, 1995, p 6). Administering futile treatment is never the goal of medicine.

The wishes of the terminal patient and his family to prolong his life mirror our attitude that the sick should not be deserted. The medical profession may take itself to have the duty to continue futile treatment simply for the sake of not deserting a single patient. That is exactly the confusion of futility of medicine and the futility of care. Care would not be futile. If we do care about patients, we should transform our care, not into futile treatment, but into assistance with establishing a proper and dignified environment for dying, such as hospice service. The terminal patient needs care, not treatment (Schneiderman & Jecker, 1995; pp. 59-63, 167-168, Twyeross, 1995; Kearon, 1995, p. 42).

IX. THE PATIENT'S RIGHT TO ACCEPT OR REFUSE TREATMENT

Futility of medicine only provides an abstract guiding principle to determine if treatment should be withdrawn from a terminal patient. Still there remain unsettled and perplexing matters. We may have consensus that treatment could be withdrawn from a patient who is considered to be in chronic coma, literally a vegetable. But what are the exact conditions for being in PVS? Even the medical profession cannot so far provide us a definition with precision. In 1994 the House of Lords in the UK issued the Walton Report (paragraph 258), indicating the need for the medical profession and society to work out a code of practice guiding the consensus formulation of the understanding of PVS and the matters surrounding the proper treatment of patients in such a state. One cardinal matter to be determined is: How long should the coma last before a patient is properly defined as being in PVS?

Given that clear consensus has not been reached regarding the proper definition of PVS, we could not on every occasion declare that prolonging a patient's life is meaningless, and that therefore the treatment is futile. We have to admit that those relatives who visit permanently unconscious patients regularly will feel uncomfortable or anxious when they cannot (Dworkin, 1993, p. 212). The Wanglie case in 1991 sheds light on this. Mrs. Wanglie was a PVS patient, and the hospital applied to the court for an order to withdraw life support. But Mr. Wanglie believed that Mrs. Wanglie would prefer to live as long as possible and opposed the hospital's application (Dworkin, 1993, p. 213). It is obvious that the notion of futile treatment has to be linked up with the patient's conception of life. Patients should have the right to opt for a certain course of action, and the medical profession should have the duty to assist the patient to reach an informed decision.

Then, what about those without the sufficient mental faculty for self-determination, like those in quasi-coma or chronic coma? The medical profession can advise terminal patients to write an advance directive before their illnesses progress too far, explicating his wish of receiving or refusing extraordinary treatment. In the event that the patient decides he cannot know in advance what his preferences will be, he may appoint a proxy to make the decision for him. The proxy or proxies could be a relative, a friend or the medical professional. Since 1976 when California enacted the Natural Death Act, all other states except three followed suit, empowering the patient to make an advance directive so as to preserve his right of self-determination (*Choices in Dying*, 1994). In December of 1991, the Patient Self-Determination Act went into effect. This is a federal statute which requires health care institutions to provide upon admission to each adult patient written information regarding his/her "legal rights to make decisions concerning medical care, to refuse treatment, and to formulate advance directives, plus the relevant written policies of the institution" (Wolf et al., 1991). In 1994 the Walton Report in the UK also recommended such an advance directive or living will. Five provinces in Canada have passed similar legislation (Gordon & Singer, 1995). Most of the states in the USA have legislation governing proxy decision–making (*Choices in Dying*, 1994). According to a recent article, all American states except Alaska have laws that permit the appointment of a proxy for health care (Capron, 1998). Advance directives are now authorized in every state of the U.S. by statutes or case law (Veatch, 2000).

But surveys in the US suggest that the number of patients exercising their power in making advance directive or living will is not impressive, less than 20% (Sach, Stockir & Miles, 1992; Stelter, Elliot & Bruno, 1992). In regard to newborns, infants or adult patients without a will, many state governments have started to enact laws for surrogate decision making (*Choices in Dying*, 1994). Such laws stipulate who would be entitled to make the decision when there is no advance directive. The laws also spell out the sequence of qualified persons, which is formulated in accordance with the proximity of relationship, ranging from parents, spouse, offspring, and friends to the medical professional. A surrogate decision is made according to the guidance imposed by law. Generally speaking, the surrogate decision-maker needs to consider the patient's views regarding his preference in the event of losing self-determination, if he has ever expressed them. If not, the surrogate decision-maker may consider the patient's views as to how he is expected to be treated in PVS. Again, if no such view is ever expressed, the surrogate decision-maker should consider the patient's moral values and religious beliefs in order to reach a decision acceptable to the patient. The decision-maker should figure out the counterfactual decision of the patient, i.e., what the patient would have chosen had s/he known that s/he would be mentally incapacitated. If none of the above works, the surrogate decision maker should make the decision in the best interests of the patient. In deciding what constitutes the best interests of the patient, the decision maker should reason like a reasonable man who is placed in the same position as the patient's (Hasting Center, 1981; Arras, 1991). In the process of surrogate decision making, the patient's choice is of fundamental importance, while the importance of the best interests of the patient are secondary, because they will be considered only when the surrogate decision-maker cannot determine the patient's choice.

X. THE HEART OF THE MATTER

Unfortunately, many people mistakenly used to use the controversial term "euthanasia" when they were discussing the less controversial matter of forgoing treatment. Some hold that ceasing or discontinuing treatment or administering heavy opiates or sedative drugs violates respect for life. In addition, the preservation of life is always a legitimate interest to be enshrined by the court. As a result, irresolvable conflicts often arise when the patient and his family are upset because prolonging life means prolonging suffering, as the case of *Cruzan v Director, Missouri Dept. of Health* in the USA illustrates.

Nancy Cruzan, 25, had been in PVS since 1983 after a traffic accident. Four years afterwards, Cruzan's parents requested the hospital to cease life-saving hydration and nutrition but the hospital refused. Cruzan's parents resorted to the courts. It was only after some years that the US Supreme Court decided to allow withdrawal of the life-saving hydration and nutrition. Cruzan's father sighed that his daughter's life had been interrupted by many strangers (medical professionals, lawyers, press, judges and protestors), but at the end of the day, only her parents would visit her graveyard and weep after the decision (Caplan, 1995, p. 68). Justice Brennan in the US Supreme Court made similar remarks (Gostin & Weir, 1991).

The court would no doubt honor and preserve life and would not accept euthanasia as the justification for withdrawing life support. But the court is more prepared for the self-determination argument for accepting a patient's decision of refusal of treatment. In the premises, ceasing treatment at the will of the terminal patient is most acceptable to the court and the society as a means of respecting self-determination. On the contrary, since the notion of euthanasia is more controversial, using it to justify the cessation of life support will likely provoke unnecessary social conflicts and make the issues more divisive.

Cruzan's case reveals the importance of making public policy on the basis of self-determination. The US Supreme Court demanded clear and convincing evidence in support of the claim that Cruzan ever indicated her wish of ceasing treatment were she ever in a persistent vegetative state. For the sake of honoring life, the slightest reasonable doubt would cause the court to reject the application for cessation of treatment. Such a stringent evidential requirement rendered Cruzan's parents almost unable to prove Cruzan's will. It is therefore argued that an effective surrogate decision making process should not put the burden of proof on the family. Rather the burden should be shifted to those suspecting and objecting to the propriety of the cessation of treatment. The remarks of Cruzan's father and Justice Brennan urge us to trust our family. The President's Commission on Deciding to Forgo Life–Sustaining Treatment explicitly holds that when those patients without the ability to make informed choices do not have an appointed surrogate decision maker, their families should make the decision. Although such a recommendation has not yet received the blessing of law, Cruzan's case has caused many other states in the US in the 90's to enact or amend the surrogate decision legislation so as to reflect the family's status in making the surrogate decision.

What has emerged is the practice of honoring the individual choices and interests of the terminal patient according to their wishes via advance directives, proxy-appointment, and surrogate decision making (Buchanan and Brock, 1990; Veatch, 1998). Conceptualizing the matters in terms of self-determination and best interests would be less exclusive and divisive, less likely to provoke social conflicts, and thus more desirable (Arras, 1991). On the contrary, conducting the matters via a discussion of euthanasia could only stir up the split views among the patient, the patient's family and the public.

X. THE PRACTICES OF SOME EAST ASIAN SOCIETIES

The above practice that has emerged in countries like the US can be called a liberal model of decision making. Although the family does have a role to play, this model is entirely patient-centered because the family only helps the patient to exercise his/her choice or to promote his/her individual interests. The family is marginalized and becomes a shadow of the patient with no independent status. So it is dubious whether the model can be fully applied to societies with a strong culture of familialism.

In Japan, the utilization of advance directives is very limited for several reasons (Ohara, 2000; Ohi, 1998; Tuschida, 1998). First, the patient is often not told by the physician or the family that she is terminally ill. There is thus no perceived need for the preparation of an advance directive. Second, truth-telling would create burdens on both sides and undermine the normal relations among family members because they could not act as if nothing had happened once the truth was disclosed. Third, verbal instruction is regarded as an adequate means of communication in a harmonious family. It is inappropriate to articulate one's wishes in writing, as this would be perceived as a sign of not trusting other family members. Fourth, the decision of an individual, even stated in a living will, can be overridden by the collective decision of a family.

In a recent field visit to a major hospital in Beijing, my colleagues and I found that the physician only breaks the bad news to the family. The patient will not be told that she is terminally ill and the family will take the full responsibility of making decisions for the patient. In another visit to a major hospital in Hong Kong, we found that although there is no single practice (as it depends on the condition of the patient and specialty of the doctor involved), it is not uncommon that the physician will first break the bad news to the family. Nor is it rare that the patient is not informed of the terminal illness if the family wants to hide the news and the patient does not take the initiative to ask the doctor. However, one major difference between the practices in Beijing and in Hong Kong is that, in Hong Kong, if the terminal patient does take the initiative to ask, many doctors believe that they should let the patient know about the diagnosis. Also, many people indeed prefer the doctor to release the information to the patient in the presence of his/her family.[2]

In another study conducted in Hong Kong in the summer of 1999, my colleagues and I ran a number of focus group discussions with elderly people, social workers and professionals contacted through elderly service agencies in Hong Kong.[3] A typical response to the question that asks about the importance of choice for them is: "It is important, but we do not know how to choose; being cared for here is good already and we have no other demands." It is quite apparent that many of the elderly are only paying lip-service to the importance of choice.

XII. THE MODEL OF FAMILIALISM

The practices of these East Asian societies seem to be based on a model of familialism. In this model, the terminal stage is seen as the last journey that the patient and his/her family members go through together, a process in which they show their mutual concern and care, but not essentially a process in which the patient exercises his/her choice or realizes his/her best interests. The liberal model ignores the fact that the preference and interests of family members are connected. I am a husband and a son, and I should not make a decision, say to move to Shanghai, based solely on what I want for myself. Similarly, an advance directive, if I really wanted to make one, should not be regarded as solely a means for me to exercise my self-determination, but should also be used to express my concern for my kin and my commitment to their well-being when I become incompetent. The directive is a means of helping them to know my voice and of facilitating the ongoing dialogue with them when I lapse into incompetency. My family members would then try to talk to me as if I were competent, but the whole point of the dialogue is not so much to figure out what I would have wanted for myself (my counterfactual choice) but rather to arrive at a family decision with my counterfactual participation. The prior directive only encodes my initial voice, and my voice, along with those belonging to my significant others, is likely to be transformed as the dialogue goes along. So the final decision need not be dictated entirely by the literal meaning of my advance directive, however clear and specific it is, though it is nevertheless an important reference for my family in the decision making process. Furthermore, I may have conveyed my view about death and dying on some intimate occasions and that may serve as a much more significant reminder of my voice than a written directive. It is likely that my intimate others may have already accepted and shared my view on those occasions. So, in the familial model of decision making, it is not necessary to institutionalize the expression of prior wishes by laws and regulations as in the United States.

By the same token, if the incompetent patient has not expressed any prior wish, instead of figuring out what the patient would have chosen for him/herself, his/her relatives will try to figure our what all the family members (including the patient) would have decided together had s/he known that s/he would lapse into incompetency. Of course, in the familial model, the other members of the family still need to know the counterfactual view of the patient as in the process of surrogate decision making, but the point of figuring that out is to enable them to engage with him/her in a dialogue so that they can arrive at a collective family decision with the presence of his/her counterfactual voice. In case they cannot figure out the counterfactual voice of the patient, the decision should be made in the best interests of the family (including the patient) rather than that of the patient alone. So surrogate decision making in the familial model carries a meaning very different from that in the liberal model.

All in all, in the model of familialism, a son, for example, will consider not only the prior/counterfactual wish and the interests of his father who has become incompetent. The son will also consider the burden of care and the feelings of his mother in going together with her husband through the last journey of his life. The mother will also consider the financial burden that her son might have to bear for his father if he (the father) were to be kept alive at all costs (Nelson and Nelson, 1995). Under the familial model, prior expressions of wishes and surrogate decision making are not the means for the patient to exercise his/her autonomy or to advance the best interests of his/her own but rather for the family to arrive at a collective decision. The decision to forgo treatments in the familial model, unlike the liberal model, is justified in terms of the autonomy and the interests of the family (including the patient) rather than the self-determination or the individual interests of the patient.

XIII.THE PROBLEM OF PERSONAL IDENTITY

The familial model also has the advantage of avoiding a problem that in the liberal model is difficult to solve. Suppose that a patient lives a joyful life with her family when she becomes demented but has made an advance directive that no treatment be offered except those needed to keep her comfortable. Now, if the demented patient is suffering from severe pneumonia, what should be done? Should she be treated in defiance of the directive? One possible way out is to argue that the demented patient is a different person (or non-person) because she is radically different from or is not psychological connected to the person who wrote the advance directive. However, the price of this solution is high because it leads to the counterintuitive conclusion that the earlier person is now dead but the family cannot bury her body, and that the family should have nothing to do with treatment decisions for the new person (non-person) (Veatch, 2000; Olick, 2001).

The other possible way out is to argue that the person can make sense of her issuing an advance directive only if she understands her being demented as a stage of *her* life, and that conversely to regard the directive as irrelevant is to deny the moral agent an authorship of a complete life (Olick 2001). But this solution will lead to the counterintuitive result that the advance directive is binding in the case in which the demented patient is quite contented with her life (Veatch, 2000).

Indeed, the common presupposition that underpins the above two paradoxical views is that the continuity of one's personhood depends upon the relevance of one's prior wish. This presupposition is problematic. In the familial model, whether the incompetent person is a different person has nothing to do with whether her/her prior wish is honored, i.e., there is no intrinsic relation between personal identity and choice. This model embodies a relational conception of personhood because individuals are embedded in a network of relations and are identified in terms of their connections with others. According to such a conception, my grandmother would still be my grandmother simply because she was related to me in a certain way; she stood in the same relation to me and would be the same grandmother both before and after she was demented.[4] Hence, whether or not she was the same person is not tied to whether her prior directive, had she written one, was valid in the period of incompetency, and so the problem of personal identity does not arise at all in the familial model.

XIV. TWO POLICY OPTIONS: WHO IS THE AUTHORITY BY DEFAULT, THE INDIVIDUAL OR THE FAMILY?

Despite the above strength, one common objection to the familial model is that it provides no adequate protection to the patient from abuse and neglect. A family can be full of conflicts or even dysfunctional and it may then be dangerous to entrust the family with decisions for the patient who may be the most vulnerable. However, there are patients who choose to leave the decision entirely in the hands of the family even when they are competent. They may even want the family members to make their own decision or a decision for the *whole* family, which is not quite the same as a proxy's executing the *individual* choice of the patient in the liberal model. It seems that the patient should be permitted to do that because people should be free to *give up* their choices.

As I said earlier, in the liberal model, autonomy is regarded as the value of making one's own choice without external interferences and personal limitations, such as inadequate information. Yet we could use a thinner notion that conceives of autonomy as "a constraint on acting against others without their consent" (Engelhardt, 1996). The patient who freely gives up her choice for treatment to the family can now be seen as an autonomous person, though in the weak sense, because the family is not acting against her without her permission. Yet she is not autonomous in the thick sense because she has decided not to exercise her own choice of treatment. The thick notion of autonomy indeed belongs to the liberal model because the treatment decision for a dying patient is equated with the execution of *her* choice (prior or counterfactual).

According to H. Tristram Engelhardt Jr., the thin notion of autonomy can serve as a side-constraint to promote mutual respect and peaceful coexistence amongst people with different value commitments, including both liberals and non-liberals. Autonomy as a side-constraint is a content-less notion while the wider notion of autonomy (autonomy as a value) is content-full and is the cardinal value of the liberal model. Adopting the liberal model as the policy framework for decision making will result in imposing a particular ethic on those who are in favor of the familial model. In contrast, using autonomy as a side-constraint as the guiding principle for dealing with the decision making problem for the terminal patient allows room for the practice of familialism to flourish.[5] Yet the principle can also safeguard the patient from abuse and neglect, for the family cannot act for her without her consent.

However, I believe that the above approach is still inadequate for two reasons. First, take the case of a patient who, while competent, neither said that she will give up her choices to the family nor asserted her endorsement of the liberal model, say by issuing an advance directive. What would be the default or preset position? Whose authority can be taken for granted, the decision of the family or the counterfactual wish of the patient? It seems that we still need to make a choice between the two.

Secondly, under the thin notion of autonomy, if the physician breaks the bad news to the family members first without the patient's prior consent, she may still be accused of intruding into the privacy of and hiding information from the patient. However, in societies with a strong familial culture, this kind of physician behavior is normally regarded as acceptable.

Of course, we should not overlook the fact that in some unusual cases, say in the case of a dysfunctional family, following the practices of the familial model can harm the patient. In order to safeguard the fundamental interests of the patient, we can stipulate that the physician should follow the familial practice unless the patient has shown her disapproval in the first place. This provides leeway for the patient to safeguard herself from abuse and neglect, and allows room for the patient to practice the liberal model. However, the burden of disapproval is on those who want to veto the familial practice. So the physician does not need to clarify this with the patient in the first place; it is the patient's responsibility to let the physician know the objection beforehand. If the patient does not do that, the physician will not be charged with malpractice. We can call the above a moderate model of familialism because the family only has default but not absolute authority in the decision making process. This is different from adopting autonomy as a side-constraint. According to this understanding of autonomy, the physician needs to seek prior approval from the patient, otherwise she could *not* follow the familial practice, such as breaking the bad news to the family in the absence of the patient. The difference between moderate familialism and autonomy as a side-constraint is akin to that of "innocent until proven otherwise" vs. "guilty until proven otherwise", and can be coined as "the family until proven otherwise" vs. "the individual until proven otherwise." It seems that by making the family rather than the individual the default authority, we can on the one hand pay due respect to the family but on the other hand protect the patient from abuse and neglect and also give room for people to practice the liberal model.

XV. THE HONG KONG SITUATION

Presently Hong Kong has no legislation legalizing the medical professional to practice euthanasia or assisted suicide. Such conduct could constitute the offenses of murder or manslaughter under the law of Hong Kong. At the level of professional ethics, the Hong Kong medical profession endorses the Hippocratic Oath, refraining from administering drugs for the patient's death or recommending anything to that effect. The International Code of Medical Ethics, which is endorsed by the profession as well, also makes it explicit that preserving life is the doctor's duty. So, from the perspectives of both professional conduct and the legal framework, Hong Kong does not endorse euthanasia.

The Hong Kong medical profession has already had consensus regarding many matters about the patient's death, though not all. The doctors prevailingly accept brain death as the patient's death, in which case any life-sustaining apparatus could be withdrawn. The medical professionals generally accept that, if necessary, high dosages of opiate or sedative drugs could be administered with the intent to reduce pain and discomfort for the terminal patient, even though such drugs may convey high risk of accelerated death. It is also recognized that the patient has the right to refuse treatment and cardio-pulmonary resuscitation. In the late 1990s, guidelines on in-hospital resuscitation decisions were issued by the Hong Kong Hospital Authority, the public hospital service provider that provides 94% of the hospital service in the territory. Whether respiration apparatus could be withdrawn from a PVS patient is also unclear but the medical professionals largely agree that prior consent from the patient's family is required.

In November of 2000, the Medical Council of Hong Kong inserted a new section, "Care for the terminally ill," in the revised *Professional Code and Conduct for the Guidance of Registered Medical Practitioners*. The new section explicitly states that the Council does not support the practice of euthanasia, which is regarded as illegal and unethical. It also maintains that the withdrawing/withholding of artificial life sustaining support for the terminal ill is not euthanasia. The decision to forgo such a treatment should be based on the principle of the futility of treatment for a terminal patient and take into account the patient's benefits, and the wish of the patient and the family. The Hospital Authority had developed a set of guidelines on life-sustaining treatment in the terminally ill under the framework outlined in the Professional Code and Conduct by the Medical Council. The Guidelines were issued to all public hospitals in April 26, 2002. What we have seen so far is that Hong Kong has basically accepted the distinction between euthanasia and forgoing futile treatments that was established in the early part of this paper.

However, as we have seen, our study in Hong Kong shows that although the family culture is strong, no single practice is followed in the decision making process for the terminally ill. Hong Kong is not a pluralistic society, but it is not a homogeneous society either. Under Western influence, some people may find the liberal model more appealing. Their views cannot be ignored. So this paper therefore recommends that the moderate model of familialism be adopted as the guiding principle in the decision making process for the terminally ill, because the model on the one hand pays due respect to the family culture in Hong Kong, but on the other hand can safeguard patients from neglect and abuse, and allow space for the liberals to follow their own practices.

Despite the on-going cultural changes in Hong Kong that make the health care system more open and accountable, the medical profession is still perceived with great respect and people in general accept a moderate level of paternalism. It is easier to build up a partnership between the medical profession, the patient, and the family. This form of paternalism and the moderate model of familialism are compatible. When the patient's family is left alone to exercise their power in surrogate decision making, they may tend to be conservative in averting blame and criticism. If the surrogate decision could be jointly made by the family and the responsible medical professionals, that will enable the family to be more capable of looking after the interests of the patient. According to Hospital Authority Guidelines on Life-sustaining Treatment in the Terminally Ill (Hospital Authority 2002), the decision making process is regarded as a *consensus*-building process among the health care professional, the patient and the family, and the healthcare profession should work towards a consensus with the family if possible when the patient is incompetent. So due respect is paid to the autonomy of the family because, other than in emergency situations, medical decisions for the incompetent patient require the consensus of the family. However, we cannot exclude the possibility that the family and the medical professionals may hold conflicting views, particularly in case where the view of the family is believed to be contrary to the best interests of the patient. According to the Guidelines, such disagreement should first be resolved by further communication. If the resolution fails, the advice of and the facilitation by the ethics committee should be sought and the committee may also serve the role of a mediator as appropriate. In case of unresolvable dispute, the decision of the court should be sought. So the authority of the family is not absolute and the practices in Hong Kong actually manifest a moderate form of familialism.

City University of Hong Kong
Kowloon, Hong Kong SAR, PRC

NOTES

1 The research related to this paper was supported by Governance in Asia Research Centre (GARC) at the City University of Hong Kong.

2 The field visits in Bejing and Hong Kong are part of the Research Project on The Principle of Informed Consent and Chinese Familialism in Health Care, a Competitive Earmarked Research Grant (CERG) project funded by the Research Grant Council (RGC) of Hong Kong. The project aims to compare the role of the family in medical decision making in Beijing, Hong Kong and Houston.

3 The focus group discussion is part of the research project "A Comparative Study of Elderly Policies Regarding Quality Care in Hong Kong, Singapore, and Britain", which is a flagship project of Centre for Comparative Public Management and Social Policy (RCPM) at the City University of Hong Kong

4 Quite a number of articles have recently developed the relational conception of personhood and argued that Western theories often over-emphasize psychological continuity, rationality and autonomy at the expense of the relational. See J. P-W. L. Tao and A. Y. H. Fung, 'Reconciling Autonomy and Connectedness in Bioethics.' Paper presented in: International

Conference of Bioethics, National University and South China Management College, Taiwan, June 16-19, 1998; and various articles by R. Qiu, D. K. S. Au, and E. Hui collected in Becker (2000).

5 This point was made by Engelhardt in a conversation that took place in May 2001.

REFERENCES

American Medical Association (1994). *Code of Medical Ethics.* Chicago: American Medical Association.

Arras, John D. (1991) 'Beyond Cruzan: Individual rights, family autonomy and the persistent vegetative state.' In Tom L. Beauchamp & LeRoy Walters (eds.), *Contemporary Issues in Bioethics, 4th ed.* Belmont, California: Wadsworth Publishing Company, 1994.

Beauchamp, Tom L. (1978). 'A reply to Rachels on active and passive euthanasia.' In Tom L. Beauchamp & LeRoy Walters (eds.), *Contemporary Issues in Bioethics, 4th ed.* Belmont, California: Wadsworth Publishing Company, 1994.

Becker, Gerhold K. (2000). *The Moral Status of Persons: Perspectives on Bioethics.* Amsterdam-Atlanta: GA. Rodopi.

Buchanan, Allen E. & Brock, David W. (1990). *Deciding for Others: The Ethics of Surrogate Decision Making.* Cambridge: Cambridge University Press.

Callahan, Daniel (1992). 'When self-determination runs amok.' In Tom L. Beauchamp & LeRoy Walters (eds.), *Contemporary Issues in Bioethics, 4th ed.* Belmont, California: Wadsworth Publishing Company, 1994.

Callahan, Daniel (1988). 'Vital distinctions, moral questions: Debating euthanasia and health-care costs.' In Tom L. Beauchamp & LeRoy Walters (eds.), *Contemporary Issues in Bioethics, 4th ed.* Belmont, California: Wadsworth Publishing Company, 1994.

Caplan, Arthur (1995). *Moral Matters: Ethical Issues in Medicine and the Life Sciences.* New York: John Wiley & Sons, Inc.

Capron, Alexander Morgan (1998). 'Advance directives.' In H. Kuhse and P. Singer (eds.), *A Companion to Bioethics.* Oxford: Blackwell.

Choices in Dying (1994). *Refusal of Treatment Legislation: 1993 Update.* New York: Choices in Dying.

Dworkin, Ronald (1993). *Life's Dominion: An Argument about Abortion, Euthanasia, and Individual Freedom.* New York: Alfred A. Knopf.

Engelhardt, H. Tristram, Jr. (1996). *The Foundations of Medical Ethics, 2nd Ed.* New York and Oxford: Oxford University Press.

Foot, Philippa (1980). 'Euthanasia.' In Marshall Cohen, Thomas Nagel & Thomas Scanlon (eds.), *Medicine and Moral Philosophy.* N. J., Princeton: Princeton University Press.

Gordon, Michael & Singer, Peter A. (1995). 'Decision and care at the end of life,' *Lancet*, 346, 163-166.

Gostin, L. & Weir, R.F. (1991). 'Life and death choices after Cruzan: Case law and standards of professional conduct,' *The Milbank Quarterly,* 69(1), 143-173.

Gromally, Luke (1995). 'Walton, Davis, Boyd and the legalization of euthanasia.' In John Keown (ed.), *Euthanasia Examined: Ethical, Clinical and Legal Perspectives.* Cambridge: Cambridge University Press.

Hardwig, John (1995). 'What about the family?' In Joseph H. Howell & William Friderick Sale (eds.). *Life Choices: A Hastings Center Introduction to Bioethics.* Washington D. C.: Georgetown University Press.

Harris, John (1995). 'Euthanasia and the value of life.' In John Keown (ed.), *Euthanasia Examined: Ethical, Clinical and Legal Perspectives.* Cambridge: Cambridge University Press.

Hastings Center (1981). 'Guidelines on the termination of life-sustaining treatment and the care of the dying.' In Tom L. Beauchamp & LeRoy Walters (eds.), *Contemporary Issues in Bioethics, 4th ed.* Belmont, California: Wadsworth Publishing Company, 1994.

Hospital Authority (2002). 'HA Guidelines on Life-sustaining Treatment in the Terminally Ill." Hong Kong: Hospital Authority.

Nelson, Hilde Lindemann & Nelson, James Lindemann (1995). *The Patient in the Family.* New York and London: Routledge.

Rachels, James (1979). 'Euthanasia, killing, and letting die.' In James P. Sterba (ed.), *Morality in Practice.* Belmont, California: Wadsworth Publishing Company, 1994.

Kearon, Kenneth (1995). *Medical Ethics: An Introduction.* Dublin: Twenty-Third Publications.

Kuhse, Helga (1991). 'Euthanasia,' in Peter Singer (ed.), *A Companion to Ethics.* Oxford: Basil Blackwell.

Ohara. S. (2000). 'We-consciousness and terminal patients: Some biomedical reflections on Japanese civil religion.' In Gerhold K. Becker (ed.), *The Moral Status of Persons: Perspectives on Bioethics.* Admsterdam-Atlanta: GA. Rodopi.

Ohi, Gen (1998). 'Advance directives and the Japanese ethos.' In Hans-Martin Sass, Robert. M. Veatch & Rihito Kimura (eds.), *Advance Directives and Surrogate Decision Making in Health Care.* Baltimore: Johns Hopkins University Press.

Olick, Robert S. (2001). *Taking Advance Directives Seriously: Prospective Autonomy and Decisions Near the End of Life.* Washington, D.C.: Georgetown University Press

Pellegrino, Edmund D. (1994). 'Euthanasia as a distortion of the healing relationship.' In Tom L. Beauchamp & LeRoy Walters (eds.), *Contemporary Issues in Bioethics, 4th ed.* Belmont, California: Wadsworth Publishing Company, 1994.

President's Commission for the Study of Ethical Problems in Medicine (1983). *Deciding to Forgo Life-Sustaining Treatment.* Washington DC: Congress of the US.

Steinbock, Bonnie (1979). 'The intentional termination of life.' In James P. Sterba (ed.), *Morality in Practice.* Belmont, California: Wadsworth Publishing Company, 1994.

Schneiderman, Lawrence J. & Jecker, Nancy (1995). *Wrong Medicine.* Baltimore, London: The John Hopkins University Press.

Sommerville, Ann (1993). *Medical Ethics Today: Its Practice and Philosophy.* London: BMJ Publishing Group.

Tao, Julia Po-wah Lai & Fung, Anthony Yin-him (1998). 'Reconciling autonomy and connectedness in bioethics,' paper presented in International Conference of Bioethics, National University and South China Management College, Taiwan, June 16-19, 1998.

Tuschida, Tomoaki (1998). 'A differing perspective on advance directives.' In Hans-Martin Sass, Robert. M. Veatch & Rihito Kimura (eds.). *Advance Directives and Surrogate Decision Making in Health Care.* Baltimore: Johns Hopkins University Press.

Twyeross, Robert G. (1995). 'Where there is hope, there is life: A view from the hospice.' In John Keown (ed.), *Euthanasia Examined: Ethical, Clinical and Legal Perspectives.* Cambridge: Cambridge University Press.

Veatch, Robert M. (1998). 'Ethical dimensions of advance directives and surrogate decision making in the United States,' in Hans-Martin Sass, Robert. M. Veatch & Rihito Kimura (eds.), *Advance Directives and Surrogate Decision Making in Health Care.* Baltimore: Johns Hopkins University Press.

Veatch, Robert M. (2000). *The Basics of Bioethics*. Upper Saddle River, NJ: Prentice Hall.

[Walton Report] *Report of the Select Committee on Medical Ethics*, House of Lords Paper 21-I of 1993-94, London: HMSO.

Wittgenstein, Ludwig (1961). *Tractatus Logico-Philosophicus.* London: Routledge & Kegan Paul.

Wolf, Susan M. et al. (1991). 'Sources of concern about the patient self-determination act.' In Tom L. Beauchamp & LeRoy Walters (eds.), *Contemporary Issues in Bioethics, 5th ed.* Belmont, CA: Wadworth Publishing Company.

CORINNA DELKESKAMP-HAYES

DISSENSUS IN THE FACE OF A PASSION FOR CONSENSUS: HOW THE JAPANESE AND THE GERMANS COULD STILL UNDERSTAND ONE ANOTHER

I.INTRODUCTION: MORAL DIVERSITY IN BIOETHICS

In making the case for the plausibility of a southeast Asian bioethics, indeed, for a Japanese bioethics, Kazumasa Hoshino has recognized the role of hidden cultural assumptions in framing the bioethics literatures of particular cultures and countries. Europeans with ease recognize that American bioethics is American and not framed from a universal human perspective. So too, Americans with ease recognize that German bioethics is German and not framed from a universal human perspective. The problem is that when Americans reflect on American bioethics, they take it to be the flawless revelation of that bioethic which should guide mankind. Lamentably the same holds for the Germans, who without any hesitation affirm that German bioethics clearly sees, as no other bioethics, the dangers of germline genetic engineering, to mention only one of the issues that divide the various national bioethics.

In this brief essay, I want to take special acknowledgement of the contribution of Hoshino to the recognition of cultural difference and its implications for bioethics. Hoshino has helped us to understand that pleadings on behalf of global bioethics are often a backhanded attempt to advance a particular bioethics under the guise of a universal moral vision. In short, one finds that what is at stake is a form of cultural imperialism in moral disguise.

Due to particular historical developments that led to an imbalance of political as well as technological power between what is generally subsumed under the heading of "the West" on the one hand and the various countries of "the South" and "the East" on the other, cultural imperialism has in the past been a specifically Western temptation. At the same time, it has been difficult for Western observers to recognize the injustice involved in such "acculturating" use of power: The presumption always was that one brought the light (of true faith, rational insight, and the universal morality of human rights and human dignity) to those sitting

H.T. Engelhardt, Jr. and L.M. Rasmussen (eds.), Bioethics and Moral Content: National Traditions of Health Care Morality, 191–201.

in darkness. Therefore, I shall first give a short summary of the cultural presuppositions which underlie the very Western propensity to the raising of universal validity claims for ethical insights, which are also shaped by those cultural presuppositions. In a second section, I shall restrict myself to the relatively homogeneous continental European portion of that Western culture. I shall expose, even within that portion, surprising differences between, as well as mutual incompatibilities among, the underlying value judgements, which are nevertheless, each in its sundry way, claimed to be universally compelling. As a particularly illuminating example I shall attend to Germany vis-à-vis its neighbor countries. In concluding, I shall show why at least the Germans have good reasons to acknowledge the right of different polities to their different bioethical cultures. Just as the Japanese have learned that they need not adjust themselves to American standards, if they wish to interact with America economically and scientifically, so Germans should understand that neither Germans nor Europeans or even Westerners in the wide sense (as far as their moral agreement can be claimed to go) should impose such adjustment on their partners in the rest of the world.

II.THE SPECIFICALLY CHRISTIAN ROOTS OF SECULAR WESTERN BIOETHICS

The Western propensity to claims of moral universality has two cultural roots: on the one hand, Christianity, and, on the other hand, a pagan rationalism, which first merely re-shaped (in the process of its philosophical reconstruction during the Middle Ages), but later thoroughly transformed (through its moralist reduction in the era of the Enlightenment) the Christian cultural framework.

On the one hand Christianity, for the last two millennia, has provided the dominant intellectual framework in the West (even though not exclusively in the West). It had in turn replaced the ethnically or politically particular accounts of morality which were endorsed by either Judaism or the ancient, polis-oriented political philosophies. Whereas the political universalism of the pagan Roman Empire was restricted to the legal sphere and tolerated religious and moral diversity (at least as long as this would not threaten political loyalty and piety), the Christianization of the Roman Empire, which started with Constantine the Great (280?-337), led to an increasing cultural homogeneity even in the moral and spiritual realm. The missionary imperative, which is central to traditional Christianity, was strongly supported by a state that increasingly derived its secular authority from its divine Christian institution. This support discouraged moral and spiritual diversity.

Yet even that missionary imperative (even in combination with the protective role the state assumed vis-à-vis the dogmatic integrity of its official religion) provides no justification for, and should never have encouraged, any aggressive cultural imperialism. The imperative after all, as pronounced by Christ himself, imposes efforts at teaching and baptizing, not at suppressing. It places the evangelizing endeavor within a context of faithfulness to His own example of gentle meekness and sacrificial service. The protective role of the state, on the other hand, was assumed only within its confines, and only in relation to warding off heresies.

If Western Christianity in effect could nevertheless be instrumentalized for imperialist goals, it was because of its combination with rationalism. When Thomas of Aquinas undertook to harmonize what was believed to rest on the authority of "reason itself" in Aristotelian philosophy with the truths of the Christian revelation, Christian moral principles were separated from their spiritual context. They were presented as results of purely intellectual research. Their value content, which had once been experienced literally (as with the Apostles) or mystically (as with some of the evangelists and the fathers of the church) through communion with God, was claimed accessible independently of the grace required for such communion. Moral principles thus were claimed to be both content rich and derivable from purely human intellectual insight. It was this transformation, which first offered a parallel system to, and later altogether replaced, those truths of faith by a secular morality. It thus came to nourish a legalistic claim for the latter's "right reasoning"-based universal validity, instead of nourishing a spiritual endeavor towards "grace-supported" universality: If all humans share the same reasoning faculty, then the same rational truths must be acknowledged by all humans who deserve to be respected under that name. Any refusal to endorse that acknowledgement could then be either counted as evidence for a lack of full humanity, or as a proof of moral perversity (rather than, as in the spiritual original, as evidence for lacking holiness among the missionaries). The use of secular imperialist violence for the imposition of those moral principles could be immunized against the charge of violating humans' rights: Either the victims were not "fully human" enough to claim such rights, or the violence justly punished their culpable refusal.

It is thus at bottom specifically Christian value commitments which underlie (after having been exposed to a thorough process of transforming and perverting adjustments) the purportedly rational Western political ethos, as well its particular bio-ethical correlate: Both invoke principles such as human dignity, the sanctity of life, individual human rights, state enforced solidarity, the supreme value of individual autonomy and the moral limits for the legitimate use of that autonomy. It is this ultimate cultural rootedness of what is claimed to be rationally compelling, which gives substance to Hoshino's diagnosis: Western claims for impartial, universally valid moral rationality, and Western attempts at global advocacy and implementation of human rights which are claimed to follow from that rationality, in fact merely serve as a cover for imposing particular cultural values on people who are culturally committed to quite different values.

III.GERMAN BIOETHICS: SOME OF THE PECULIARITIES

Quite independently of their generalizing claims, Westerners are never very disturbed by the fact that among themselves they rank the various and often incompatible elements of their purportedly rational faith differently. They are strangely oblivious to the fact that they endorse quite heterogeneous varieties of their supposed single "universally compelling" morality. State-enforced solidarity is considered irrational among those who are committed to the specifically American tradition of protecting individual freedom and responsibility, while it is considered a reasonable policy by the overwhelming majority of Europeans. Of course, even among Europeans the meaning of such solidarity is not uniformly understood: in Great Britain the public's obligation to furnish medical care is limited by economic considerations to a much greater extent than in, say, Germany: Whereas Germans take the universal right to health care to encompass everything that is considered medically necessary, and to include the right to be cared for rather immediately, Britons restrict certain more expensive services to the young, withhold other services from all, and impose heavy waiting periods on many. Surrogate motherhood, as well as sperm- and ova-donation are considered acceptable ways of realizing family values in the United States, but violations of human dignity (of the future child) by Europeans. Germ line therapy and genetic engineering seem beneficial ways of using medical knowledge to Americans, while for Europeans such techniques constitute a violation of the sanctity of human life and a door opener for the instrumentalization of future humans. Genetic screening in the United States is regarded as a resource of useful knowledge for responsible decision making, whereas Europeans mostly attend to the risks involved for the protection of informational privacy and of the right to beneficial ignorance, as well as for the danger of social and economic discrimination.

Regardless of their ultimately common Christian roots, the separation of these roots from their tightly spiritual context and origin in a life of ascetic striving toward holiness has exposed the contents of Christian morality to multifaceted mutilations. From these, different and even incompatible interpretations of what it means to be rational have been derived.

Thus, while the moral opposition to genetic engineering appeals to a "sanctity" of life that combines a supposedly rational supposition of some "ultimate cause" of all existence with revealed accounts of divine creation, the acceptance of genetic engineering rests either on secularly rational doubts concerning the knowability of such ultimate causes, or on the (admittedly non-rational) revealed imperative to use God's creation within Divinely established constraints for beneficial purposes. Or human dignity (and thus the legal entitlement to human rights concerning protection and respect), insofar as it is derived from revelatory accounts of God's having created man in His image and likeness, while often thought to encompass all human life, is sometimes restricted only to those specimens who have a potential for ("still again", or "ever at all") realizing the goal set by that creation. While some rational accounts attribute such dignity to every instance of life that has some "interest" in itself and its wellbeing (thereby including higher vertebrates), other rational accounts restrict that dignity to morally responsible persons. Moreover individual autonomy, insofar as it is understood as a leading principle, is sometimes reasonably invoked to have freedom rights extend to the sale of one's organs and agreements to physician-assisted suicide or voluntary euthanasia, (all of which are generally opposed by Christians, though accepted by some secularized specimens of rationality who rest their case on post-modern pluralism), sometimes that autonomy is severely restricted by reference to a (Kantian-style, and therefore philosophically rational) "universal" obligation towards humanity as embodied in human persons, which is taken to impose a duty towards preserving one's life and bodily integrity.

Even among continental Europeans, there are noticeable differences. Perhaps the most illuminating example is presented by Germany, which (along with Poland and Belgium, but for significantly different reasons) refused to sign the pan-European *Convention for the Protection of Human Rights and Dignity of the Human Being with regard to the Application of Biology and Medicine* of Oviedo in 1997 (Council, 1997a). The German perception of adequate levels for ethical justifiability is more rigorous and demands noticeably greater restrictions on the freedom of medical research and economic gain as well as private self-determination than what its neighboring countries would endorse.

Thus the German law for the protection of the human embryo (*Gesetz zum Schutz von Embryonen, Dec. 13th, 1990)* forbids any interventions that seek to modify the human genome (*§5)*, whereas the *Convention* permits such interventions for preventive, diagnostic or therapeutic purposes, as long as the aim is not to introduce any modification in the genome of any descendants (*Art. 13*). That same German law limits the fertilization of human ova to the number of those actually to be transferred to the mother's womb (maximally 3, *§ 1, (1), 2.-5. and (2)*). It thus excludes the creation (and cryoconservation) of those very surplus embryos, the existence of which the *Convention* tacitly presupposes (in *Art.* 18, which permits their use in research under the rather unspecified condition of their "adequate" protection). The German law further excludes practices such as surrogate motherhood (*§ 1 (1) 1., 6., 7. and (2))* and the fabrication of embryos for the development of organs or tissue for siblings (*§ 2)*, which the *Convention* leaves unregulated. Thus also, German standards for the protection of non-competent subjects in therapeutic and non-therapeutic medical research *(BGB § 1904, in connection with § 1901)* were considered incompatible with – in the first case (*Art. 17.1*) – the *Convention*'s engaging a very vague understanding of what should count as acceptable probabilities for "potential" real and direct benefits, and – in the second case (*Art. 17.2*) – its permitting such research at all. Thus finally, German standards of privacy rights (*Bundesdatenschutzgesetz, Jan. 21st, 1977*) with regard to genetic information were considered incompatible with what the *Convention* left un-considered in its main articles and with the *Explanatory Report*'s allowing (in # *84*, # *85*) "health-related" data to be passed on to or to be required by employers or insurances (Council, 1997b).

To be sure and formally speaking, the *Convention*'s restriction of its decisions to the establishment of mere minimum standards, and its explicit toleration of nationally set higher protection (Article 27), should not have rendered it impossible for Germany to sign the *Convention*. The commitment to higher standards, after all, at least logically includes the endorsement of lower standards.

Germany's refusal becomes even more astounding, when the motive behind its restrictive policy is considered: Germans understand their moral obligations as a nation in the context of the atrocities committed during its 12 year period of National Socialism. Since German physicians under that regime committed crimes against non- consenting, non-informed research subjects in the name of (poor) medical research, so they argue, Germans today must be particularly on their guard against any reappearance of such injustice. Since national socialist German physicians practiced euthanasia with respect to the handicapped, Germans today must be particularly committed to safeguarding handicapped individuals' rights to life and bodily integrity. This is why even pre-natal diagnosis, as it usually results in the abortion of fetuses that are not up to the standards of normality, is highly disputed among the German public: National as well as regional associations of the handicapped have expressed their fear that, if a social consensus is created which renders the existence of handicapped humans an accident that ought to have been avoided, even currently existing handicapped individuals' right to continued existence (as well as societal support for their professional and social integration) will be threatened. Representatives of these associations have appealed to the Kantian foundation of the German constitution according to which (as this foundation is generally understood) already the very classifying of human beings according to their "person-" or "non-person-" status is immoral. This is also why the recent liberalization of both voluntary and involuntary euthanasia in the Netherlands and in Belgium is being intensely criticized in the German media. Since, moreover, National Socialism, on the basis of a racist ideology, had ventured into breeding experiments with "racially desirable" individuals (and had committed mass murder in order to exterminate racially – or behaviorally – "undesirable" portions of its own as well as other countries' populations), therefore Germans today feel called to be particularly critical against gene-technological endeavors at human enhancement. Finally, since Germany experienced a totalitarian system that disregarded privacy rights, such rights, especially with regard to sensitive genetic information, are taken very seriously.

It is this admitted particularity of German recent history, which lies at the root of Germans' bioethical tutiorism. At the same time however, they tend to consider that particularity not as their "privately" national affair. Had they done so, there would have been no reason not to sign a *Convention* that left other, not so historically compromised nations free to be more daring in their research and therapeutic projects, and to leave more space for individual autonomy in patients, parents, and physicians. The fact that Germans refused to sign indicates that they interpreted their admitted historical particularity as a historical challenge that rendered them merely more alert with regard to the demands of a morality which they consider universally valid and obligatory for all. Due to their particular historical experiences, so it must be concluded, Germans understand their calling as one of universal moral forerunner-hood in the cause of human dignity and human rights.

The fact, on the other hand, that most of Germany's European neighbors did sign the *Convention* indicates that they do not share Germany's perception of her superior moral authority. As a result, even within the comparatively homogenous European continent, most countries have ruled that the protection of non-competent research subjects should be weighed against these subjects' supposed interest in the advancement of research that will benefit those in the same age- and illness-categories, whereas Germany insists that such weighing is morally wrong. Most countries do not take fertilized human eggs to be bearers of human dignity, so that these eggs (or embryos) may under carefully specified conditions be instrumentalized in the interest of future or present bearers of human dignity, whereas Germany considers fertilized ova as future persons and thus as bearers of human dignity, and entitled to full legal protection. Moreover, some European countries take their legalizing voluntary as well as (under very carefully restricted conditions) non-voluntary euthanasia as an indication of respect for autonomy (in the first case) or for reconstructed autonomy and of humane mercy (in the second), whereas Germany takes human life to lie outside of humans' rightful self-determination. It considers humans as not being "owners" of their (or others') lives in a sense that would permit them to dispose of these lives. Such practices are thus in Germany classified as profoundly immoral

Kazumasa Hoshino's observation that any attempt to enforce a content rich understanding of human rights and medical ethics globally would amount to the proclaiming something particular as universal, can thus be rendered even more radical: any even merely imaginable attempt to enforce such an understanding even just within continental Europe would amount to the cultural imperialism Hoshino opposed.

IV. SOME CONCLUSIONS REGARDING BIOETHICS CULTURAL IMPERIALISM

In spite of all this, recent discussions concerning stem cell research have shown that there is hope. These discussions suggest that perhaps Germany could join Japan in refraining from, and at the same time objecting to, any attempt at global (or even regional) content-rich bioethics enforcement.

Even though the German law for the protection of the embryo declared that human life from the moment of fertilization is to be understood as an embryo (*§ 8)*, and even though the German *Bundesgerichtshof* has always considered human embryos as bearers of human dignity, and thus as entitled to unconditional protection of life and bodily integrity, nevertheless the German public no longer to any large extent supports that interpretation. Changes in the German abortion law *(StGB § 218 a)*, while retaining the illegality of abortion, have rendered it non-punishable under certain conditions: either some "ethical advising" must be documented to have taken place, or the attending physician must decide that the physical or psychological health of the pregnant woman is endangered by continued pregnancy or by the burden involved in the raising of – especially a handicapped – child. The result has been, among large parts of the population, a loss in moral sensitivity with regard to the right to life of unborn humans. The accepted practice of technology-assisted reproduction, even though severely limited, in some cases still involves the loss of embryos. Even in Germany, some human life is being created only to enable other specimens of human life to live, or some human life is being instrumentalized. The increasingly accepted practice of pre-implantation diagnosis and its implied selection of normal fertilized eggs at the expense of "unnormal ones" has introduced additional occasions for such instrumentalization.

As a result, it has proven to be quite difficult to create a public consensus against the instrumentalization of fertilized eggs for the production of stem cells. Research on these stem cells was advertised as promising great therapeutic benefits for present and future patients. Also, even much more developed forms of human life, and even in its native biological environment, had come to be quite routinely left to pregnant women's interpretation of whether they constitute a "burden … so serious and extraordinary that it exceeds the reasonable limits of sacrifice" (*StGB § 219)* and physicians' ranking of the embryo's right to life against threats to the mother's emotional wellbeing. Thus the German laws' fastidiousness with regard to protecting artificially fertilized ova has lost its intuitive compellingness even within Germany.

Moreover, public concern about the economic consequences of a restriction on research that would develop into a crucial resource for international competition (loss of chances for pharmaceutical development, loss of academic skill, loss of technological innovation) are placing a heavy burden on any attempt to uphold Germany's favored moral scrupulousness. In the end, a compromise was reached that permits research on human stem cells but restricts it to a limited number of cell lines that are already available in certain non-European countries. It is easy to foresee that a legal commitment to the unconditional protection of beginning human life cannot very well be upheld, if one legally permits profiting from violations of that commitment, provided these are perpetrated on human life that had been imported from abroad.

In other words, Germans are in the process of learning that even within Germany there are no longer universally acknowledged, content-rich moral principles that could justify enforcing of what some hold morally obligatory for all on those of a different moral creed. The late Spanish conquerors of South America could still make themselves believe that the native Indians, as their behavior did not fit into the Christian rational mold of decency and probity, should be colonized, in order to protect them from their native immorality (such as cannibalism, lack of pants for men and blouses for women, idolatry, sexual promiscuity, unwillingness to work for their colonizers, unwillingness to stay in stone buildings, and sodomy). Since they were excluded from the class of those rational beings who are entitled to respect, their not consenting to the violent methods employed for their acculturation could be considered morally insignificant. By contrast, present-day Germans, quite irrespective of their confessed faith in their collective and history-sanctified moral mission, must face not only their native, post-modernity induced moral pluralism. They also have to pay the price which an underdeveloped national pride imposes on the chances for persuasively inviting immigrants' voluntary acculturation. As a result, increasing numbers not only of such immigrant groups, but even of their own native progeny, can no longer be drafted into any ethic solidarity of guilt-shouldering, which might have motivated them to share the moral heritage of Germany's past.

Quite on the contrary: with at least some of these groups seeking not only their economic but also their respectively diverse cultural, religious, and moral futures, Germany will have to give more space for moral diversity and for the market, which, in engaging nothing but the respective participants' consent, represents the only truly universal, but thereby also contentless, (meta-)moral procedure.

As that process continues, Germans will have a chance of foregoing the arrogance of claimed moral superiority, and of extending tolerance towards moral difference – within their own polity as well as within Europe and the larger Western culture, way over to the Asian realm as well. Perhaps it will one day even join Japan, and her particularly forceful spokesman, Kazumasa Hoshino, in advocating that, among partners on a global scale, one has no moral choice but to modestly leave each country to its own moral resources.

International Studies in Philosophy and Medicine
Freigericht, Germany

REFERENCES

Council of Europe (1997a). *Convention for the Protection of Human Rights and Dignity of the Human Being with regard to the Application of Biology and Medicine: Convention on Human Rights and Biomedicine,* Oviedo, 4. IV. 1997.

Council of Europe (1997b). *Explanatory Report to the Convention for the Protection of Human Rights and Dignity of the Human Being with Regard to the Application of Biology and Medicine: Convention on Human Rights and Biomedicine.* Strasbourg: Directorate of Legal Affairs.

BGB (2002). *Bürgerliches Gesetzbuch.* Baden Baden: Nomos Verlag.

Strafgesetzbuch (2001). K Lackner and K. Kuehl (Eds.). München: Beck Verlag.

PART IV

GLOBAL BIOETHICS AND ITS CRITICS

LISA M. RASMUSSEN

MORAL DIVERSITY AND BIOETHICS CONSULTATION

I. INTRODUCTION

In the United States, bioethics consultation has become a necessary facet of health care. The reasons are multiple. First, and most practically speaking, the Joint Commission on the Accreditation of Healthcare Organizations mandates that accredited institutions have some provision for the discussion of ethical issues that arise in the hospital. However, as no exact requirements are given, this mandate may be satisfied in a number of ways, including 1) hiring an independent "bioethics consultant"; 2) establishing a bioethics committee comprised of various people (who do or do not work for the organization), or even 3) determining that a risk management department will discuss cases that arise.

Second, bioethics is a growth industry in the United States, as evidenced by the fact that the number of degree programs in bioethics is growing and that the press seeks out bioethicists for a sound bite whenever a new technology surfaces or a medical ethics issue becomes a hot topic.[1] What exactly fuels the popularity of the field is certainly an open question, but in part it may be due simply to a growing awareness of ethical issues raised in medicine, brought about by a number of historical events and trends.[2] It may also be due, as Engelhardt has pointed out, to a search for secular moral authority in a post-modern, post-traditional culture (Engelhardt, 1996; 2000). Whatever the reason, with increasing public awareness of the existence of bioethics and bioethicists, a corresponding increase in demand for their services in the hospital would not be unexpected. Many hospitals have responded by securing some form of bioethics consultation to serve patients, their families and hospital staff.

Third, and directly to the point of this *festschrift* for Kazumasa Hoshino, the international clientele of many hospitals has led to culture clashes over questions of medical treatment, which the bioethics consultant or committee regularly addresses. This has inspired the publication of many articles (Freedman, 1998; Tan Alora & Lumitao, 2001; Toombs, 2001) addressing the question of cultural values that clash

H.T. Engelhardt, Jr. and L.M. Rasmussen (eds.), Bioethics and Moral Content: National Traditions of Health Care Morality, 205–214.

with the established "common morality" espoused by many American or Western bioethics writers. Another question raised indirectly by the consideration of foreign cultures is whether bioethics consultation would look different in another country than in the United States. To that end, I take a hypothetical look below at bioethics consultation in Japan, after a brief discussion of the state of the field in the United States.

II. BIOETHICS CONSULTATION IN THE UNITED STATES

Despite the nearly three decades we have had to work on the question of just what bioethics is, there is no clear agreement on the subject, especially when it comes to the question of bioethics consultations. As I will argue in this section, there is no consensus in the field regarding either the goals or the success standards of bioethics consultation. Moreover, the many goals that have been advocated are mutually incompatible and offer very different conceptions of the bioethics consultant's job.

A. Division in the field

Currently there are many competing models for bioethics consultation, which do not agree on the appropriate goals of the activity (cf. Ackerman, 1987; 1989; Fletcher, 1989; Freedman, 1994; 1998; Moreno, 1991). Additionally, the recent statement on the field (*Core Competencies for Health Care Ethics Consultation*) by the Task Force of the Society for Health and Human Values (which was subsequently included in the new American Society of Bioethics and Humanities) suffers from underdevelopment and a lack of clarity. Unsurprisingly, then, there seems to be little agreement on how one ought to behave in order to be a successful bioethics consultant.

Consider the contrast between the models proposed by Terrence Ackerman and Benjamin Freedman. Ackerman argues that bioethics consultants ought not to function as upholders of the right, but rather, as consultants who come when a doctor calls them. Their purpose, he argues, is to facilitate in such a situation, and help the physician to answer whatever questions arise.[3] Freedman, on the other hand, and diametrically opposed to Ackerman, argues that bioethicists *should* function as upholders of the right. He sees bioethics consultation as a "forum for expressing moral commitments, as other professions may provide a forum for expressing intellectual, aesthetic, utilitarian, or other commitments" (1994, p. 123). Moreover, for him it is a calling:

> ... I suspect my own experience is usual: choosing bioethics at a time of rising social demands that the academy be socially and politically relevant, under the spur of a need to fulfill personal moral commitments and needs without abandoning academic interests and predilections (1994, p. 123).

Though not all bioethicists disagree quite as directly as do these two over the role of the bioethics consultant, there is nevertheless deep disagreement between the various models proposed.

The *Core Competencies* document does not help to clarify matters. While the Task Force has begun to sketch out the favored model for bioethics consultation (something they call "ethics facilitation"), this model is far from able to ground a profession either philosophically or practically. The problem is not just that their terminology is ambiguous and their examples vague. The deeper problem is that once these terms are analyzed in depth, it becomes clear that they can cut in several directions, with very different implications for bioethics consultation.

For example, one of the goals cited for the bioethics consultant is the identification of a range of "morally acceptable options within the context" (*Core Competencies*, p. 6). However, attempts to shed light on what counts as "morally acceptable" are weak. As part of defining "moral acceptability", the Task Force emphasizes both "an inclusive consensus-building process" and respect for patients' rights to act according to their values, in the context of "societal values, law, and institutional policy, often as discussed in the bioethics literature", which "have implications for a morally acceptable consensus" (p. 7). What might be done when the "inclusive consensus-building process" fails, and the ways in which it is appropriate to arrive at consensus, are only briefly discussed. For example, in a section entitled, "What if consensus among the involved parties cannot be reached?", the Task Force notes that often the best answer is to determine who should be allowed to make the decision, and concludes that "[s]ocietal values often indicate who should be allowed to make the decision in the absence of consensus" (p. 8). The matter of "societal values" is problematic; it is not clear that there is anything to which the term refers. "Society" might agree that it is good to avoid doing bad things, and that it is good to be a good person, but everything depends on one's definition of "bad things" or "good person". In the end, the Task Force has left a great deal unsaid by referring simply to "societal values". As a result, "moral acceptability" – and the side-constraints on action that it might dictate – is crucially underdetermined.

B. The Roles of the Bioethics Consultant

In a larger project, I have identified at least a dozen different roles that a bioethics consultant might play, including detective, priest or spiritual advisor, moral policeman, facilitator, educator, mediator, patient advocate, risk manager, etc. (Rasmussen, in preparation). Without such careful identification of intertwining roles, any consideration of the appropriate goals of the bioethics consultant will be incomplete; as we have seen from the examples above, brief treatments miss important distinctions. I will not here examine all of the abovementioned roles, but I will consider three in order to show that the way in which we understand the role of the bioethics consultant has important implications for the practice guidelines that might result. In addition, this prepares the ground for a consideration of how bioethics consultation might appropriately differ in, for example, Japan.

Often the bioethics consultant functions as a risk manager. This role is never, to my knowledge, made explicit. However, data in the last 10 years or so have suggested that patients and their families who feel that they had good communication with their caregivers were less likely to sue (Shaprior, Simpson, Lawrence, Talsky, Sobocinski & Schiedermayer, 1989; Valente, Antlitz, Boyd et al., 1988; Buller & Buller, 1987). As a bioethics consultation provides even more communication time, it is certainly reasonable to speculate that it would help to decrease the likelihood of suit. It is not unreasonable of institutions to include bioethics consultants in the clinical encounter as a way of mitigating their risk. However, at the same time it is unclear, first, whether bioethics consultants *ought* to function as risk managers, and second, if such a role is permissible, whether there are any side-constraints.

By itself, playing this role need not be morally problematic for a bioethics consultant. However, if a bioethics consultant felt herself to be hired in large part for litigation mitigation, she might decide that this was an inappropriate use of her skills and intentions. More importantly, the performance of this role might (either directly or indirectly) be in tension with the performance of one of the other roles she might play. For example, if a bioethics consultant were also to play the role of patient advocate, there would certainly be times at which risk management and advocacy clashed: the point of the first role is to protect the institution, and the point of the second is to protect the patient. Determining which takes priority and why is crucial to defining any coherent practice of bioethics consultation. The justification given for the inclusion of risk management in the bioethics consultant's job will also help to determine the side-constraints, if any, on the practice.

Consider again the role of patient advocate. Is this a role or the primary role that a bioethics consultant ought to play? The history of bioethics in the United States certainly includes movements designed to protect patients from zealous researchers or paternalistic physicians, so this role has the right pedigree. However, in some quarters the sentiment has changed; Ackerman, for example, regards the bioethics consultant as an advisor to physicians, not patients. The physician is the one who ought to call the consultation, and is the one who determines whether it is successful. Provisions for patient advocacy are not made in Ackerman's model.

If we accept this role for the consultant, however, what is the goal or standard for successful performance? As in the legal system, ought the consultant to fight for her patient's needs and rights loyally and exclusively? Or does patient advocacy rather imply that the consultant is there to ensure that the patient has a chance to voice his preferences and have them taken seriously? Again, the justification offered for this role will help to answer these questions, the question of what to do when roles conflict, and the side-constraints on the performance of a role.

Finally, consider the role of mediator. Mediators can function both as intermediaries between opposing parties and as independent parties whose job it is to obtain a settlement. A bioethicist as mediator can perform many tasks: she can simply ask the right questions and let the parties voice their opinions; suggest solutions to the problem; use persuasion to effect agreement; or even unilaterally determine which party's wishes will be followed. Which is the appropriate manner in which the bioethics consultant ought to perform her role?

Again, the justification offered for the role in the first place will help to answer these questions. If the reason bioethics consultants are to act as mediators is because all parties to a disagreement deserve to be heard, her task will be simply to ensure that they are in fact heard. If upon an airing of everyone's views no one changes his mind, there is nothing more for the bioethics consultant to do on this conception of the role. On the other hand, if the justification for the role of mediator is that the consultant is a moral expert, then perhaps it will be within the scope of the consultant's job either to express her expert opinion or even to ensure that it is followed, depending on the authority granted to her expertise.

Defining the job of bioethics consultation is very complicated. Because there is little to no discussion of the justification for the job as a whole or the roles involved in the performance of that job, the models proposed are too vague to ground the practice in any deep sense. Until we know what the underlying justifications for our roles are (which help to define the goals of the practice), bioethics consultation will be, to a certain extent, a blind groping for purpose.

III. MORAL DIVERSITY IN BIOETHICS CONSULTATION: A HYPOTHETICAL EXAMPLE

If I began a private bioethics consultation firm, would I be able to practice in Japan in the same fashion as I would in the United States? That is, would my roles be different there than they are here? There are reasons to think that the answer is yes.

Take, for example, the role of patient advocate. In American bioethics, this is a role with historical precedent. After all, among the roots of bioethics in the US are research scandals involving abuse of patients, as well as the influence of the civil rights movement, which together with the cultural climate of the 1960s led many to question traditionally accepted authorities. For this and other reasons, the attempt to speak on behalf of the patient, or to ensure that the patient herself has a voice, is a task bioethics consultants regularly perform.

This is not likely to be a common task in Japan. First, as Hoshino points out, Japanese may not accept, or may not accept in the same way, that autonomy is a critical value in bioethics: "Most Japanese patients tend to think they are asking a favor of the physician to take care of their medical problems. They, thus, try to be as good and obedient a patient as possible. Generally, patients in Japan do not care much about their civil rights" (Hoshino, 1997b, p.14). The idea of inviting a stranger (the bioethics consultant) into the clinical encounter in order to defend a patient's rights simply does not coincide with such views.[4] Additionally, the concept of *wa* ("conciliation, concord, unity, harmony, submission, and reconciliation" (Hoshino, 1997b, p. 19)) is very important in Japanese culture. Often advocacy can become confrontation, a value opposed to that of *wa*. Again, the dominant cultural values in Japan suggest that advocacy would be unwelcome, rude, and even simply wrong.

Second, again as Hoshino points out, "[t]here is a famous Japanese proverb, 'manaita no ue no koi,' which means that the patients are resigned to their fate" (Hoshino, 1997b, p. 15). In other words, not only is the exercise of individual autonomy not necessarily important, but additionally the pursuit of health simply does not have the same priority in Japan as it does in the United States. One might accuse the Japanese of "false consciousness" or enslavement to old-fashioned traditions in their declining vigorously to pursue health, but this accusation would simply beg the question of values. This resignation to fate can hold a very important place in the moral life of many people, not just Japanese. For example, as Engelhardt has pointed out (2000), preparing for and engaging in a "good death" can be one of the most important tasks a Christian faces. One may be resigned to one's fate in an autonomous, morally defensible manner. If these are the values held by a particular patient, advocacy will be unnecessary, or at least take on a quite different form.[5]

It is also not clear whether mediation would ever be a task for bioethics consultants in Japan, as it is in the United States. Given the fact that, according to Hoshino, "[t]here is, in fact, no concept in the mind of the Japanese that one of the family members has such individual rights [i.e., to autonomy, self-determination and privacy] independent of the family" (1997b, p. 17), it is less likely that dissension between patient and family would be explicitly acknowledged. Moreover, since in many cases the very expression of familial love is protecting the patient from harmful information, there would be less opportunity for it to arise at all. This is not simply tradition, though it is that as well. It is also not simply family love, though it certainly is that. The idea of families making decisions together is grounded in practical considerations that patients in the United States would do well to consider. As Hoshino points out,

> When one member of the family becomes sick, it is the responsibility of the entire family to look after him. ... The family knows that the care of the sick member is a family matter. In these circumstances, it seems rather natural for the family first to decide on the medical procedures and to care for him .... On such occasions, the patients typically leave the final decision to the family so that the family may take into

> consideration not only realistic medical factors but also the family's own convenience (1997b, p. 16).

Since the family pays the cost of a patient's decision by sacrificing and working hard to take care of him, it makes sense from more than a Confucian or traditional Japanese perspective that the family ought to be able to make decisions regarding his care. Again, given this cultural background, a bioethics consultant might rarely play the role of mediator, in contrast to what she might do in America.

IV. CONCLUSION

Certainly, I do not mean to suggest that there are no values Japanese and Americans share in considering their health care choices. Nor do I mean to suggest that a bioethics consultant can practice only one role; each consultation might involve the performance of a half-dozen or more of these roles. I have argued only two points: First, in order to understand the function of a bioethics consultant, one must assess all of the roles that he can perform in order to understand what the goal of the outcome is, which roles take priority when performed in combination, and the side-constraints on action. Second, it might very well be the case that a bioethics consultant practicing in the United States performs radically different functions than she would in Japan, based on the moral and cultural milieu. If this is the case, the training and accreditation requirements for bioethics consultants in different countries might vary widely.

Rice University
Houston, Texas, U.S.A.

NOTES

[1] See also the web site <www.bioethics.net>, whose byline for a time read "Where the world goes for bioethics". Among the features on this site, in an easy-to-read format, one finds "Bioethics on NBC's ER", in which ethical issues raised by a popular television show set in an emergency room are analyzed.

[2] Various authors give divergent accounts of the history of bioethics (cf. Jonsen, 1998; Stevens, 2000 and Rothman, 1992), but each cites several historical events or trends as giving

rise to the bioethics we experience in the United States today, including the Nuremberg Trials, various research scandals, the Karen Ann Quinlan case, and the civil rights movement.

3 There is much to say about both Ackerman's and Freedman's theories, and I say it in a larger project (Rasmussen, in preparation). Of relevance here is the fact that stipulating "facilitation" as the bioethics consultant's goal says next to nothing. Since "facilitating" simply means "making things easier", a very wide variety of activities (some of which we would certainly want to prohibit) fall under this rubric. For example, coercion of the patient or his family by the bioethicist might make it much easier to make treatment decisions, but if there is any consensus about the point of bioethics consultation, it certainly includes the determination that coercion is wrong.

4 Related to this is a perhaps more aesthetic point. Hoshino gives the example of ordering food in a restaurant. In the United States (in many cases), the guest chooses everything that he wishes to eat; in Japanese restaurants the side dishes, sauces, etc. are chosen by the chef "in order to avoid interfering with the cozy atmosphere at the dinner table" (Hoshino, 1997b, p. 15). In a similar fashion, a Japanese patient might wish to have his medical decisions made by a good and virtuous doctor in collaboration with his family. Usually a scene around someone's death bed is not "cozy", to be sure, but there is a similar sense of intimacy and privacy that would be broken by a great deal of intervention, especially by strangers.

5 Of course it is possible that there are many Japanese patients who only behave complacently because they feel pressure to do so, when what they really want is to be able to demand (or at least request) particular treatments. In this case, advocacy would be important to protect the interests of these patients and to ensure that they are heard. However, my main point is to suggest that in a given context, where there are definite cultural tendencies, the role of the bioethics consultant might take on a very different form.

REFERENCES

Ackerman, T. (1987). 'The role of an ethicist in health care.' In: Garmy R. Anderson and Valerie A. Glesnes-Anderson (Eds.), *Health Care Ethics: A Guide for Decision Makers* (pp. 308-320). Rockville, MD: Aspen Publications.

Ackerman, T. (1989). 'Moral Problems, moral inquiry, and consultation in clinical ethics.' In: B. Hoffmaster, B. Freedman, & G. Fraser (Eds.), *Clinical Ethics: Theory and Practice* (pp. 141-160). Clifton, NJ: Humana Press.

Buller, M.K & Buller, D.B. (1987). 'Physicians' communication style and patient satisfaction.' *Journal of Health and Social Behavior*, 28, 375-388.

Fletcher, J.C. (1989). 'Standards for evaluation of ethics consultation.' In: J.C. Fletcher, N. Quist and A. R. Jonsen (Eds.), *Ethics Consultation in Health Care* (pp. 173-184). Ann Arbor: Health Administration Press.

Freedman, B. (1994). 'From avocation to vocation: Working conditions for clinical health care ethics consultants.' In: F. Baylis (Ed.), *The Health Care Ethics Consultant* (pp. 109-132). Totowa, NJ: Humana Press.

Freedman, B. (1998). 'Offering truth.' *Archives of Internal Medicine*, 153, 572-576.

Hoshino, K. (Ed.) (1997a). *Japanese and Western Bioethics: Studies in Moral Diversity*. Dordrecht: Kluwer Academic Publishers.

Hoshino, K. (1997b). 'Bioethics in the light of Japanese sentiments.' In: K. Hoshino (Ed.), *Japanese and Western Bioethics: Studies in Moral Diversity* (pp. 13-23). Dordrecht: Kluwer Academic Publishers.
LaPuma, J. and Scheidermayer , D. (1991). 'Ethics consultation: Skills, roles and training.' *Annals of Internal Medicine* 114, 155-160.
La Puma, J. and Scheidermayer, D. (1994). *Ethics Consultation: A Practical Guide*. Boston: Jones and Bartlett Publishers.
Moreno, J. (1991). 'Ethics consultation as moral engagement.' *Bioethics* 5, 43-56.
Rasmussen, L. (in preparation). *A Critical Assessment of the Practice of Bioethics Consultation.*
Shapiro, R. S., Simpson, D.E., Lawrence, S.L., Talsky, A.M., Sobocinski, K.A., & Schiedermayer, D.L. (1989). 'A survey of sued and nonsued physicians and suing patients.' *Archives of Internal Medicine*, 149, 2190-2196.
Tan Alora, A. and Lumitao, J. (Eds.). (2001). *Beyond a Western Bioethics: Voices from the Developing World.* Washington, DC: Georgetown University Press.
Toombs, K. (Ed.) (2001). *Handbook of Phenomenology and Medicine*. Dordrecht: Kluwer Academic Publishers.
Valente, C.M., Antlitz, A.M., Boyd, M.D. et al. (1988). 'The importance of physician-patient communication in reducing medical liability.' *Maryland Medical Journal*, 37, 75-78.

DAVID C. THOMASMA†

THE CHALLENGE OF DOING INTERNATIONAL BIOETHICS

"In my book, if you're going to touch someone, you must only do it with intent to heal."

– Tim Cardigan, S.J. (Nalty, 1994, p. 49).

"Men are free when they belong to a living, organic, believing community, active in fulfilling some unfulfilled, perhaps unrealized purpose."

– D. H. Lawrence (Rorty, 1995, p. 86).

"Mankind was my business. The common welfare was my business; charity, mercy, forbearance, and benevolence were all my business. The dealings of my trade were but a drop of water in the comprehensive ocean of my business."

– Marley's Ghost to Scrooge (Irving, 1990, p. 238).

In both national and international bioethics there is a distortion of the nature and scope of our bioethics conversation. This distortion impedes the fruitfulness of initial discussions and efforts to build international bioethics consensus. As I will argue, the distortion lies in the assumption about the nature of human persons that affects so much of our thinking. In this essay in honor of Dr. Hoshino, I want to explore the impediments to and make some recommendations for international moral discourse. This will be done first by examining American bioethics discourse, then international critiques of our discourse, some characteristics of Japanese culture that can assist the international bioethics discussion, and finally, some recommendations.

H.T. Engelhardt, Jr. and L.M. Rasmussen (eds.), Bioethics and Moral Content: National Traditions of Health Care Morality, 215–234.

I. AMERICAN MORAL DISCOURSE

In general, American medicine suffers from an abundance of means and a poverty of ends. We have many interventions and technologies, but little or no unanimity about how and when to employ them. Characteristically, because of this lack of unanimity, Americans accompany their dialogue with firmness without conviction, and take a strong stand without sufficient moral analysis of that stand, or even of the other competing ones. Despite America's fabled "melting pot" ideology, there is very little multicultural analysis, at least in our philosophy, although this is now becoming rectified (Parens, 1995; Veatch, 1989).

Further, many ethical issues are debated on psychological and even emotional grounds. If the discussion becomes "too abstract," then it is "trumped" by someone who can tell a personal story. Indeed, our media reflect this trend. There must be an angle, or some outrageousness that grabs the reader or viewer. To be in the middle on an issue is not newsworthy, so more attention is paid to polarized views, the extremists on either side. Ironically, this has the effect of enhancing the judgment that our culture is too pluralistic to reach moral consensus, even though we pay little attention to multicultural analysis itself.

Some television programs in the United States entertain by simply bringing two or more people together who have been hurt by one another (but who suffer genuine moral quandaries, e.g., betrayal), and letting them argue and emote publicly. If things get too calm, then the "moderator" (a strange word for this role) provokes further disagreement. The audience, like the Romans at the Coliseum games of old, hoot and holler and egg the participants on. In one case, a moderator and talk-show host twice suffered a broken nose from this kind of provocation (Anonymous, 1995, p. 2).

I suggest that these "media events" are all too often a metaphor for the larger cultural and international dialogue. Witness the enormous demonstrations of world-wide solidarity provided by the United Nations on important moral topics like human rights, reproductive rights, human development (in Denmark), and most recently women's rights (in China). Unfortunately most of the news we receive is dominated by those who disagree rather than those who agree. For example, at a human development meeting in Denmark, the media focused on how charming Fidel Castro was to everyone; panoramic pictures of heads of state were also provided, all of them enjoying their time together, it appeared. I would not want to gainsay the benefits of putting the world's leaders together in a neutral environment, of course. But the point remains. Serious thinking is often replaced by what we call "sound bites," or "photo opportunities," in effect pictures and sounds masquerading as the harder work of ethics, politics, and being about the business, as Marley's ghost says, of "the common welfare".

The reason for this distortion in ethical conversation is not hard to find. There is precious little agreement on the fundamentals. So instead, the debate shifts to the means rather than the ends, the points and counterpoints of the debate leading to intractable and often unresolvable disputes (MacIntyre, 1984). Yet our contemporary moral disputes cover incredibly important human and social values, about abortion, euthanasia, reproductive rights, the moral status of embryos, and so on. People get caught up in what John Paris and Richard McCormick call the "casuistry of means"(Paris and McCormick, 1987). Some examples:

A pair of conjoined twins were born at Loyola University Chicago where I teach, and the debate about separating them took hold throughout the United States for over a year. The debate focused on whether it is moral to take one twin's life to save the other's, even when "saving" meant that the surviving twin would lie in an iron lung for almost a year and then die of respiratory failure, as one could predict from the early days of their care (Thomasma and Marshall, 1995, pp. 80-84). This case revealed a lack of vision about the goal of health care and its role in society, especially at the cutting edge of new technological interventions and surgeries. What was the goal of care for Amy and Angela Lakeberg?

A second instance of this means/ends gremlin arose when a Catholic priest in Alabama placed an advertisement in a newspaper advocating killing an abortionist on the grounds that taking one "guilty" life would save many other "innocent" lives. His bishop, thankfully, ordered him to withdraw the ad because moral teaching has never permitted using immoral means to accomplish moral ends.

Yet another example of the means/ends gremlin: a woman on a television talk-show offered to get pregnant and then abort her fetus at the end of the second trimester so that its brain tissue could be used to help her father who had Parkinson's disease (actually one needs about 6 or more fetuses for such a procedure). The father, also on the program, shook violently. (One might have hoped his shaking was due more to the outrageousness of his daughter's suggestion than to tremors from his disease.)

There are many other causes of the *moral collapse of our culture*, of course. Americans are particularly fond of, and famous for, practical, pragmatic, procedural resolutions to ethical dilemmas. Yet these, too, often fail, because they do not properly respect the fact that human beings are related to one another in very complex ways.

Particularly fine compromises, for example, the requirement that institutions ask persons about advance directives, partially fail because the average person does not understand the meaning of the terms themselves, and the institutions are reluctant to "push" the person, soon to be a patient, to develop them because it will appear that they expect that person to succumb to horrible circumstances while under their care.

In other words, even when clear moral and legal rights are established, the community (in this case, care givers in a hospital or other health care setting) is actively counseled *against* helping individuals accomplish these important rights and responsibilities because it may *appear* that there is a conflict of interest between the care they offer and a patient's decision, with their help, to limit that care. This strikes me as absurd enough to warrant further examination.

II. INTERNATIONAL MORAL DISCOURSE

International discussion of the first case would reveal a host of other problems that Americans ought to address. Most often, colleagues from other countries find families pushing the limits of medicine quite appalling. Because they do not emphasize autonomy to the extent Americans do, the case would exemplify the way persons "hold the doctors hostage" But there are deeper issues. In South America, for example, a critic might point to the need to eliminate infections in the young population as an overriding moral concern, such that the expenditures in the Lakeberg case would be truly unfathomable. European commentators would stress the importance of following rational standards of care in a National Health Plan that would not permit such an intervention. And among other points, a Japanese ethicist might stress the importance of stoic and dignified acceptance of one's lot, that there are limits, not just to medical care, but to the nature of intervention itself. This is particularly true of malformed infants, since Japanese culture supports the treatment of disabilities less than other cultures. It would make no cultural sense to "rescue" a child to this extent, given the real attendant problems of developmental and physical disabilities as the best-case scenario.

About proposals like gunning down abortionists and gestating fetuses for transplant purposes, other countries have their extremists, too. No culture is exempt from such thinking. But peaceable discussion, as Engelhardt calls for (1986; 1996), among colleagues from other cultures, reveals just how skewed the above-instanced thinking really is.

Sometimes our disputes assist in our natural human propensity to lose sight of the important, larger questions, in favor of more "manageable," concrete and pragmatic projects or conduct. Small wonder, then, that as the *means/ends gremlin* is transported worldwide in bioethics, a similar danger is posed to international bioethics. Let us briefly examine some of the challenges by considering a different culture, that of Japan.

III. JAPANESE CULTURAL PRINCIPLES

It isn't easy to characterize an entire people. Regularly, ethnographers warn us of the dangers of characterizing an ethnic group as a "community," as in "African-American community," or "Asian-American community." These supposed communities are, in reality, conglomerates in the scientist's or the observer's mind, and do not exist in reality.

Yet some truths about an entire people emerge with quiet regularity in response to crises in their history. Traditionally, the Japanese have taken pride in their sense of order and civility. This sense of order was borne out when Kobe suffered a devastating earthquake on January 17, 1995, when hundreds of thousands of people were displaced, and thousands were injured and died. In the midst of the terror and the aftershocks, the people coped with the disaster with quiet pride. Even though most stores were destroyed or closed, when one grocery store opened, people stood in line patiently waiting for some milk or bottled water. There was no grousing, no price-gouging, no rioting, no looting.

The primacy of community and tradition was made salient by the offense they suffered as a result of government tardiness responding to the crisis, but also in other remarkable ways. A man who worked for the American Consul General in Osaka, a neighboring city, remarked that his newspaper was delivered the next morning at 7:15 AM, exactly on time as usual (Komarow, 1995, 3A).

The solidarity of the family is a central feature of Japanese, as well as other cultures. Rather than individual autonomy, these cultures stress solidarity with one another. This is a major bioethical decision-pathway that is virtually unexplored in American-influenced bioethics, except perhaps as a "problem" within the larger analysis of a case. Family decision-making should itself be at least as primary a principle as autonomy, since each of us is shaped by the values conveyed in a family (or replacement family) unit.

In Japan, such devotion to family values was shown by Kenzaburo Oe, the winner of the Nobel Prize for literature, who announced at the ceremony where he received the Nobel Prize in Stockholm that he would stop writing fiction. He had resolved, he said, some thirty-one years ago to speak for his severely brain-damaged son, and his son now had found his own voice through music. Oe's son has two compact discs devoted to his classical compositions. All of his writing is based, Oe said, "on our life together, the communion with my son" (Remnick, 1995, p. 38).

Within this broad characterization there are many variations. And once again it should be noted that all cultures are too complex to single out a primary feature that governs all interactions within a given culture. Of course this is not accurate. Oe himself says that the West knows only a mask, created by the Japanese themselves for the West to admire, "masks of Japanese modesty or technological strength" (Remnick, 1995, p. 43). He wants to enter the arena of public debate in Japan because he sees that arena, now Westernized, as "a happy wasteland, self-satisfied, money-crazed, unreflective." It is a culture preoccupied with the images and contentments of a post-adolescent subculture (Remnick, 1995).

Kai Hoshino characterizes Japanese culture with respect to autonomy in this way:

> Japanese social systems are based on familiarity, collectivism, and totalitarianism, depending on the size of the group, and a unified opinion is always the goal in each group. People are discouraged from making autonomous decisions, or speaking out with their personal opinions even when they do not agree. Group members are expected to follow the group consensus, and individualistic attitudes based on autonomy and self-determination are basically incompatible with that aim.
>
> Group consensus is more likely to be determined by the dominant opinion expressed by the group leader, rather than determined by

democratic means ... Japanese society is still basically feudalistic (Hoshino, 1995, p. 72).

Hoshino notes the contrast between American and Japanese societies by these sayings: In America one says that "the squeaky wheel gets the oil." In Japan, with its focus on group consensus and obedience to leaders, the saying is "the nail that sticks out gets pounded down" (Hoshino, 1995).

IV. THE CLASH OF CULTURES

When C.P. Snow wrote about the clash of two cultures, he underlined the problems that existed between science and the liberal arts, between a scientifically-based culture and a humanistic culture. Surely this has been one of the most difficult problems the West has faced in the past century. Consider, for example, the criticism of medical education, that students are taught early on that primarily their focus should be the scientific understanding of cellular and microbiological processes, only secondarily, organ systems, and thirdly, down the line, the persons who are patients (Vernacchio, 1995). This has been called "scientific materialism." The principal feature of such a materialism is the conviction that problems can be understood, can be solved, by breaking them down into their component parts, and then by putting the elements together again. The lack of an underlying, cohesive structure in this model requires that the scientific investigator him- or herself put the puzzle back together, not the person or family from whom the puzzle was derived.

Further, in the international arena, there is a clash between Western and Asian value systems that shows up continually when the cultures meet. As Oe observed, to Asians, Western culture can look like a post-adolescent uninvolvement with the common good. Although he was too kind to say it, this picture of Western, and especially American culture, emerges from our focus on autonomy and individual rights.

The West, and especially the U.S., emphasizes individual freedom and human rights, while Asians traditionally honor social order, family, and the community itself. In America the Western liberal tradition in politics was wedded to the frontier. Although the importance of the frontier in American thought recently has been disputed, there is no question that "the frontier spirit" has significantly modified Western emphases on freedom (Axelrod and Phillips, 1992). It has done so by focusing on the individual, isolated but proud, who alone faced the terror of the vastness of nature and the attacks of indigent native Americans on his or her encroachments.

The frontier was such a powerful force on the consciousness of Americans, that on July 12, 1893, at the Art Institute of Chicago as part of the Columbian Exposition taking place in the city, Professor Frederick Jackson Turner announced that the frontier was "closed," and discussed the ramifications of this closure on the American spirit. His argument was that the "restless energy" and rugged individualism of Americans would seek an outlet elsewhere, in new challenges. This perception was later picked up by Woodrow Wilson, then President of Princeton University, who later incorporated it into world political action (Axelrod and Philips, 1992).

One can see the assumptions about autonomy percolating in international relations in recent years. President Clinton underscored the right to autonomy in a trip to Indonesia in 1994, following up on the UN Conference on Human Rights in Vienna the year before. The objection that workers there did not crave human rights and liberty as much as other people struck him, and most Westerners, as absurd. Yet Asian leaders like to argue that socioeconomic rights and community rights are just as important as political and civil rights. Lee Kuan Yew, a Singapore advocate of "order first, democracy second," attributed Singapore's economic success to: "cultural backdrop, the belief in thrift, hard work, filial piety and loyalty in the extended family ..." (Editorial, 1994).

This description of values, however, might readily apply to the American Midwest or to any more rural civilization. Indeed, the ultimate clash of cultures seems not to lie between Western and Eastern or any other geographic delineation, but between more industrial and more rural civilizations. As the family unit is sacrificed for economic opportunity, and persons are forced together in the workplace in new ways, their interests change. The common denominator of persons with many backgrounds and many different family and cultural traditions is their autonomy.

That is why autonomy is seen as "post-adolescent" self-engagement by a community-based culture. It is a nemesis from that point of view. But from the point of view of human rights and social development it is essential. In fact, a key feature of Western civilization, in its art and music, is the restless energy of development and growth, a kind of "urgency for progress" (Griffiths, 1995, pp. 101-102).

Let me return to bioethics with this account in hand.

V. THE ROLE OF AUTONOMY

Many American bioethicists have become comfortable with both principlism and the primacy of the principle of autonomy. This is perhaps a natural result of success, but it does produce smug assumptions. Principlism is an analysis of ethical dilemmas in terms of at least four (sometimes competing) ethical principles: autonomy, benefice, non-maleficence, and justice. Resolution of cases and problems can be brought forth through a sophisticated "balancing" of those principles, "weighting" them differently in each case according to their relative merits (Graber and Thomasma, 1989). The earliest advocates of this view of bioethics were Tom Beauchamp and James Childress (Beauchamp and Childress, 1994).

The primacy of autonomy within that balancing procedure came more and more to be viewed as a condition of the possibility of ethics itself, a position argued and formulated by H. Tristram Engelhardt, Jr. in *The Foundations of Bioethics* (Engelhardt, 1996). Engelhardt in that work viewed autonomy as a "side constraint," a kind of condition for the possibility of ethics in a pluralistic society, since the starting point of all "peaceable discussion" in such a pluralistic environment is that nothing can be assumed to be agreed upon *a priori.* Thus, the only *a priori* must be respect for the individual's own self-determination as he or she comes to the table for the discussion and resolution of an issue (Engelhardt, 1991; 1996). No one position could predominate over another without consensus among the equal partners in the dialogue.

Gradually, the goals of the healing process in medicine (about which we cannot agree) are replaced by the importance of the means (about which we can agree), the respect shown the person. The worst-case scenario of capitulation to autonomy occurs when bioethicists promote the "ethics of caring" without spelling out how to care or what to care about. As Erich Loewy argues in a *reductio ad absurdum*, even the Nazis "cared" about what they were doing (Loewy, 1995). The lack of consensus about goals casts a wide net over all assumptions (even those that Pellegrino and I, in our books on philosophy of medicine, have argued are *a priori* assumptions for the accomplishment of the healing goals of medicine, such as equality of treatment; consistency irrespective of race, religion, or social class; respect for persons; and beneficence, acting in the best interests of the patient) (Pellegrino and Thomasma, 1981; 1988; 1993). The "consensus" that has long been assumed in health care turns out to be a chimera. The assumption requires argumentation and support instead.

Clinicians and other bioethicists have been consistently critical of both principlism and the primacy of autonomy, claiming that principlism does not respect the particularities and emotional, personal, professional, and cultural content of ethical cases and dilemmas, and that the primacy of autonomy is foreign to the primary principle of beneficence in medicine ('Beyond Autonomy,' 1995). That criticism has led to widespread dissatisfaction with autonomy-based ethics, and to a growing discussion of alternative bioethical theories, such as virtue ethics, narrative ethics, situation ethics, feminist ethics, caring ethics, and the like. It is hard to predict where this discussion will go. Most certainly it will lead to a refinement of principlism that will continue to help it develop in the 21st Century.

Add to this discussion the vigorous questioning of the American cultural content mixed with both principlism and the primacy of autonomy, and a more international and culturally-sensitive bioethics should emerge for truly cooperative work on important bioethical and ethical concerns throughout the world.

VI. RIGHTS AND AUTONOMY

While particularities of culture will continue to be stressed, one cannot help but perceive that international bioethics will depend upon at least two major actions. First, a respect for persons as enculturated with their own value systems; and, second, a baseline arrived at through international dialogue about fundamental human rights in health care, much as the UN Charter does for broader human rights issues.

The greatest challenge will be to search for a rights-based bioethics that could be accepted in all cultures, even those like traditional Asian cultures that stress community over individualism. Other bioethics theories are equally to be welcomed, yet for appeal to objective standards in disputes, it seems that a rights-based bioethics would be required.

Nonetheless, preoccupation with autonomy and self-determination in Western bioethics, especially among U.S. bioethicists, is indicative of the extent to which cultural values influence our orientation to biomedical morality. Our beliefs about personhood and autonomy inform every aspect of our medical transactions, including notions about informed consent and confidentiality in the patient-physician relationship.

In the United States and other Western nations, the individual is identified as the locus of decisional capacity for informed consent. Yet this concept is virtually meaningless in societies that stress the overriding importance of an individual's relationship to family and community. In these contexts, decisional capacity is socially, not individually expressed. As Hoshino notes in his discussion of bioethics in Japan, although the traditional relationship-centered ethics of the physician's virtuous duty to patients was altered by events after World War II, "the traditional ethics, though altered, still lingers ... Despite the general post-War trends, therefore, the Japanese social ethos still permits medical paternalism to go largely unquestioned" (Hoshino, 1992, p. 380). There has been some progress in the Japanese courts, mandating that explanations to patients be a duty for doctors, but progress in this regard is slow (Morikawa, 1994).

Similarly, the notion that one's privacy and confidentiality ought to be respected is thought to be a shared ideal in Western cultures. However, this does not necessarily constitute a universal value. Social science research on beliefs and norms associated with the cultural construction of the self indicates significant variability concerning the relative importance of privacy (Gergen, 1990). Thus, the American emphasis on the primacy of autonomy does not constitute a resolution in international bioethics, but part of the deepest problematic for most cultures.

VII. TECHNOLOGY RECONSTRUCTING THE COMMON GOOD TRADITION

Technology in medicine has a life of its own. As a result, as more and more cultures adopt a Western mode of medical delivery, cultural disjunctions must of necessity occur. This causes the kind of value clashes that virtually guarantee backlash, often called religious fundamentalism, that decries not only the effects on values of the new technology, but the whole Western vision of life itself.

What is that "Western value set" that provokes such a response? Primarily it is the objectification of persons to such an extent that persons become objects for manipulation. Such dominion replaces the highest power or God in many cultures and religions.

An alternative to over-emphasis on autonomy as the basis of human rights and bioethical resolutions is to reconstruct the common good tradition that influenced Western thought from the time of Aristotle. In this tradition, individual good and rights coincided with the community's good (Weisstub and Smith, 1979). One could not have one without the other. Rather than pitting autonomy against communitarianism, both could be synthesized in a new common good methodology of bioethics analysis.

The reluctance to wholly succumb to a communitarian model, and our love of tragic stories of outlaw heroes like Robin Hood, is due to our ambivalence about civilization itself; we may feel that we have sacrificed too much natural and individual vigor for the sake of public order. Some cultures are more tolerant of this sacrifice than others. Most likely, however, it is the advance of a technological civilization and its requirements for a coordinated and committed work force that give rise to a more secularized, urban culture that creates conflicts with traditional home, family, social, and religious values in any civilization. The same problems faced in the past century by other industrialized nations are now being faced by those who have accepted this notion of human development and have industrialized their economies.

Recognition of pluralism, too, can move in two different directions. In the first, there is a book-burning, heavy-handed reaction. There can be only *one* way of coping with the challenge, and that is to reassert the traditional value system. Most often such an assertion, when combined with political authority, leads to despotism. The other way of confronting pluralism is to fragment into parties, interests, caucuses, and the like, each scrambling for power and each imagining that it possesses the truth without taking the other splinter groups seriously. This too is a political solution to a profoundly personal and familial problem. Following these two responses, we are left with either a coerced unity or a series of isolated camps, both dominated by claims to certitude to the exclusion of other valid viewpoints.

A *via media* suggests itself in any clash of cultures. If one can be self-possessed enough to carefully analyze the sources of morality, one can readily see that the reactions to change that occur throughout human history are based on a complex of personal proclivities, fears and hopes, family and social values, traditional coping mechanisms embedded in one's culture and religion, and, more importantly for this essay, both an ethics and a philosophy that either incorporates change or development, or does not.

In any case, the ethical and religious sources of morality stress the fact that reality is transactional, that it requires individuals and other persons who rub shoulders with one another and are shaped by one another. Even the authoritarian or despotic culture is doomed to fail because it must receive gifts from "the other," other individuals who do not accept the idea that there is only one way, or from other cultures with which it must trade and do business. These "gifts," however unwelcome, are not only the undoing of any monolithic response to change, but themselves may lead to demands for change. As Walter Brueggemann has argued:

> In our time, it has been the voices of suffering and marginality that have kept available for us the urge that well-lived life is inescapably transactional ... the transactions of respect, dignity, and openness between rich and poor, between "superpower" and "colony," between the powerful and the weak, between parent and child. And when that transaction ceases to operate, when it dysfunctions or gives up on respect, dignity, and openness, both parties, not only the weaker, are deeply diminished, placed under threat, and driven to brutality. It is not hidden from us that the refusal of such interaction leads in a jagged line to brutality and abuse in the life of both parties (Brueggermann, 1995, p. 8).

My own conviction is that communitarian ethics must rejuvenate bioethics discussion that has become too complacently reliant on standard analysis in terms of autonomy. While communitarian ethics can mean many things, the main features are:

1. A corrective to an over-emphasis on individualism, usually employed by stressing the role of relationships, family, and community, in bioethics decision-making.

2. A conviction that values are culturally embedded, and cannot be taken in isolation from the cultural assumptions that shaped them.

3. An appeal to the context or "story" of the principals within a moral quandary or dilemma, rather than to abstract principles and rules, thus employing sociology, history, economics, politics, and other disciplines in the fabric of ethics and public policy.

4. Often, a preference for the common good over individual good, or rather, an appeal to the moral principle that, when faced with a conflict, it is better to preserve the common good rather than promote an individual good to the detriment of the common good.

5. The basis of morality in communitarian ethics is led away from the purely personal and rational will (freedom of choice), to qualities or instincts of compassion and empathy with all living creatures. A good example of this kind of work can be found in Erich Loewy's efforts to ground ethics in the physiological capacity to suffer (Loewy, 1991).

Opening up the parameters of the bioethics debates in this way will ensure that international bioethics will continue to grow. Consensus on issues may not always be feasible. However, several conditions for international, intercultural discourse about biomedical ethics are essential for effective development of an international bioethics discipline.

1) The first of these must be a simultaneous appreciation of another's culture coupled with a suspension of total acceptance (i.e., a suspension of total abandonment of one's own culture for the other). This is difficult to say the least. If one abandons one's culture and accepts the insights of the other, say "the Navajo Way" of seeing the world, then one's critique of one's own culture winds up being supplanted with yet another total way of thinking that may or may not be as good as one's original culture (Orona, Koenig, and Davis, 1994). On what basis does one make inter-cultural judgments? Is the standard by which one judges what is good or better lie within one culture, or does it transcend all cultures? Does a person then become "a-cultural," in making comparative judgments? How is this possible? Would not that person be like "the Flying Dutchman," a person condemned to wander the seas without an anchor in identity?

In order to carry out this step there must be a commitment to discerning cultural context. Bioethicists can be the beneficiaries of the richness that characterizes cultural diversity if opportunities are created to experience the challenge of transcultural dialogue. Yet this challenge will require a new and perhaps uneasy acceptance (for some) of pluralism. As Marshall, Bergsma, and I have argued (Marshall et al., 1994), an attempt would be made to reach *minimal agreement* regarding the language, meaning and value of ethical concepts and processes of moral reasoning. This will require explicit self-critical attention to the meaning of concepts and their cultural context in ways that have not yet been present in the international dialogue. As Marshall points out:

> One person's truth is another's conundrum ... this perhaps is the key to understanding the subjective phenomenology and cultural diversity in questions of medical ethics. Whose judgment is correct? Where does the ownership of legitimacy reside? At the individual level, the answers to these questions are easier: the 'right' morality is an expression of the heart as much as it is the head, and here we can all claim authority. But in matters of public policy, both nationally and internationally, the answers become distressingly clouded and ambiguous. Individuals may experience an abandonment of their particular 'truth', and the struggle for ethical dominance and control over medical discourse and technology becomes voluble (Marshall, 1992, p. 62).

Anthropologists have engaged in prolonged debates about the theoretical and social utility of ethical relativism as it relates to cultural context (D'Andrade, 1984; Hatch, 1983; Fabrega, 1989; Spiro, 1986; Douglas, 1983; Geertz, 1984). The problem of pluralism is a major challenge to cross-cultural bioethics (Brown, 1992). A full discussion of the issues, however, is beyond the scope of this paper.

2) Second, as argued so far, the primary principle of international bioethics should not be autonomy, or community, but a type of dialectical respect for persons and enculturated values. This dialectical respect would be constructed in a way similar to Dewey's methodology of "reflective equilibrium," a method of balancing values without topping one with another *a priori.* Negotiation should not require that people abandon their cultural traditions and replace them with some other culture's successes, but rather that their cultural traditions assist them and others to circumscribe an action or initiative with the values they profess.

There is a trend in American culture of abandoning our traditions, themselves among the youngest cultural traditions in the world, in favor of a search for other people's. This is a necessary accompaniment to the first stages of correction for cultural myopia. Many Americans are just now able to begin their journey along the pathways of cultural hegemonies, Western and other cultural systems, and are just beginning to face the inevitable conflicts. Although we are neophytes in this effort, we are certainly farther along than persons in other cultures who think that any single difference from their own is anathema. These are the fundamentalists of any society. What is repulsive about them is their lack of cultural sensitivity, of self-critical assessment, of awareness that there are other, perhaps better ways of perceiving things.

This trend of openness to other cultures should be encouraged, but not to the point that the cultural tradition of Republican Democracy is abandoned, since that tradition has much to offer international debates in bioethics. In particular, it should be stressed internationally that such a democracy is not about rights but about compromise.

In this respect there should be a conscious effort to suspend Romanticism of all stripes. In an age of anxiety about the future, there is a tendency to romanticize the past and to characterize it as simpler or more fundamentally secure than the present. In this essay I have targeted two mainstream romanticizations about America: Libertarianism and, to a lesser extent, Communitarianism. Although these are set against each other, the former stressing individualism and the latter stressing the community, ironically as Christopher Lasch has pointed out, both are grounded in a false understanding of the human person (Lasch, 1995, p. 86, pp. 263-278). Liberals begin with a false assumption, Lasch holds, that human beings are like a nugget or bundle of needs and rights. Their communities exist merely to insure both the fulfillment of the needs and to respond properly to their rights. Communitarians hold that communities exist to be compassionate to all citizens, although they tend to think, rather romantically in fact, that the last innocents on earth are the lower working classes.

3) Third, from this dialectical version of Engelhardt's "peaceable dialogue," an effort must be made to craft international accords in bioethics that would emerge from lengthy considerations of many points of view. More serious philosophical work therefore must be done on transcultural structures in human behavior and existence. Some of these can be uncovered in exposures of violations of human rights (Unknown, 1993a, b).

In this regard, recall the first conference on human rights in 25 years, sponsored by the United Nations in 1993 in Vienna. Some countries like China argued that nations with a different, more communal tradition, should be exempt from now-standard international expectations about respecting human rights. China argued, for example, that human rights should be secondary to the needs of the state, such as law and order. This objection was roundly rejected by the majority of countries in the world (Unknown, 1993c). In fact, the conference ended with a proposal that the U.N. establish an office of high commissioner to protect and promote human rights around the world. The conference reaffirmed the universality of human rights against a concerted effort to subordinate them to the state or to cultural considerations (Washington Post News Service, 1993, A10). The same conference recognized that "women's rights are an inalienable, integral and indivisible part of universal human rights" (Washington Post New Service, 1993, A10).

Such widespread theoretical acceptance of fundamental human rights around the world demonstrates that, to a large degree, our international expectations regarding individual rights help shape progress in developing our conceptions about how these rights are to be implemented. Is there a basis in the structures of human existence for such rights? Just as the Roman Empire developed the Stoic theory of natural rights into a system of law, so too must we develop a newer and more sophisticated theory of "natural law" for the modern era.

4) Fourth, as a consequence of the above conditions, discourse about biomedical ethics must have some *a priori* commitments present on the table. These are "experiential conditions" because they may not be metaphysically defensible, *per se*. Instead they arise from the past experience of a culture whose history demonstrates the evil effects of ignoring these commitments. Among candidates for such conditions might be the goal of assisting individuals to enhance their autonomy in the context of their family, to enhance their moral personhood in decisions to be made. Another would be the rights of all women in the world to control their own reproductive gifts and not to be used as objects These are some developing international human rights that could inform medical ethics. Still other conditions might include those that emerge from our collective experience in reaching a consensus about actions through ethics committee deliberations or national policy committees.

5) Finally, some major principles or rules could be formulated from this dialogue for all cultures. These can be developed inductively from cultural and bioethical experience. Many could emerge from the process just noted in point 4, above. But others can be the result of sifting through common experience in helping and healing. I opened with a quote from a young biology research fellow, who is also a Jesuit priest. It would make a good start for developing principles of international health care:

One should not lay a hand on another without the intent to heal.

Another possible principle might be:

Any objectification of life should include provisions to care for the vulnerabilities produced by that objectification.

VIII. CONCLUSION

I am pleased to have the opportunity to honor Dr. Hoshino by reflecting on the difficulties of doing international bioethics. Besides articulating those difficulties, I have tried to propose a few steps in developing an international platform for reaching a consensus about fundamental human rights in health care. Dr. Hoshino's interest in modifying American notions of autonomy in the Japanese cultural setting prompted me to think about the boilerplate necessary for such a cultural interaction in bioethics. His efforts have inspired many of us.

NOTE

† The Editors, with great sorrow, note the passing of a friend, colleague, and contributor to this volume. David Thomasma died in April, 2002.

REFERENCES

Anonymous (1995). 'Fight erupts on Geraldo set; nose broken again.' *The Chicago Tribune,* May 16, Sec 1:2.

Axelrod, A. and Philips, C. (1992). *What Every American Should Know About American History.* Holbrook: Bob Adams Publishing Co, Inc.

Beauchamp, T. and Childress, J. (1994). *The Principles of Biomedical Ethics*, 4th ed. New York: Oxford University Press.

'Beyond Autonomy' (1995). *Cambridge Quarterly of Healthcare Ethics* 4, a thematic issue.

Brown, K. (1992). 'Death and access: Ethics in cross-cultural health care.' In: E. Friedman (Ed.), *Choices and Conflict.* Chicago: American Hospital Association.

Brueggemann, W. (1995). 'Othering – Random thoughts on covenant,' *Explorations* 9, 8.

D'Andrade, R.G. (1984). 'Cultural meaning systems.' In: R.A. Shweder and R. Levine (Eds.), *Culture Theory: Essays on Mind.* Cambridge: Cambridge University Press.

Douglas, M. (1983). 'Morality and culture.' *Ethics* 93, 786-791.

Editorial (1994). 'Pushing human rights in Asia.' *Chicago Tribune* Nov. 18, Sec 1:28.

Engelhardt, H. T., Jr. (1986). *The Foundations of Bioethics*, 1st ed. New York: Oxford University Press.

Engelhardt, H. T., Jr. (1991). *Bioethics and Secular Humanism.* Valley Forge: Trinity Press International.

Engelhardt, H.T., Jr. (1996). *The Foundations of Bioethics*, 2nd ed. New York: Oxford University.

Fabrega, H. (1989). 'Cultural relativism and psychiatric illness.' *Journal of Nervous and Mental Disease* 177, 415-424.

Geertz, C. (1984). 'Anti Anti-relativism.' *American Anthropologist* 86, 263-278.

Gergen, K. (1990). 'Social understanding and conceptions of the self.' In: J.W. Stigler, R.A. Shroder, and G. Herdt (Eds.), *Cultural Psychology*. Cambridge: Cambridge University Press.

Graber, G.C. and Thomasma, D.C. (1989). *Theory and Practice in Medical Ethics*. New York: Continuum Books.

Griffiths, P. (1995). 'Now Beethoven. Musical events.' *The New Yorker* Oct. 2, 101-102.

Hatch, E. (1983). *Culture and Morality: The Relativity of Values in Anthropology*. New York: Columbia University Press.

Hoshino, K. (1992). 'Bioethics in Japan: 1989-1991.' In: B.A. Lustig, H.T. Engelhardt, Jr. and L.B. McCullough (Eds.), *Bioethics Yearbook*, 2nd volume. Dordrecht: Kluwer Academic Publishers.

Hoshino, K. (1995). 'Autonomous decision making and Japanese tradition.' *Cambridge Quarterly of Healthcare Ethics* 4, 71-74.

Irving, J. (1990). *A Prayer for Owen Meany*. New York: Ballantine Books. (Originally quoted from Charles Dickens, *A Christmas Story*.)

Komarow, S. (1995). 'Grief, quiet pride amid "Museum of Destruction".' *USA Today* Jan. 18, 3A.

Lasch, C. (1995). *The Revolt of the Elites and the Betrayal of Democracy*. New York: W.W. Norton.

Loewy, E. (1995). 'Care ethics: A concept in search of a framework.' *Cambridge Quarterly of Healthcare Ethics* 4, 56-63.

Loewy, E. (1991). *Suffering and the Beneficent Community: Beyond Libertarianism*. New York: University of New York Press.

MacIntyre, A. (1984). *After Virtue*, Notre Dame, IN: University of Notre Dame Press.

Marshall, P.A. (1992). 'Anthropology and bioethics.' *Anthropology Quarterly* 6, 49-73.

Marshall, P.A., Thomasma, D.C. and Bergsma, J. (1994). 'Intercultural reasoning: The challenge for international bioethics.' *Cambridge Quarterly of Healthcare Ethics* 3, 321-328.

Morikawa, I. (1994). 'Patient's rights in Japan: Progress and resistance.' *Kennedy Institute of Ethics Journal* 4, 337-344.

Nalty, K.H. (1994)., 'Studying God's creation: Jesuit profile.' *Georgetown Magazine* 26, 49.

Orona, C.J., Koenig, B.A. and Davis, A.J. (1994). 'Cultural aspects of nondisclosure.' *Cambridge Quarterly of Healthcare Ethics* 3, 338-346.

Parens, E. (1995). 'The pluralist constellation.' *Cambridge Quarterly of Healthcare Ethics* 4, 197-206.

Paris, J.J. and McCormick, R.A. (1987). 'The Catholic tradition on the use of nutrition and fluids.' *America* May 2, 356-361.

Pellegrino, E.D. and Thomasma, D.C. (1981). *A Philosophical Basis of Medical Practice*. New York: Oxford University Press.

Pellegrino, E.D. and Thomasma, D.C. (1988). *For the Patient's Good: The Restoration of Beneficence in Health Care*. New York: Oxford University Press.

Pellegrino, E.D. and Thomasma, D.C. (1993). *The Virtues in Medical Practice*. New York: Oxford University Press.

Remnick, D. (1995). 'Reading Japan.' *The New Yorker* 70, 38-44.

Rorty, R. (1995). 'Two cheers for elitism.' *The New Yorker* 70, 86-89.

Spiro, M.E. (1986). 'Cultural relativism and the future of anthropology.' *Cultural Anthropology* 1, 259-286.

Thomasma, D.C. and Marshall, P.A. (1995). *Clinical Medical Ethics: Cases and Readings*. Rockville: University Press of America.

Unknown (1993a). 'Human rights took a beating in 1992: Group condemns 100 nations for torture.' *The Chicago Tribune* July 9, Sec 1:2.

Unknown (1993b). 'U.N. paper on rights is criticized.' *The Chicago Tribune* June 3, Sec 1:14.

Unknown (1993c). 'Conference resolves dispute over rights.' *The Chicago Tribune* June 20, Sec 1:14.

Veatch, R.M. (1989). *Cross Cultural Perspectives in Medical Ethics: Readings*. Boston: Jones and Bartlett Publishers.

Vernacchio, L. (1995). 'Depersonalizing the medical student.' *America* Feb. 25, 16-18.

Washington Post News Service (1993). 'U.N. Parley backs human rights office.' *The Sacramento Bee Final* June 26, A10.

Weisstub, D. and Smith, J.C. (1979). 'The evolution of Western legal consciousness.' *International Journal of Law and Psychiatry*, 215-234.

JONATHAN CHAN

TAKING MORAL DIVERSITY SERIOUSLY: A DISCUSSION OF THE FOUNDATIONS OF GLOBAL BIOETHICS

I. INTRODUCTION

This paper addresses the question of how to establish a theoretical framework for global bioethics capable of resolving moral conflicts over bioethical issues. By 'moral conflict', I mean the clash of validity claims regarding moral issues. Moral conflicts arise on the global level mainly because of the fact that people from different ethnic groups or cultures hold conflicting comprehensive doctrines, each with its own conception of morality. I shall call this the fact of 'moral pluralism'. The notion of moral pluralism I use here is a descriptive term describing certain human conditions rather than expressing a philosophical thesis about morality. It means no more than that different ethnic or cultural groups hold conflicting comprehensive doctrines, each with its own conception of morality, and that this human condition will continue to exist for a long time or even permanently.[1] It is instructive to note that, although the fact of moral pluralism is a logically contingent anthropological or cultural fact, this fact taken as a permanent feature of human condition has significant implications for how we understand the nature of moral reasoning.

It is chiefly this permanent feature of the human condition that results in moral conflicts among different ethnic or cultural groups. A Catholic society, for instance, may deem using contraceptives as immoral, whereas a Buddhist society may regard using contraceptives as morally permissible. This clash of validity claims as to the morality of using contraceptives is evidently due to the fact that these two societies hold conflicting conceptions of morality. One way to resolve the moral conflict is for one of the societies to adjust its moral perspective so that its moral position on using contraceptives is not substantively different from, or at least not in opposition to, that of the other. Nonetheless, the question is whether there is any good reason for the society to do so. Unless we can provide a reason for society to adjust its moral perspective, the parties involved do not have the rational means to resolve the conflict.

H.T. Engelhardt, Jr. and L.M. Rasmussen (eds.), Bioethics and Moral Content: National Traditions of Health Care Morality, 235–250.

One important view is that there exists a certain set of moral principles that is either universally shared or capable of being demonstrated as universally valid through some rational method. On this view, moral conflicts over bioethical issues can be resolved not only on the societal level but also on the global level, for people from different ethnic or cultural groups can then appeal to a set of moral principles that are either universally shared or demonstrably capable of resolving their conflicts. Accordingly, some form of global bioethics, above and beyond the moral traditions to which people adhere, is not only possible but also inevitable. Let us call this view 'the global view'. It is this view that enabled the Nuremberg Tribunal, which consisted of three American judges, to convict the "Nazi doctors" of "crimes against humanity" in a Second World War crimes trial (i.e., the 1946-1947 Nuremberg "Doctor Trial"). If we take the opposite view, then the conviction would be deemed groundless.[2] In what follows, I shall focus on three major theories that have been used to support the global view, namely, the 'essentialist theory', the 'convergence theory' and the 'contract-based theory'. I shall argue that they are all in one way or another flawed, and, therefore, none of them can lend support to the global view. However, it is instructive to note that it is not the view of the present paper that the opposite view should prevail. For even if my critiques of these theories were to succeed, that fact would not exclude the possibility of finding a more adequate theory that will offer strong support for the global view.

II. THE ESSENTIALIST THEORY

I shall begin with the essentialist theory. The essentialist theory is the theory that morality is essentially determined by the true nature of some aspect of the world. On this theory, the moral order is no more than a manifestation of the way the world is. The moral order is an extension of the natural order, and human morality thereby reflects the nature of things. It follows from this view that morality must be universal. Bioethics also must be global; there is no such a thing as local bioethics. For if the moral order is itself a part of the natural order which, in turn, is universal, then morality must be universal too. Accordingly, the true moral principles that govern the moral order also must be universal, thereby being able to serve as a sound theoretical basis for global bioethics.

Confucianism is a prominent example of a philosophical system that embraces the essentialist theory. To capture the essentialist feature of Confucianism, we may begin by looking at the moral order fleshed out by the Confucians. It is a commonplace of Confucianism that the Confucian moral order is characterized in terms of five basic human relations (*wulun*): ruler-minister/ruled, father-son, husband-wife, elder brother-younger brother, and friend-friend. In this moral order, each of us has certain definite moral obligations derived on the basis of the foregoing human relations. These relation-based moral obligations usually are summed up by the principles of *ren* (or humaneness) and *yi* (or appropriateness and righteousness). From the Confucian point of view, these moral obligations, and thereby the related moral principles, are not merely social conventions. They are no more conceived merely as social conventions than the five basic human relations are conceived merely as products of our social construction. For the Confucians, both the five basic human relations and their corresponding moral obligations, and thereby the related moral principles, manifest some respects of the natural order.[3]

Mencius, for instance, maintains that the moral virtues and obligations that correspond to the basic human relations have roots in human nature:

> The way benevolence [*jen*] pertains to the relation between father and son, duty [*yi*] to the relation between the prince and subject, the rites to the relation between guest and host, wisdom to the good and wise man, the sage to the way of Heaven, is the Decree, but therein also lies human nature. That is why the gentleman does not describe it as Decree (*Mencius* VIIB: 24, trans. Lau).

In another passage, Mencius assigns an ontological ground to these basic moral virtues and obligations:

> The heart of compassion is possessed by all men alike; likewise the heart of shame, the heart of respect, and the heart of right and wrong. The heart of compassion pertains to benevolence, the heart of shame to dutifulness, the heart of respect to the observance of the rites, and the heart of right and wrong to wisdom. Benevolence, dutifulness, observance of the rites, and wisdom do not give me a lustre from the outside, they are in me originally (*Mencius* VIA: 6, trans. Lau).

Thus, for Mencius, moral obligations and principles reflect the nature of our 'heart'. Since all men alike possess this 'heart', moral obligations and principles that reflect the nature of the 'heart' must be universal. Hence, Mencius say

> [A]ll palates have the same preference in taste; all ears in sound; all eyes in beauty. Should hearts prove to be an exception by possessing nothing in common? What is it, then, that is common to all hearts? Reason and rightness. The sage is simply the man first to discover this common element in my heart (*Mencius* VIA: 7, trans. Lau).

Another example of the essentialist view also can be found in Neo-Confucianism. A Neo-Confucian such as Chu Hsi, following the classical Confucians, took the principle of *ren* (or humaneness) and the principle of *yi* (or appropriateness and righteousness) as the fundamental moral principles. Chu Hsi assigned the metaphysical status of the principle of Heaven (*T'ien Li*) to these moral principles. Further, every kind of thing in the universe has its own *Li* and there are none that do not have *Li*. As soon as a thing exists, the *Li* is inherent in it and constitutes its nature (Chu, 1963, pp. 593-597). In consequence, our moral actions also have their own *Li*. And it is this *Li* that makes moral actions what they are. It is, then, clear that the *Li* of moral actions and the moral principles (in this case, the principles of *ren* and *yi*) are identical. One of the logical consequences of this essentialist theory is that actions that are not in line with the *Li* or the principles of *ren* and *yi* cannot be moral actions. Accordingly, the moral principles must be transcendent and universal in the sense that they are beyond and above all traditions. On this theory, there is no such a thing as local bioethics; bioethics must be global because the moral principles on which bioethics are based must be global. Examples of the essentialist theory also can be found in the history of Western philosophy. Plato's theory of Ideas, Roman natural law theory and John Locke's theory of rights are paradigms of this essentialist theory. All these theories assume that what makes an action moral is the 'essence' or the 'true nature' of some aspect of the world.

One major defect of these essentialist theories is that they all beg the question, for they all presuppose that morality has an unvaried 'essence' or that there is such a thing as the 'true nature' of certain aspects of the world on which morality depends. However, it is exactly this presupposition that the essentialist moral philosophers need to prove. Given the fact of moral pluralism, how could we tell what that 'essence' or that particular 'true nature' would be? As different traditions will come up with different interpretations concerning the 'essence' or the 'true nature', it is unlikely that we can identify a set of properties that can be said to determine indisputably the 'essence' or the 'true nature' on which the right conception of morality depends. Hence, the burden is on those essentialists to prove the truth of the above presupposition.

The Confucians such as Mencius and Chu Hsi attempted to ground the above essentialist presupposition in certain metaphysical views. As we have seen earlier, these Confucians posited either a certain human faculty (the "heart") or a certain law-like principle (*T'ien Li*) as the sole source of moral authority for human morality. However, the fact of moral pluralism makes the idea of positing such a human faculty or law-like principle implausible. Since people from different moral traditions perceive morality differently, the hope that we can identify a certain human faculty or law-like principle as the sole source of moral authority for human morality is illusory. For if people from different moral traditions perceive morality differently, that fact constitutes a good reason to doubt that there is such a human faculty or that a law-like principle will constitute the sole source of moral authority for human morality. It simply is begging the question to posit the existence of such things without an adequate explanation of the existence of a huge moral divergence among different cultures and nations.

The comment that I have made so far, although focusing on the essentialist feature of Confucianism, is not confined only to the essentialist theory presupposed by Confucianism. It can be extended to other essentialist theories such as the Natural Law theory or human rights theory. For all of them have the following tendency: they do not take the implicative feature of the fact of moral pluralism seriously. The fact of moral pluralism as a permanent feature of the human condition imposes certain epistemological constraints on how the foundation of morality is to be understood. It requires us to take a less presumptuous approach to how such a foundation is to be fleshed out. We are required not to take for granted a certain moral conception of a particular culture or tradition when fleshing out such a foundation. The essentialist theories, however, do not take this implicative feature of the fact of moral pluralism seriously enough when they posit certain things or properties as the unvaried 'essence' or the 'true nature' of morality, which, in turn, are merely cultural constructions of a particular culture or tradition.

III. THE CONVERGENCE THEORY

A global view theorist might argue that the global view does not necessarily presuppose the essentialist theory. According to bioethicists such as Beauchamp and Childress, although people hold different ethical theories as well as rules and particular moral judgements, there is a convergence at the level of principles (Beauchamp et al., 1994, pp. 100-111). These philosophers maintain that some principles of bioethics are universally valid for different traditions or cultures. And these universal principles of bioethics can serve as a foundation for global bioethics. Let us call this view 'the convergence theory'. The convergence theory defined above is not a first order moral theory but only a second order theory because this is a theory about how the notion of universal principles of bioethics can be entertained or defended. However, some clarification is needed regarding the formulation of the theory. The theory can be formulated in two different ways. First, the theory can be understood as the descriptive thesis that there are principles of bioethics *in fact* held by all traditions or cultures. Second, the theory also can be understood as the normative thesis that there are some principles of bioethics that *should be* adopted by all traditions or cultures.

Nevertheless, no matter how the theory is formulated, one major problem this theory encounters is the task of finding a set of non-controversial principles of bioethics that can be said to be universally valid, either in the descriptive sense or normative sense, for all traditions or cultures. Childress and Beauchamp assert that there are four – the principle of respect for autonomy, the principle of nonmaleficence (a norm of avoiding the causation of harm), the principle of beneficence, and the principle of justice (Beauchamp et al., 1994, pp. 37-38). The claim that these four principles are universally valid, either descriptively or normatively, it seems to me, begs the question.

As a descriptive thesis, the claim seems to neglect the fact that there are traditions that do not embrace the above principles, or at least not all of them. Oriental philosophers have consistently pointed out that some of the principles listed above have never been important principles of moral conduct in societies with strong Oriental traditions such as Japan, Korea and China. They argue that some of the principles are even inconsistent with the moral traditions of these societies. For instance, Kazumasa Hoshino, a distinguished Japanese bioethicist, has argued this point with regard to the acceptance of Western bioethics in Japanese society. He wrote:

> Japanese people in general seem to be insensitive to or even subconsciously reluctant to accept the vital importance of autonomy, self-determination and individualistic freedom in decisionmaking; all of which are indispensably valuable principles in Western bioethics (Hoshino, 1997, p. 12).

and

> In general, Japanese people are not accustomed to making medical decisions regarding their own diseases by themselves without consulting the family. This is because of their deep regard and respect for the opinions and feelings of the family. When one member of the family becomes sick, it is the responsibility of the entire family to look after him ... In these circumstances, it seems rather natural for the family first to decide on the best medical procedures and to care for him ... There is, in fact, no concept in the mind of the Japanese that one of the family members has such individual rights independent of the family (Hoshino, 1997, p. 16-7).

and

> Each member of the family seems to be connected individually with each of the other members perhaps not only by love or affection ... but also by a certain kind of spiritual tie in this collectivistic society of Japan. This type of spiritual tie appears to be based upon the long lasting traditions, culture, and ethos of Japan (Hoshino, 1997, p. 18).

From the foregoing citations, it is clear that Japanese bioethicists such as Hoshino decline to accept all the important principles of Western bioethics without questioning or modification. If Hoshino's foregoing observation about Japanese society is correct, then it is obvious that principles that express liberal moral values such as autonomy, self-determination and individual rights, as presented in Western bioethics, is at odds with the ethical tradition of Japanese society.

Even if we grant that the principles proposed by Beauchamp and Childress might play some role in different traditions, the moral force and content of these principles in different traditions are still not on a par. Different traditions may impose different theoretical constraints on the formulation, as well as the use of these principles. To adopt a Kuhnian term, these principles are all "theory-laden". They are all subject to theoretical interpretation. This being so, the universality of these principles is suspect, and they are therefore too flexible to serve as a descriptive basis of global bioethics.

As a normative thesis that all cultures or traditions should adopt the four principles, it is exactly this universal status of the principles that their proponents need to prove. The burden is on the proponents of these principles to show us the mechanism for deriving their normative universal status. Without supplying an adequate mechanism or framework for deriving the universal status of these principles, to claim that they are the principles that every one should follow, no matter what tradition he or she comes from, simply begs the question.

Recently, Beauchamp and Childress have argued for a theory of common-morality as the basis for the four principles:

> A common-morality theory takes its basic premises directly from the morality shared in common ... common-morality ethics relies heavily on ordinary shared moral beliefs for its content, rather than relying on pure reason, natural law, a special moral sense, and the like .... An important function of the standards in the common morality ... is to provide a basis for the evaluation and criticism of actions in countries and communities whose customary moral viewpoints fail to acknowledge basic principles. A customary morality, then, is not synonymous with the common morality. The latter is a pretheoretic moral point of view that transcends merely local customs and attitudes (Beauchamp et al., 1994, p. 100).

If there exists such "a pretheoretic moral point of view that transcends merely local customs and attitudes," that point of view may well be used as a basis for deriving basic principles as well as "for the evaluation and criticism of actions in countries and communities whose customary moral viewpoints fail to acknowledge basic principles." However, it is exactly the existence of such a moral point of view that is suspect. To argue for the basic principles on the basis of such a moral point of view is begging the question. Furthermore, if a country's or community's customary moral viewpoints fail to acknowledge basic principles, then that is a good reason to doubt the existence of a common morality or of a sufficient set of commonly shared moral beliefs that serve as the basis of the common morality.

IV. THE CONTRACT-BASED THEORY

In view of the pluralistic nature of global morality, some bioethicists have made serious efforts to develop a theoretical framework for global bioethics based on the model of contract or negotiation (Baker, 1998b). In using such a model, these bioethicists claim that they are able to construct a transcultural or cross-cultural moral order for global bioethics. The model has a strong theoretical linkage to the contractarian tradition. This tradition treats a norm as binding only for those who have consented to this norm. On this view, people's consent or agreement is both a necessary and sufficient criterion for the justification of a moral norm.

In order to appreciate the force of this view of moral legitimacy, we need to probe a little deeper into the philosophical motivation of the contractarian theory. The contractarians recognize that the interests of people are naturally in conflict, yet some form of cooperation is necessary between agents with conflicting principles and interests. For the contractarians, the important challenge to moral philosophy is to flesh out a moral order that enables the agents to resolve their conflicts in a peaceful way so that they can enjoy the advantages of their mutual cooperation. The contractarians meet this challenge by making people's mutual consent or agreement the sole source of the moral legitimacy of a norm. People can appeal to an agreed upon moral order to govern their social interaction and cooperation. Or, if there is no such agreed upon moral order, people may create one through negotiation. For the contractarians, a negotiated moral order is the only legitimate moral order for agents whose principles and interests conflict with each other. In addition, this is the only kind of moral order with a built-in motivation for agents to adhere to its norms.

In applying this view of moral legitimacy to global bioethics, one might argue that a transcultural or cross-cultural moral order is possible since different ethnic or cultural groups, through negotiation, may come up with a consensus or agreement on a certain moral order. Insofar as this moral order is the one agreed upon by different ethnic or cultural groups, it has transcultural or cross-cultural moral legitimacy. People from different ethnic or cultural groups can appeal to this agreed upon or negotiated moral order to govern their interaction and cooperation. I shall hereafter call this theory of global bioethics the 'contract-based or negotiation-based theory'.

One major problem this theory encounters is: Why does the mutual consent of the people have such a justificatory force? According to one interpretation of contractarianism, the answer lies in the fact that a moral order based on agreement is mutually advantageous (Gauthier, 1985, pp. 251-269). On this interpretation, morality is viewed as a cooperative venture of mutual advantage. A moral order is no more than a set of social conventions upon which contracting parties agree or would agree simply out of self-interest. This being so, a moral order based on agreement must be rational from the perspective of each contracting agent to the extent that the agreement is the best possible option he or she can ask for in order to advance his or her self-interest. An agreed upon moral order is then rational from the perspective of a contracting agent so long as he or she finds that the moral order enables him or her to pursue his or her own advantage more effectively than were he or she to act without that order. Accordingly, moral norms that are justified from the perspective of each individual are norms for governing people's interaction and cooperation which are agreed upon by rational individuals, each of whom seeks to cooperate with fellow contractors in order to maximize his or her own utility. It is then evident that the idea of morality as a cooperative venture for mutual advantage links rational collective choice with moral legitimacy. The moral legitimacy of a norm is simply derived from the fact that the norm is the result of a rational collective choice.

However, in order to show that a collective choice is rational, some interpretation of the choice situation is needed. We need to determine in advance which factors we will allow agents to consider when making a choice. To choose a plausible interpretation of the choice situation for reaching agreement on a certain moral order is itself a controversial philosophical issue. What factors can be assumed in the choice situation in question highly depends on our philosophical theories. For instance, we may design the choice situation similar to the Hobbesian state of nature, in which people have complete freedom to do whatever they like, and 'morality' simply does not exist. Even if, unlike Hobbes, we allow that each person may have his or her own prior moral conception in the choice situation, such "a prior moral conception has no place except insofar as it may happen to enter into and to inform considered preference" (Gauthier, 1986, p. 202). Under this choice situation, there are no moral constraints as to how negotiation ought to be carried out. A person may take full advantage of his bargaining power to influence, manipulate or even force others to accept a certain agreement. There is no question of fairness as to how the agreement is made. Indeed, the agreement is deemed fair insofar as it is what people have agreed upon, no matter how that agreement was reached. Nevertheless, a theory that allows people to use force to compel others or to manipulate others to reach a consensus is not an account of justification, and certainly not an account of moral justification. A justification, if genuine, must be based on reason or persuasion by virtue of better argument, rather than force or manipulation. A religious believer who uses force to make others agree to the belief of the existence of God is not providing a justification for that belief. We can never justify a belief by forcing or manipulating others to agree to it.

One might object that the above criticism illegitimately begs the question, because it assumes the existence of a certain standard of morality that can tell us whether a moral justification can be counted as a justification or not. However, the whole point of the Hobbesian contractarian theory is to challenge that assumption. A quick response to this rejoinder is that the above criticism does not rest on the assumption that there exists a prior standard of morality. Rather, it rests on our minimal understanding of what the term "justification" means. In other words, it is our linguistic assumption, not our moral assumption, that defies the Hobbesian account of moral justification.

A contract must be made under fair conditions if it is to have any justificatory force. That is why some contractarians try to impose constraints on the choice situation so that unequal bargaining power would not affect the fairness of the contract being made. The problem for these contractarians becomes one of identifying a set of constraints that each contracting agent will deem fair. Nevertheless, no matter how the set is identified, the aforementioned contractarians have to face the following dilemma: either the set of constraints identified has no moral import or a prior moral conception is presupposed. It must have some moral import, exhibiting at least a certain degree of fairness. Otherwise, there is no guarantee that the contract being made is fair. However, if it does have moral import, then it must presuppose a prior moral conception, thereby rendering the whole idea of contract as a method of moral justification superficial. The contractarians may, like John Locke, identify the set with a set of basic human rights, or they may identify the set with something like the veil of ignorance and a list of primary goods specified in Rawls' original position (Rawls, 1972). In either case, a prior moral conception is presupposed. This move renders the idea of contract superficial and, therefore, defeats the whole purpose of using the contractarian approach to flesh out a foundation for morality.

One might argue that the contractarian projects pursued by Locke and Rawls fail chiefly because they read into the bill of rights or the list of primary goods the Western liberal goods or values. If we allow the contracting agents to define their own bill of rights or list of primary goods, then the contractarian project may be able to avoid the foregoing charge of smuggling the Western liberal goods or values into the agreed upon moral order. This is the line pursued by Robert Baker when he attempts to flesh out a theoretical framework for international bioethics by reinterpreting the central cannons of the contractarian tradition. In a recently published article, he argued for the following (Baker, 1998b, p. 233): (1) International bioethics can be rationally reconstructed as a negotiated moral order that respects culturally and individually defined areas of non-negotiability. (2) The theory of a negotiated moral order is consistent with traditional ideals about human rights, is flexible enough to absorb the genuine insights of multiculturalism and postmodernism, and yet is strong enough to justify transcultural and transtemporal moral judgments. In what follows, I shall examine critically his argument for the above theses.

I shall summarize the structure of Baker's argument as follows:

(1) A legitimate moral order can be fleshed out in terms of two things – (a) agreement through negotiation and (b) areas of non-negotiability.

(2) The condition (a) is important to all contractarian theories "[b]ecause contractarians look to the assent of those who would be bound by a moral norm as ultimately the sole source of a norm's legitimacy" (Baker, 1998b, p. 234).

(3) The condition (b) is also important "because agents embroiled in conflict will *not* sacrifice everything that they value in order to enjoy the advantage of mutual cooperation. Some goods, principles and values are nonnegotiable" (Baker 1998 (b), p. 235). In other words, the moral order agreed upon, if it is to be legitimate, must respect those areas of nonnegotiable primacy recognized by each contracting agent.

(4) Each party is free to define his or her list of "rights" or "primary goods," i.e., areas of non-negotiability. For "it is irrelevant which items are on anyone's list of rights or 'primary goods,' what matters is that each party negotiating morality holds some goods, interests, or values to be so fundamental that he or she will not accept any norm that intrudes upon them" (Baker, 1998b, p. 240-241). In consequence, for any set of agents, some areas will be considered nonnegotiable, but these areas may vary from agent to agent.

(5) A rights violation is said to have occurred "if any good considered primary [i.e., one's areas of non-negotiability] by a (rational or capacitated) agent is violated." As the content of what is considered primary may vary between and within cultures, what counts as a rights violation also may vary. However, "rights violations, in the sense of violations of primary goods, are impermissible in any possible moral framework and in all cultures" (Baker, 1998b, p. 241).

In the above, I have outlined Baker's argument for a contract-based theory of international bioethics. If that argument were to succeed, it would provide a very attractive theoretical framework for international bioethics that "is consistent with traditional ideals about human rights, is flexible enough to absorb the genuine insights of multiculturalism and postmodernism, and yet is strong enough to justify transcultural and transtemporal moral judgments." However, a number of critical points need to be raised with respect to this argument. To begin with, Baker stipulates that violations of primary goods, i.e., the self-defined areas of nonnegotiable primacy, amount to rights violations. But why do we need to accept such a stipulation? Baker asserts that "[w]illful trespasses on aspects of life considered so primary that they are nonnegotiable always will violate the fundamental presuppositions of morality because such trespasses always will be unacceptable to the persons whose primary goods are being violated" (Baker, 1998 (b), p. 242). However, he nowhere argues for why respecting others' areas of nonnegotiable primacy is the "fundamental presupposition of morality." It is true that trespasses on a person's areas of nonnegotiable primacy would be unacceptable to that person. But why does this amount to violating the "fundamental presupposition of morality," and whose morality?

Furthermore, the stipulation that violations of "any good considered primary by a (rational or capacitated) agent" are rights violations is counterintuitive. For instance, a radical feminist may consider the good of a 'pornography free' society primary. But why does violation of this subjectively defined 'primary good' amount to a rights violation? The notion of rights does refer to some interests that normally are considered primary by individuals. However, it does not follow that whatever an individual considers primary is a right. Nor does it follow that violation of such primacy is a rights violation. The radical feminist in our example may deem works of pornography morally unacceptable. Nevertheless, the feminist has no 'right' to say that they are genuine cases of rights violations. A fundamentalist religious believer may consider a 'heresy free' society a primary good. But he or she does not have the right to such a subjectively defined 'primary good'. Nor does the fundamentalist have the 'right' to say that violation of such a good is a genuine case of a rights violation.

Suppose the contractarian makes the following rejoinder. The radical feminist or the fundamental religious believer in the above examples may not want to insist that they have the rights to such goods. For if they insist on having and thereby exercising such rights, the conflict between the believer and the non-believer, for example, could be resolved only through intractable power struggles. However, nobody will be the 'winner' in such power struggles. For the costs of energy, time, and resources needed to gain hegemony over the struggles would probably outweigh the presumed benefits of 'winning'. But if this rejoinder were to be accepted, then it follows that one's primary goods or areas of nonnegotiable primacy are subject to negotiation and thereby negotiable. That being the case, the contractarian could rescue his notion of rights violation only by paying lip service to his notion of the areas of nonnegotiability.

V. CONCLUSION

In the above, I have gone through three major theories of global bioethics, namely, the essentialist theory, the convergence theory and the contract-based theory. I also have argued that all these theories, in one way or another, are flawed. The above analysis reveals that these theories, even if in the most updated forms, are defective. Both the essentialist theory and the convergence theory are defective mainly because they do not take the implicative feature of the fact of moral pluralism seriously. As I showed earlier, the fact of moral pluralism as a permanent feature of the human condition has implications for how we understand the nature of moral reasoning. Hence, any moral theory that neglects the implicative feature of this fact is bound to be logically defective. The contract-based theory is defective not because it fails to appreciate the challenge posed by moral diversity, but because it rests upon the metaphor of contract that either lacks justificatory force or already has smuggled in Western liberal goods or values. In either case, the metaphor of contract is hardly an acceptable device for fleshing out a sound theoretical framework for global bioethics.

Hong Kong Baptist University
Hong Kong SAR, PRC

NOTES

1 John Rawls takes the fact of moral pluralism as "a permanent feature of the public culture of democracy" (Rawls, 1993, pp. 36-37). However, it is my view that this fact constitutes a permanent human condition of our ethical world.

2 The opposite view is that each society has its own standard of morality and standard of practical rationality and that there does not exist a higher standard by which a society's standards of morality and practical rationality can be judged to be superior to another society's. On this view, people can resolve their moral conflicts only within a morally homogenous ethnic or cultural group. Within a morally homogeneous ethnic or cultural group, people can resolve their moral conflicts by appealing to a set of commonly shared moral principles that, in turn, can be agreed to be valid by referring to the standards of morality and practical rationality of the group. However, on the transcultural level, since there does not exist a set of commonly shared standards of morality and practical rationality, it is unlikely that people from different ethnic or cultural groups can resolve their moral conflicts in a mutually acceptable manner (MacIntyre, 1981, 1988). Then, as in the example mentioned above, neither the Catholic nor the Buddhist society can come up with a rational account to persuade the other to adjust its own moral perspective so as to avoid the conflict, for the standards of morality and practical rationality embodied in their moral perspectives are very different.

3 Jiwei Ci has given an excellent explanation as to how the five basic human relations and thereby the corresponding moral obligations are naturalized (Ci, 1999).

REFERENCES

Baker, R. (1998a). 'A theory of international bioethics: Multiculturalism, postmodernism, and the bankruptcy of fundamentalism.' *Kennedy Institute of Ethics Journal* 8(3), 201-231.

Baker, R. (1998b). 'A theory of international bioethics: The negotiable and the non-negotiable.' *Kennedy Institute of Ethics Journal* 8(3), 233-273.

Beauchamp, T. L. (1999). 'The mettle of moral fundamentalism: A reply to Robert Baker.' *Kennedy Institute of Ethics Journal* 8(4), 389-401.

Beauchamp, T. L. & J. Childress (1994). *Principles of Biomedical Ethics*, 4th edition. New York: Oxford University Press.

Ci, J. (1999). 'The Confucian relational concept of the person and its modern predicament.' *Kennedy Institute of Ethics Journal* 9(4), 325-346.

Chu, S. (1963.) 'A treatise on *jen*.' In: W. T. Chan (Trans. And Comp), *A Source Book in Chinese Philosophy* (pp. 593-597). Princeton: Princeton University Press, Princeton.

Engelhart, H. T., Jr. (1996). *The Foundations of Bioethics*, 2nd edition. New York: Oxford University Press.

Gauthier, D. (1986). *Morals By Agreement*. New York: Oxford University Press.

Gauthier, D. (1985). 'Justice as social choice.' In: D. Copp and D. Zimmerman (Eds.), *Morality, Reason and Truth: New Essays on the Foundations of Ethics* (pp. 200-213). Totowa, N.J.: Rowman & Allanheld.

Hoshino, K. (1997). 'Bioethics in the light of Japanese sentiments.' In: K. Hoshino (Ed.), *Japanese and Western Bioethics: Studies in Moral Diversity* (pp. 12-23). Dordrecht: Kluwer Academic Publishers.

Lau, D.C. (trans.) (1984). *Mencius*. Hong Kong: The Chinese University Press.

MacIntyre, A. (1981). *After Virtue*. London: Duckworth.

MacIntyre, A. (1988). *Whose Justice? Which Rationality?* London: Duckworth.

Rawls, J. (1972). *A Theory of Justice*. New York: Oxford University Press.

Rawls, J. (1993). *Political Liberalism*. New York: Columbia University Press.

MARK J. CHERRY

COVETING AN INTERNATIONAL BIOETHICS: UNIVERSAL ASPIRATIONS AND FALSE PROMISES

I. FALSE CLAIMS TO MORAL CONSENSUS

As a field of inquiry, bioethics covets an international political stage. Bioethics lays claim to a universal account of proper moral deportment, including the foundations of law and public policy, as well as the moral authority for national and international institutions to guarantee uniformity of practice. The challenge, as Kazumasa Hoshino rightly notes, is that religious and cultural moral diversity is very real. The national and international political landscape compasses persons from diverse and often fragmented moral communities with widely varying moral intuitions, premises, evaluations, and commitments. Policy must be created to span a diverse set of individuals, cultures, and communities. Yet, such policy is never neutral. It inevitably promotes the social and moral acceptance of certain practices, endorsing particular moral values and metaphysical understandings over others. Political struggles regard both the form and content of what will become the prevailing medical, moral, and social ethos.

As Hoshino observes, such disputes are often substantial: "There are many subtle and overt racial, national, social, cultural, and religious differences among divergent societies, such as Japan and the United States. Such differences may explain the difficulties that the Japanese and other cultures have in accepting many Western principles of bioethics" (1997a, p. xi; see also 1995a). As he notes, Western bioethical reflections have, for better or worse, been imported into Japan, altering traditional Japanese understandings.[1] Yet, unlike the West, Japan remains in large measure a traditional society, with shared, non-Western, understandings of value and strong ties to culture, community, and family (Hoshino, 1997a; 1997b). The Japanese moral perspective draws on cultural and religious understandings that are often at odds with the conclusions that Western bioethicists endorse. Moral understandings, particular accounts of human flourishing, accepted social roles, including appreciation of gender and sexuality, expressed in often taken-for-granted norms of

H.T. Engelhardt, Jr. and L.M. Rasmussen (eds.), Bioethics and Moral Content: National Traditions of Health Care Morality, 251–279.

human form, behavior and grace, mark the conceptual frameworks that underlie public policy.

This chapter continues the critical exploration that Hoshino so successfully engaged throughout his distinguished and notable career as one of Japan's preeminent bioethicists. Hoshino's detailed analytical insights shed light on the significant differences between Japan and the West, drawing attention to the complexity of framing universal biomedical and health care policy. In a similar vein, I begin with a conceptual geography of contemporary bioethical analysis and its often stark contrast with the values, assumptions, and moral understandings of traditional cultures and religions. Whereas a global bioethics offers the hope of a communality binding all persons and the resolution of biomedical moral controversies through universal moral norms, as I argue, such a hope is chimerical. The cosmopolitan liberal vision of contemporary bioethics offers only the false promise of a global moral consensus, while failing to acknowledge the deep divisions between traditional religious and cultural moral communities and its own post-modern, post-traditional universal aspirations. In response to such challenges, I then turn to a reconsideration of the justified foundations for health care policy.

As Hoshino appreciated, foundational understandings of the meaning and significance of birth, reproduction, and death, expressed in debates regarding the character of human dignity, the sacredness of human life, the centrality of the family, and the nature of the good life, in turn frame the justifications of particular practices, such as abortion, embryo experimentation, and stem cell research, assisted-suicide, and euthanasia. Given divergent foundational metaphysical, epistemological, and axiological presuppositions, different medical goals and political objectives will appear as not merely morally permissible but politically obligatory.

II. THE FALSE PROMISES OF A GLOBAL CONSENSUS

Rather than social space for expression of diverse religious and moral beliefs, bioethics has sought top-down guidance framed in terms of a rationally discoverable vision of proper conduct, which authorizes state authority to constrain and direct citizens, groups, and communities. This is Kant's vision of a universal legislator, who derives from a particular account of moral rationality and rational volition, an understanding of appropriate human choice. Consequently, bioethics has come to have a national socialist, liberal, statist character, seeking protection of individual autonomy (understood as acting in accord with right reason and moral consensus, rather than in accordance with one's own wishes and desires), equality in the provision of health care with uniform national and international standards, and individual choice freed from the influence of traditional family, religious, and cultural power structures.[2]

Citing objective, rational analysis, freed of the particularities of religious belief and cultural practice, bioethics endorses basic rights to prenatal diagnosis, selective abortion, and physician-assisted suicide. Similarly, claiming the existence of "global moral consensus", bioethics seeks universal declarations on cloning, embryo experimentation, third-party assisted reproduction, organ procurement and transplantation, and so forth. In short, bioethicists claim for themselves moral expertise with authority to guide individual choice and clinical decision making, court judgment, public deliberation, and legislative action.

Choosing other than in accord with "right reason" and the purported "moral consensus", whether in adherence to traditional religion or culture, or to advance diverse secular accounts of the good, is characterized as acting under a false consciousness or as the victim of exploitation or social, cultural or patriarchal despotism. For example, regardless of the underlying reasons or likely personal advantages, selling human organs for a profit is held to be exploitative and degrading, morally analogous to slavery, and incompatible with basic human values (such as human dignity) and important social goods (such as equality and a spirit of altruism). The human body, it is argued, should not be treated as property (Scott, 1981; 1990). Financial incentives are believed to coerce the poor into selling parts of their bodies. In 1970, the Committee on Morals and Ethics of the Transplantation Society held that "the sale of organs by donors living or dead is indefensible under any circumstance" (1970), and the World Health Organization's "Guiding Principles on Human Organ Transplantation" prohibits giving and receiving money for organs. Moreover, the WHO urges member states to legislate forbidding the commercial trafficking of human organs (WHO, 1991). In the United States, Title III (Section 301) of the federal "National Organ Transplant Act" makes it unlawful for any persons knowingly to acquire, receive, or otherwise transfer human organs for valuable consideration. Morally acceptable uses of the body are those that are viewed as protecting "... a central element of the undefined, yet widely endorsed demand for respect for the human body and for human dignity" (Nuffield Council on Bioethics, 1995, para 6.4).[3] Similar considerations are mustered in support of legislation prohibiting commercial surrogate motherhood, genetic engineering, and human cloning. Such state-enforced biomedical restrictions are not characterized as limiting legitimate moral diversity or individual liberty but rather as returning individuals, families, and communities, to the appropriately objective standards of rationally disclosed morality. Supported with claims to "global moral consensus" on such issues, national and international legalistic regulation denies the existence of real moral difference, while providing the secular equivalent of orthodox belief; bioethical disagreement is to be at least shunned, if not actively persecuted.

The dominant strategy for addressing biomedical moral controversy has been the interdisciplinary search for common ground – standards of reasoning or universal principles, such as compassion and love, solidarity and human dignity – which provides moral content for individual choice while also guiding law and policy formation. Such approaches seek universal standards for understanding and protecting the dignity of the human person as well as for creating and maintaining the common good. Such dialogue, however, inevitably adopts a fully secular language. To frame bioethical issues in common terms requires the evacuation of any moral content not justifiable in general secular rational terms. Traditional Christians, Japanese, and others may not simply affirm their religious beliefs or cultural practices as true.[4]

To be acknowledged, to have a voice in bioethical debate – whether regarding the moral status of embryos, fetuses, and so forth, or of particular acts, such as assisted suicide, or third-party assisted reproduction – one's claims must either be evacuated of all particular religious or cultural content, or be affirmed as merely one possible moral perspective among many. Cultural, moral and religious diversity may only be affirmed as akin to variations in aesthetic tastes: at best the expression of personal or group idiosyncrasy. Real disparity of belief threatens the possibility of reaching content-full agreement. True believers, i.e., those who denounce others as wrong, attempt to convert, or refuse to see central religious or moral beliefs as the appropriate subject of political compromise, are perceived as dangerous and threatening. To forge consensus, different religious perspectives may not appear to have an exclusionary character.

While often referring to the goods of moral pluralism, this perspective embraces a fully secularized understanding of religion and culture, in which the search for meaning is fully individualized, all spiritually generic and interchangeable, with all cultures and religions affirmed as equally valuable. In its attempt to liberate morality from traditional viewpoints, cultural practices, and religious beliefs, it seeks a binding universal vision of autonomy in which individuals free themselves from what are perceived as the superstitions and illiberal constraints of the past.[5]

For example, while the family plays a central role in traditional cultures and religions, its role in modern Western medical decision making has been marginalized. Where the family in traditional culture and religion is typically hierarchical, patriarchal, and paternalistic, health care policy and law, especially in the United States and Western Europe, is framed in terms of individualistic consent to ensure adequate opportunity for persons to free themselves from what are perceived to be the illiberal constraints of the past.[6] While informed consent in Japan is typically paternalistic and family-oriented, where patients may not even know their own diagnosis, much less personally consent to treatment, Western bioethics seeks legal requirements for patient-oriented confidentiality and informed consent to protect individual autonomous control over decision making, shielding personal information from spouses, children, parents, and other relatives.

Here one might consider the focus on education as the means to spread AIDS awareness, and thereby to slow transmission. In its 1986 report, "Confronting AIDS," the National Academy of Sciences argued that education is the most efficient and effective means to stem the tide of HIV infection. The Surgeon General of the United States concurred in his "Report on AIDS." Yet, what information was to be conveyed, who was its audience, whose moral views and which social values should be incorporated? Education is not neutral.

Debate concerned whether to teach abstinence, fidelity within heterosexual marriage, and refraining from drug use, or rather, to utilize graphic images and descriptions of "safe" sex practices (e.g., condom use), the means to avoid infection while injecting narcotics (e.g., cleaning and refusing to share needles), and the means to avoid bearing infected children (e.g., perinatal testing and elective abortion). The Task Force on Pediatric AIDS recommended that an important component of the anticipatory guidance pediatricians provide to young teens should include information about HIV transmission, implications of infection, strategies for prevention, and safer sex options for those electing to be sexually active. Parental permission was seen as desirable but unnecessary (1993; Committee on Adolescence, 1993).

More traditional Christians objected to the teaching of sexual pleasure outside of heterosexual marriage and the encouraging of women to seek abortions if they become pregnant. Moreover, they objected to the use of public resources, e.g., tax dollars, to endorse such practices. Critics retorted:

> It is unthinkable that religious, educational, and social institutions whose mission is to prepare youth to be good citizens and responsible adults and to be informed in the exercise of their moral agency, would be permitted to deprive them of knowledge essential to that mission and more important, knowledge that might save their lives (Bell, 1991, p. 150).

Such criticism, though, misses the point. While public awareness of safe sex practices, easily accessible, elective abortion, and needle usage appears to present value neutral medical information, such "instruction" inherently promotes the permissibility of certain practices, endorsing particular moral values over others.

It is not that religious communities do not understand the utility of such education; rather, its message is clearly very effective propaganda in support of values and practices contrary to their traditional beliefs. It combines a particular secular moral viewpoint with state resources and the powerful endorsements of the medical community and governmental institutions to promote social and ethical practices that are contrary to the survival of those cultural and religious communities.

Indeed, it even coercively taxes those very communities to advertise such alternative life-styles. Taxation to support what one knows to be deviant moral visions impoverishes one's ability to sustain one's own traditional religious understanding. As Lord Acton noted, writing in the late 19th century, private property is central to the preservation of liberty. It protects one's liberty of conscience regarding the use of oneself, one's talents, and abilities. Even when defense of conscience does not directly arise, property is always exposed to interference; it is the constant object of public policy (Acton, 1988, p. 572). To paraphrase John C. Calhoun, it enriches and strengthens those hostile to traditional cultures, practices, religions, while impoverishing and weakening those who would wish to pursue such ways of life (1992, p. 19).[7]

Proponents are fully aware of such civic education's significant propaganda potential. As Amy Gutmann comments:

> Some kinds of social diversity … are anathema to political liberalism. Civic education should educate all children to appreciate the public value of toleration. The basic political principles of liberalism, those necessary to protect every person's basic liberties and opportunities, place substantial limits on social diversity. … The limits on racial and gender discrimination, for example, enable many people to pursue ways of life that would otherwise be closed to them by discriminatory practices at the same time as they undermine or at least impede some traditional ways of life (1995, p. 559).

State-based education of children is viewed as crucial for redressing religious assumptions and moral viewpoints that are incompatible with the understanding of personal autonomous choice.

Similarly, Rawls argues:

> … a long and historic injustice to women is that they have borne, and continue to bear, a disproportionate share of the task of raising, nurturing, and caring for their children. … These injustices bear harshly not only on women, but also on their children and they tend to undermine children's capacity to acquire the political virtues required of future citizens in a viable democratic regime. Mill held that the family in his day was a school for male despotism: it inculcated habits of thought and ways of feeling and conduct incompatible with democracy. If so, the principles of justice enjoining democracy can plainly be invoked to reform it (2001, p. 166).

According to Rawls, state re-education of children is required to prepare the young "to be fully cooperating members of society and enable them to be self-supporting; it should also encourage the political virtues so that they want to honor the fair terms of social cooperation in their relations with the rest of society" (1993, p. 199). The political virtues, Rawls argues, include toleration and mutual respect, together with a sense of fairness and civility (1993, p. 122).[8] Such education teaches children "…such things as knowledge of their constitutional and civic rights … to insure that their continued membership [in their parent's religion] is not based simply on ignorance of their basic rights or fear of punishment for offenses that do not exist" (1993, p. 199).[9]

The family must be subject to significant governmental regulation to ensure proper attitudes and beliefs. As Rawls urges, the concern to support equal worth of liberty through fair equality of opportunity tends towards the dissolution of the family:

> The consistent application of the principle of fair opportunity requires us to view persons independently from the influences of their social position. But how far should this tendency be carried? It seems that even when fair equality of opportunity (as it has been defined) is satisfied, the family will lead to unequal chance between individuals .... Is the family to be abolished then? Taken by itself and given a certain primacy, the idea of equal opportunity inclines in this direction (1999, p. 448).

The dominant social and bioethical ethos begins with the presumption of the sovereignty of the individual, rather than the family, which in traditional forms, whether Christian or Japanese, and so forth, is pejoratively caricatured as an institution of repression, injustice, and despotism.

The challenges facing the sustaining of a particular bioethics, whether Christian, or Japanese, etc., based on traditional assumptions regarding the family, the place and significance of gender, sexuality, birth, copulation, and death, are readily apparent.

III. BIRTH, SEX, AND DRUGS

Despite its universalistic aspirations and promises of moral consensus, contemporary bioethics and biomedical analysis is characterized by marked departures from the moral conclusions of traditional cultures and religions. Rather than drawing peoples together though rational reflection and moral consensus, in its failure to recognize significant moral diversity, the liberal cosmopolitan political agenda of Western bioethics has widened the cultural and moral gap between the traditional and the post-traditional.

There is growing evidence, for example, that the reeducation endorsed by the liberal cosmopolitan vision has had a significant impact on traditional moral communities. Consider: In a 1999 survey by the *National Catholic Reporter*, approximately 72% of Catholics responded that one could be a good Catholic without following the Vatican's teaching on birth control; 65% believed that one could be a good Catholic without following the Vatican's teaching on divorce and remarriage; and 53% responded that one could be a good Catholic without following the Vatican's teaching on abortion. Nearly 50% reported that individual choice should be the final arbiter of the morality of abortion, homosexual activity, and sexual relations outside of marriage more generally. Indeed, 23% reported that one could be a good Catholic without even believing that Christ rose from the dead, and 38% without believing in the Transubstantiation of the Eucharist (D'Antonio, 1999). This data represents a striking departure from traditional belief and practice.

Two recent encyclical letters of the Pope of Rome signal recognition of these significant cultural shifts. In *Veritatis Splendor* the Roman Pontiff characterizes the anti-traditional character of much of contemporary moral reflection as marked by "an overall and systematic calling into question of traditional moral doctrine, on the basis of certain anthropological and ethical presuppositions" (1993, p. 8). In *Evangelium Vitae*, John Paul II places this difficulty within a major cultural crisis and a shift in the presuppositions of moral theory. "In the background there is the profound crisis of culture, which generates skepticism in relation to the very foundations of knowledge and ethics, and which makes it increasingly difficult to grasp clearly the meaning of what man is, the meaning of his rights and his duties" (1995, p. 21). As the Roman Catholic Pope recognizes, the result has been a significant transformation and fragmentation of culture, a fragmentation that sets the stage for the emergence of fundamental moral differences that divide morality into not merely different, but mutually antagonistic accounts of proper moral conduct.

To some degree such changes are due to shifting cultural attitudes regarding human reproduction, family life, and individual freedom, resulting in a new cultural climate that encourages embryo experimentation and third-party assisted reproduction, including use of donor gametes, embryo wastage, and elective abortion for fetal reduction or simple relief from unwanted children. More profoundly, such practices are generally perceived and publicly touted as compassionate and just. Each is endorsed in the name of scientific advancement, relief of suffering, reproductive choice, and individual fulfillment.

Abortion and infanticide, for example, are ever more cited as morally appropriate choices for parents regarding hemophilic or otherwise disabled newborns. Peter Singer has argued, for example, that life should be understood as a journey and that when the current prospects for that journey are seriously unfavorable it may be better for parents to choose not to let that journey continue. As a matter of compassion and dignity, they ought to be permitted to kill the fetus or infant and wait for a time when the outlook is more favorable. "Parents will grieve when a newborn child dies, just as when a pregnancy miscarries at a late stage, but in most cases they will be able to have another child, and if that child's prospects are better, both they and 'their child' will be better off in the long run" (Singer and Ratiu, 2001, p. 48). Certain lives are simply judged as not worth living.[10]

Prenatal diagnosis of Down's syndrome and hemophilia in many countries is nearly invariably followed by elective non-therapeutic abortion.[11] Moreover, failure to inform pregnant women of the possibility of non-therapeutic abortion has exposed genetic counselors to civil liability under the law of torts (Milunsky and Annas, 1976). Such suits typically allege malpractice on grounds of either "wrongful life" or "wrongful birth". Civil claims for "wrongful life" involve parental suit on behalf of the child alleging that his nonexistence would have been preferable to his current existence with defects, such that his existence is a wrong done to him as a result of the negligence of the genetic counselor. Under a wrongful birth civil suit, the parents allege emotional and financial harms associated with caring for a defective newborn, whom they would have chosen to abort if they had been informed of the appropriateness of the option. Such legally supported torts, require counselors to encourage patients to seek abortions based on quality-of-life judgments, even if in violation of deeply held religious convictions (Atkinson and Moraczewski, 1980, pp. 27-29).[12]

Such sentiments echo much contemporary United States law. In *Planned Parenthood v. Casey* (505 U.S. 833, 857-859 [1992]), the court held that in *Roe v. Wade* the significance of individual control over the self and to personal bodily integrity has been correctly applied to a woman's right to choose abortion: "… if *Roe* is seen as stating a rule of personal autonomy and bodily integrity, akin to cases recognizing limits on government power to mandate medical treatment or to bar its rejection, this court's post *Roe* decisions accord with *Roe's* view that a state's interest in the protection of life *falls short of justifying* any plenary override of individual liberty claims." Concerns to preserve the unborn living fetus, even in cases of late term, partial birth abortion, which require that enough of the fetus' head be delivered to allow its brain to be vacuumed out, prior to removing the now dead fetus, failed to satisfy the burden of proof necessary to override the significance of individual authority over one's body. Respect for individual freedom, they argued, is of greater significance than preserving life.

Unfettered access to abortion, including late-term partial birth abortion, has become central to arguments for gender equality:

> Would any of these men want to put the matter of their own reproductive organs in the hands of a woman's political caucus? ... Women who choose to end unwanted pregnancies deserve to be cared for with the same regard for their needs and their dignity as anybody else who seeks medical care. They needn't have to answer to the value judgments of others. Their decisions about their own bodies should be honored.
>
> That's precisely what I do. I honor and care for patients who want to end pregnancies. I'm an abortion doctor, and I refuse to mask my work in qualifications or apologies. What I do is right and good and important. Perhaps my story will appall some, but it also may inspire others, particularly the young women who need to know that the struggle between feminism and the patriarchy has not been in vain (Poppema, 1996, pp. 10-11).

Many contemporary Christian moralists have adopted a similar stance. As Beverly Harrison describes the challenges of abortion:

> We are only at the beginning of the public political dispute over procreative choice in human history. If we do not obliterate ourselves with other life-destructive technologies in the meanwhile, the abortion debate probably will continue in one form or another for decades, perhaps for generations. This is because all of the intricate social systems that characterize human life – our institutions, mores, and customs and all the varied religious sacralization of these systems through all recorded history – have been shaped inherently to control women's procreative power. This control will not be relinquished without a struggle (1983, p. 3).

The abortion debate is no longer about the beginnings and endings of life, or of the moral status of the embryo. Abortion has been fully recast within the guise of human dignity, social justice, and gender power struggles.

Maguire and Burtchaell argue, in addition, that the anti-abortion statements of the ancient traditional Christian Church must be placed fully within a particular cultural context:

> (1) All occurred before the beginning of any formal theology on abortion. (2) They rose from a period of ignorance of the processes of generation, the ovum having been discovered only in the nineteenth century. (3) They came at a time of under population. (4) They came in a time of notable sexism and negativity to sexuality. (5) Abortion was often condemned as a violation of the procreative nature of sex and not as murder (1998, p. 589).

This moral tradition, they urge, can only be adequately understood as part of a regrettable history of the oppression of women.

Indeed, openly affirming abortion to be intrinsically evil has come to be characterized as a form of social oppression.

> I understand oppression to mean any social situation that systematically requires heroism on the part of a class of people based on gender, race or other such identification. Given the gendered structure of society at present and the resultant lack of communal support for women, the absolute prohibition on taking the life of the fetus, however protective of the right to life of that fetus, remains oppressive of women (Whitmore, 1994, p. 14).[13]

Traditional metaphysical assumptions regarding the deep nature of reality, and their significant moral implications, are discounted, marginalized, set aside, and explained away.

Embryos and fetuses, even late term fetuses, cannot be experienced as persons from a general secular perspective, thus their interests are placed within and understood as instrumental to the interests of persons.[14] Thus, abortion, embryo wastage, research and disposal are generally sanctioned and nearly universally endorsed by the international bioethical community, as well as encouraged by governmental health care policy. Human embryo research has been heralded as very likely leading to significant new treatments for diabetes and Parkinson's disease, immunodeficiences, cancer, metabolic and genetic disorders, and a wide variety of birth defects, as well as being useful in generating new organs or tissues.[15] The necessary embryos are typically either generated through *in vitro* fertilization in the laboratory strictly for research purposes or are leftovers from IVF fertility treatments. Since such basic science will likely save lives, reduce suffering, and help to cure disease, from a general secular perspective, it appears decidedly immoral to fail to engage in such research.

In contrast, from a traditional Christian perspective, employing human embryos in research is a difficult and complex issue that is not resolved through such seemingly straightforward cost/benefit analysis. *In vitro* fertilization for the purpose of forming embryos, whether for procreation or research is morally illicit. As Engelhardt argues, "such fertilization removes the procreation of human life from the intimacy of marriage…." Moreover, "embryo research involves direct actions against an instance of human life. Although it may not be clear how to regard early embryonic life before it is or could have been in the womb, such life cannot be understood as merely disposable" (2000, p. 261). To treat embryos as merely instrumental and thus disposable is to engage in grave moral evil.

Employing material from dead embryos raises somewhat different issues. The use of embryonic tissues and cells from dead embryos is governed by similar moral considerations that govern the use of tissue from adult human beings.

> Under circumstances that allow the use of tissues and organs from persons who die accidentally, it is appropriate to use tissues and organs from fetuses who die accidentally. Under circumstances that allow the use of tissues and organs from persons who were murdered, it is similarly allowable to use tissues and organs from fetuses who have been aborted ..., from 'excess' embryos stored in *in vitro* fertilization clinics, or from embryos that have been formed to produce tissues and organs (p. 261).

Similar concerns are raised regarding use of knowledge derived from such research. One may not employ evil means, encourage their use, or avoid their condemnation; however, insofar as the information exists one may use it to good ends, provided that one is careful neither to endorse nor to encourage such illicit means. Regardless of the hoped for benefits, from a traditional Christian standpoint, one is never permitted to engage or encourage illicit circumstances or means. Here the social and political clash between the tradition and the post-traditional is stark and forceful.

Likewise, there is a growing endorsement of physician-assisted suicide and euthanasia to reducing human suffering and preserving human dignity. This call ranges from assisted-suicide for the terminally ill, to promotion of its availability for anyone who competently requests such treatment, to both voluntary and non-voluntary euthanasia for patients in a permanently vegetative state. Even optimal curative and palliative care cannot resolve all loss of personal control and all perceived loss of human dignity. As Gunderson and Mayo note, as a discipline bioethics generally holds that competent individuals have the right to determine their own fates. "The autonomy-based argument for physician-assisted death is straightforward: as illness begins to seriously compromise the quality of a person's life, few issues could be more profound and personal for that person than determining the point at which his or her life is no longer worth living" (2000, p.18). Analogous sentiments were expressed by the Ninth Circuit Court with respect to Oregon's Death with Dignity Act: "Those who believe strongly that death must come without physician assistance are free to follow that creed, be they doctors or patients. They are not free to force their views, their religious convictions, or their philosophies on all other members of a democratic society, and to compel those whose values differ from theirs to die painful, protracted, and agonizing deaths" (*Compassion in Dying v. State of Washington* 79 F 3d790 (9th cir 1996): 810-839 at 839). Compassion and love are emphasized as justifying physician-assisted killing in the face of irremediable and severe suffering. Such deaths are presented as alleviating the physical pain and mental anguish of those beyond effective therapy. Adversity can drain a person's life of meaning, and from this perspective the individual appears to have a right to determine when to end his own life.

While traditionally Christianity has always condemned suicide and assisted-suicide, as with abortion many contemporary Christians have begun following secular bioethics in adopting this non-traditional stance. In one survey of Protestant pastors, 17% supported laws in favor of assisted-suicide, with over 33% of those surveyed who were also associated with the National Council of Churches in favor (Christian Century 2000, pp. 948-949). According to Frasen and Walters, if quality of life is sufficiently minimal, assisted-suicide may be permissible since "... the traditional concept of life after death would seem to question the value of eking out every moment of life when the whole of existence goes far beyond temporal death. The Bible portrays a God who values quality of life" (2000). Or as Karen Lebacqz argues:

> And yet I am also a Christian. I know that death is not the last word, not the greatest evil. Failure to live, to care, to enact justice, to be in proper relationship – those are greater evils. Death can serve evil or it

> can serve the values of life. As a way of bringing about death, active euthanasia can serve evil or it can serve the values of life. When it serves the values of life, it can be morally justified (1998, p. 667).

Episcopal Bishop John S. Spong also favorably regards assisted suicide:

> My conclusions are based on the conviction that the sacredness of my life is not ultimately found in my biological extension. It is found rather in the touch, the smile, and the love of those to whom I can knowingly respond. When that ability to respond disappears permanently, so, I believe, does the meaning and the value of my biological life. Even my hope of life beyond biological death is vested in a living relationship with the God who, my faith tradition teaches me, calls me by name. I believe that the image of God is formed in me by my ability to respond to that calling Deity. If that is so, then the image of God has moved beyond my mortal body when my ability to respond consciously to that Divine Presence disappears. So nothing sacred is compromised by assisting my death in those circumstances (1996, pp. 3-4).

The Presbyterian Church (USA) has stepped back from absolute condemnation of euthanasia:

> "Active euthanasia" is extremely difficulty to defend morally. There are, however, extreme circumstances in which we may have to at least raise the question of a fundamental conflict of obligations. There is an analogy between such cases of "active euthanasia" and abortions, questions that are based on the circumstances of the fetus. There is an accompanying prejudice against the taking of life in both cases, since the conflict between doing no harm and protecting from harm has reference to one and the same individual. The ambiguity of this situation serves to reinforce what has already been said about cautious and consultative decision making (1981, p. 41).

In response to two cases, one involving a woman who committed suicide, the other a woman with seemingly suicidal intent who sought to end all medical care so that she would die, though with treatment she would likely live another fifteen to twenty years, a Presbyterian Minister stated: "But should we not also respond compassionately to a Diane or an Elizabeth, not condemning, but valuing a different kind of courage and faithfulness?" (Bay, 1995, p. 35). Death with dignity is likened to putting an animal out of its misery. Since we would surely aid an animal in pain, the argument concludes, we should extend the same compassion to human beings.

Incorporating a largely materialistic calculation of costs and benefits to assess quality of life, such conclusions accept without argument that the focal point of the moral life is autonomous self-determination, where liberty, as the celebration of free individualistic choice, is integral to the good life for persons. Endorsing freedom from constraint imposed on the pursuit of self-satisfaction and individual fulfillment, it simply accepts Western secular axiology: affirming no deep meaning to pain, disease, disability, suffering and death, beyond the firing of synapses, the collapse of human abilities, and the mere end of life. Human life is valued as at best instrumental, with meaning only to be found in the pleasures, beauty, and engagement of this life. From such a perspective: (1) elective abortion and infanticide protect social justice and the dignity of women; (2) embryo research reduces suffering, postpones death and promotes the "common good"; and (3) when life ceases to have significant individual meaning, physician-assisted suicide to limit suffering and preserve human freedom is simply a common sense compassionate solution that protects patient "dignity". Suffering can only be experienced as surd.

This is the central reason why most contemporary bioethical accounts are remarkably thin. Populated with the jargon of duty and obligation, autonomy, virtue, and beneficence, equality and social justice, but divorced from the metaphysical and epistemological foundations through which traditional religions and cultures ground deep meaning to life, suffering, and death, they encourage expansion of choice, elimination of suffering, and reduction of death, but are unable authoritatively to determine what choices to make, what kinds of suffering to eliminate, or which deaths to postpone.

IV. UNDENIABLE FOUNDATIONAL MORAL PLURALISM

The central challenge to the universal pretensions of bioethics is that the acrimonious bioethical controversies, such as abortion, cloning, embryo experimentation, and health care resource allocation, illustrate that within medicine there exists, as always, foundationally different accounts of the moral life. To ignore such differences so as to claim universal "moral consensus" and thereby to impose a particular moral vision, engages in what might be termed coercive moral colonialism. James Heisig notes, for example:

> On the face of it, there seems little to object to the establishing of general norms to insure distributive justice in critical medical care. On the one hand, we have the basic dignity of the human life; on the other, particular individuals of every shape and stripe, but all equal in their humanity. Hammer and anvil, these are, it would seem, tools enough with which to forge moral values of service to the whole of the human community. The only problem is, concrete human beings do not exist as particular examples of a general equation, and human life is nowhere to be found among the haphazard of items that make up the world. The particular and the universal are everywhere mediated by the specificity of human society, which cannot be abstracted from without forfeiting the concreteness of that which is being moralized about (2002, p. 303).

Here Hegel's account of why determinative moral content requires the specification of a particular context is illustrative: "Because every action explicitly calls for a particular content and a specific end, while duty as an abstraction entails nothing of the kind, the question arises: what is my duty? As an answer nothing is so far available except: (a) to do the right, and (b) to strive after welfare, one's own welfare, and welfare in universal terms, the welfare of others" (1967 [1821], § 134). Nothing particular follows from the general notions of duty, the right, and so forth.

Thus political struggles inevitably concern not merely which policies will best achieve desired objectives, but which objectives are themselves desirable; that is, which moral understanding should be established (e.g., pro-life or pro-choice, individualistic or family-oriented approaches to health care decision-making), utilizing which school of practice (allopathic, homeopathic, naturopathic, chiropractic, and so forth), at what standard of care (e.g., guaranteed equal access for all, or with regional deviations and varying levels of insurance coverage). Even to sort useful information from noise, one must already possess a moral sense, standards of evidence and inference. That is, one must first specify a particular moral context within which to make decisions. Removing or ignoring the theological and cultural particularities which mark religious and moral differences thereby eliminates any context for understanding and assessing the content and veracity of moral claims.

How then should public policy be crafted? Should one simply acquiesce to the personal preferences or deep moral intuitions of academic bioethicists, current biomedical convention, or claims to global moral consensus? Or should one seek moral content to guide public policy through appeal to intuitions, consequences, casuistry, the notion of unbiased choice, game theory, or middle-level principles? All such attempts, as Engelhardt has demonstrated, confront insurmountable obstacles: one must already presuppose a particular morality so as to choose among intuitions, rank consequences, evaluate exemplary cases, or mediate among various principles, otherwise one will be unable to make any rational choice at all. As he points out, even if one merely ranks cardinal moral concerns, such as liberty, equality, justice, and security differently, one affirms different moral visions, divergent understandings of the good life, varying senses of what it is to act appropriately (Engelhardt, 1996; 2000). In general secular terms, it is impossible to break through the seemingly interminable bioethical debates to univocal truth.

Claims to "global moral consensus" or to rationally discoverable moral truths are, therefore, implausible. Outside of an appeal to an all-encompassing moral and metaphysical viewpoint, outside of a particular moral context, moral truth appears deeply ambiguous. Without the presupposition of particular content, morality cannot distinguish among different accounts of the nature of the good life, much less provide definitive guidance on how to proceed when the right and the good conflict. Thus, the imposition of any particular moral content as the foundation of public policy begs the question. The inevitably post-modern character of contemporary bioethics is simply the recognition of the foundationally irresolvable character of such moral pluralism in general secular terms. Given such circumstances, the universalistic aspirations of contemporary bioethics simply beg the question.

Its aspirations are, however, especially insidious because they are subtly invasive, suggesting that one ought to side with the claims of "rationality", "expertise", and "consensus", i.e., with general secular bioethical "orthodoxy", over against what one may know in the fullness of a particular moral community to be true, while, at the same time, utilizing national and international legal coercion to eliminate the possibility of significant moral, religious, and cultural diversity in health care.

V. NEW FOUNDATIONS: INDIVIDUAL FREEDOM AND RESPONSIBILITY

The experience of post-modernity is the recognition that general secular reason does not transcend the diversity of moral visions, establishing one as uniquely true. Thus, substantial moral diversity inevitably defines the context for contemporary medical ethics and health care policy. The more general secular reason is unable to disclose a universal, coherent, content-full moral understanding of health care, or the justification for political authority to impose such a vision, the more one must seek alternative foundations.

One possibility is to ground secular moral authority in freedom as permission – i.e., freedom as a side-constraint. Resolution of moral controversies in medicine and health care policy will turn on whether the parties to any particular transaction have given consent. Here moral authority is not drawn from assertions of so-called "moral consensus," ideal theories of rational action, or even deep moral intuitions regarding consequences, human rights, or cardinal moral concerns, but rather from the agreement of the parties to collaborate. Collaborators need not agree regarding the background ranking of values or moral principles, cultural or religious assumptions; they need only affirm the content of their agreement. No value standard or order must be presumed, just the recognition that collaboration is possible through agreement. Agreement or permission is the ground of the moral justification of such collaboration.

Here the market is central for understanding authoritative human interaction. Market transactions and contractual relationships draw moral authority from the consent of the participants to be bound by their agreement. The parties to the transactions, themselves, freely convey authority to the enforcement of the specified conditions. Moral authority to interfere in the free interaction of consenting persons is created by, and thus limited to, the actual agreements of actual persons. Freedom as a side-constraint, as expressed in the existence of significant forbearance rights, where persons are free to venture with others, open to the possibility that one's choices may lead to success or failure, will support the existence of a free-market in health care. Forbearance rights create strong protections against battery, i.e., nonconsensual touching or use of one's person or property, defining a sphere in which one is morally immune from interference, protecting self-interest and self-preservation in the private use of person and property. Such rights describe side-constraints prohibiting nonconsensual interference, which hold against other persons, as well as society and state.

Such an understanding of freedom grounds significant property rights, where persons have exclusive control of their property, subject only to the constraints of prior agreements and the avoidance of using persons, and their property, who do not choose to participate.[16] Alienation, whether through abandonment, donation, exchange, or sale, is morally licit only if freely chosen. Provided that both vendor and purchaser freely agree to the transaction, property may be utilized for fun, beneficence, or profit, including the financing and purchase of health care. Absent actual agreement, rights as side-constraints defeat the claims of others, persons and governments, to have any entitlement to the time, talent, or property of individuals. Particular values or special considerations, such as fair equality of opportunity, benefits to others, or judgments of irrational choice, fail to establish moral authority either to create universal health care systems or to forbid consensual transactions for various types and standards of health care, shaped by varying moral commitments and taken-for-granted background assumptions.

For example, individuals, families, or communities would be free to contract for (1) various types of health care (e.g., allopathic, homeopathic, naturopathic, chiropractic, etc.), with (2) particular standards of care (e.g., regional variations and varying levels of insurance coverage), (3) shaped through divergent moral commitments and (4) framing presuppositions regarding health care practices (e.g., individual vs. family or community oriented consent, or varying concepts of health and disease (Cherry, 2000b; Sadegh-Zadeh, 2000). Imposition of all-encompassing uniform systems of health care, guarantees of equality in the provision of health care services, and the search for global standards regarding the foundations of health care policy violate such basic human freedoms and forbearance rights expressed as market rights.

The rights of persons will foreclose what many envision to be worthwhile goals. Forbearance rights recognize persons as only entitled to their own private resources and those additional resources that they are able peaceably to convince others to donate or sell to them. Basic human rights to health care, much less to the general amelioration of losses due to bad luck, individual choice, disease, ill health, or other misfortunes, do not exist.[17] Seen in this light, financing personal health care choices through coercive taxation, clearly forces those with substantive ethical commitments or content-full understandings of the good life, religious or secular, to be complicit in the purchase of health care services which they hold to be at best deviant (e.g., chiropractic or naturopathic health care), if not evil (e.g., abortion or embryo-research). Insofar as freedom is not merely one value among others, or a good which may be valued more or less along with other goods, but rather functions as a side-constraint, one may not injure, steal from, tax, defraud or otherwise coerce unconsenting others, even to produce good consequences. This would violate their status as free and responsible agents. One may not utilize persons, absent actual permission, as the means to benefit others.

Governments, even democratically elected majorities, do not possess moral authority to enforce uniform standards, to finance universal access or to regulate equal distribution of health care. Morally authorized statutes are confined to the protection of persons' rights to forbearance, protection of individuals from battery, and to those additional policies to which actual persons give actual consent. Persons, and organizations of persons, may be held responsible for nonconsensual acts of violence, fraud, and breach of contract, since such actions violate the rights of persons not to be touched or used without permission.[18] Governmental authority created by the express agreement of those governed is also limited to the extent of such agreement. So grounded, the state would have the general character of a limited democracy. It would have no general moral authority to interfere in the medical marketplace. Forbearance rights make implausible interventions to forbid persons from freely using personal resources with consenting others, including the purchase of various types and levels of health care. Note, though, that the market is not being endorsed as a good in itself, nor are free choice and moral diversity celebrated in themselves as special goods. Rather, the market defines social space for peaceable consensual human interaction in all aspects of life. It is a marketplace of ideas, moral visions, and understandings, in which one peaceably pursues what one perceives as good with free and consenting others.

Respecting the freedom of persons defaults to protecting liberties of association, contract, conscience, and religion, and thereby to protecting the possibility of substantial moral diversity. Freely chosen, market-based health care financing, procurement, and distribution, respect the liberty of persons to pursue their own deep moral commitments. Unlike the cosmopolitan lip-service paid to the value of moral pluralism, freedom as a side-constraint carves out and protects social space for the possibility of moral diversity in health care. Blanket prohibitions on health care practices among consenting individuals, universal bioethical declarations, violations of foundational religious and cultural beliefs, and paternalistic governmental decisions – in short, the tyrannous imposition of a particular secular bioethical orthodoxy – are unjustified. Such restrictions straightforwardly beg the question, assuming the very moral content that they must prove. They thereby foreclose rather than enhance the possibility of moral diversity in health care, making it impossible to develop or sustain, as many might wish, a particular bioethical understanding, whether Christian, Japanese or so forth.

St. Edward's University
Austin, Texas, USA

NOTES

[1] The continuing influence of Western bioethics on traditional Japanese bioethics can be seen, for example, in the approach to HIV and AIDS treatment. Consent is becoming much more individual, rather than family, oriented. "HIV+ and AIDS patients seldom disclose the nature of their illness even to their family and intimate friends in Japan. They thus feel very lonely and need a great deal of support medically, physically, mentally, emotionally, socially and economically. Those who do not wish to disclose their illness cannot take advantage of their medical insurance benefit because the type of illness is stated in insurance records. There is no guarantee of confidentiality with the transaction of insurance records" (Hoshino, 1995b, p. 308).

[2] Its authoritative judgment is sought on nearly all aspects of life: from copulation and birth, to appropriate diet, sexual behaviors, and methods of child-rearing, to abortion, infanticide, suffering, and death. This is often referred to as the medicalization of life (Skrabanek, 1994, p. 146).

[3] For more detailed analysis of a market in human organs for transplantation see Cherry 2000a.

[4] For instance, Namihira, citing traditional understandings of personal and bodily identity, remarks that there exists significant resistance to organ procurement for transplantation in Japanese culture. "In the case of a cadaver organ transplant, an organ must be removed from the body before those procedures by means of which the identity of the body in life is altered by cremation and the family of the dead openly acknowledge the metamorphosis and decay of the body. ...for Japanese people the cremation is not only the way of disposing of a dead body, but also a way to change the identity of the body from living to dead. In traditional Japanese thinking cremation is a way of changing the life time identity rather than disposing of it. Therefore, for Japanese people, removing an organ from a dead body before such procedures have taken place represents a failure to create a new bodily identity for the dead person" (Namihira, 1997, p. 68).

[5] Consider the increasing integration of the religion-non-specific, denominationally neutral, generic chaplain into the health care services of many hospitals. As Engelhardt documents:

"They have been hired to provide spiritual care, but the nature of that care is left strategically under-defined. Were the spiritual care specifically defined in denominational terms, it would take on a particular religious, that is, exclusionary character. But the latter is not the care sought from chaplaincy services by many hospitals. Instead, the chaplain is expected to attend to a patient population drawn from many religions, Christian and non-Christian, as well as those fully unchurched. Ministers who were once ordained in particular religions are reprofessionalized into trans-denominational roles" (Engelhardt, 1998, p. 32). Institutional expectations reshaped content-full vocational commitments into the content-empty role of generic chaplains.

6 For detailed analysis of informed consent within traditional cultures, see Alora and Lumitao (2001).

7 John C. Calhoun noted that "The effect, then, of every increase is, to enrich and strengthen the one and impoverish and weaken the other. This, indeed, may be carried to such an extent, that one class or portion of the community may be elevated to wealth and power, and the other depressed to abject poverty and dependence, simply by the fiscal action of the government; and this too, through disbursements only – even under a system of equal taxes imposed for revenue only. If such may be the effect of taxes and disbursements, when confined to their legitimate objects – that of raising revenue for the public service – some conception may be formed, how one portion of the community may be crushed, and another elevated on its ruins, by systematically perverting the power of taxation and disbursement, for the purpose of aggrandizing and building up one portion of the community at the expense of the other" (1992, p. 19).

Taxing traditional Christians for support of abortion rights, civic education to support political liberalism, toleration for alternate lifestyles, and so forth, enhances the liberty of those who oppose traditional Christianity at the expense of the Christian community.

8 Here one might also consider Habermas' position that the creation of egalitarian universalism requires institutionalized procedures and protections that go beyond and bind even nation states. "Of course, the conditions for political action must be fulfilled. And this requirement can give rise to doubts about even such a solution. Under the privileged economic and social conditions of the post-war period, the citizens of the OECD countries may in fact have had and used the opportunity to commit themselves to a project which was in *harmony* with the principles of the *existing* constitutional order. This was the project of realizing the equal value of equal liberties for everybody. But Hegel's problem returns in a different form, when we consider those societies where the immaculate wording of the constitution provides no more than a symbolic facade for a highly selective legal order. In such countries social reality controverts the validity of norms which cannot be implemented for lack of the material preconditions, and the necessary political will. ...This will happen if we do not produce a new balance between globalized markets and a politics which can extend beyond the limits of the nation state, and yet still retain democratic legitimacy. ...A solution can be expected only from a constellation in which the institutionalized principles of an egalitarian universalism could acquire sufficient impetus" (1999, p. 153; see also 2000).

9 An editorial in the Roman Catholic periodical *America* argued in the same vein that traditional Christianity, which casts Mary as the ideal feminine, contributes to the oppression and subservience of women:

> … the tradition that casts Mary as the ideal feminine paradoxically does a disservice to women. In the traditional model (which relies heavily on the notion of complementarity), men are viewed as essentially intelligent, assertive, independent and decisive, and

therefore equipped by nature for 'leadership in the public realm.' Women, on the other hand (drawing on traditional Marian imagery), should be possessed of a nurturing, gentle nature fit primarily for the 'private domain' of childrearing, homemaking or caring for the vulnerable. One weakness of this model is that it denies women the possibility of developing a personality that could include other characteristics – for example, those necessary for leadership in the community. ... There is, Professor Johnson argues, no essential feminine nature. One could conclude that women are as free as men to serve in leadership roles ("A Church of Women", editorial June 17-24, 2000).

Traditional knowledge and respect of Mary as the Theotokos is evidently to be shunned by the post-modern, post-traditional Christian.

10 In response to a possible counter-example in which being born male in a particular society was sufficient to ensure that a child will lead a miserable life, a life judged not worth living, Peter Singer stated: "But if this were the case – and there were nothing one could do about it – then I would indeed accept that the parents of newborn males should be allowed to kill them painlessly, so as to be able to raise a girl" (1993, p. 162).

11 While British Cypriot families had once chosen to remain childless or ceased reproduction after the birth of a child affected with thalassaemia major, following the introduction of prenatal diagnosis in 1975, virtually normal reproduction was resumed by at-risk families. Genetic testing coupled easily with abortion (Bobrow and Manners, 1994, p. 23).

12 Consider, for example, *Tina Smedley Reed, et al. v. Mary Campagnolo, et al.* Civil no. 1-91-512, United States District Court for the District of Maryland (810 f. Supp. 167; 1993 U.S. Dist. lexis 245) in which the plaintiffs sought damages resulting from the birth of their child who suffers from genetic birth defects. The plaintiffs contended that the physicians failed to inform Mrs. Reed of the existence and need for prenatal testing, which would have revealed the child's defects in utero. Mrs. Reed's claim was that she would have then terminated her pregnancy.

In *Phillips v. United States*, 508 F. Supp. 544 (D.S.C. 1981), the court held that based on "both the trend of authorities and the applicable policy considerations," (at 551), a claim predicated upon the alleged failure to provide adequate genetic counseling and prenatal testing did present a viable cause of action predicated upon negligence or medical malpractice. See also *Robak v. United States*, 658 F.2d 471 (7th Cir. 1981) (applying Alabama law); *Gildiner v. Thomas Jefferson Univ. Hosp.*, 451 F. Supp. 692 (E.D.Pa. 1978); *Turpin v. Sortini*, 119 Cal.App.3d 690, 174 Cal.Rptr. 128 (Ct.App. 1981); *Schroeder v. Perkel*, 87 N.J. 53, 432 A.2d 834 (1981); *Berman v. Allan*, 80 N.J. 421, 404 A.2d 8 (1979); *Becker v. Schwartz*, 46 N.Y.2d 401, 386 N.E.2d 807, 413 N.Y.S.2d 895 (1978); *Jacobs v. Theimer*, 519 S.W.2d 846 (Tex. 1975); *Dumer v. St. Michael's Hosp.*, 69 Wis.2d 766, 233 N.W.2d 372 (1975). In short, the court held that "society has an interest in insuring that genetic testing is properly performed and interpreted" (*Gildiner v. Thomas Jefferson Univ. Hosp.*, 451 F. Supp. 692, 696 [E.D.Pa. 1978]).

13 "Women need the freedom to make reproductive decisions not merely to vindicate a right to be left alone, but often to strengthen their ties to others: to plan responsibly and have a family for which they can provide, to pursue professional or work commitments made to the outside world, or to continue supporting their families or communities" (West, 1990, p. 104).

14 On the strict secular sense of being a person see Engelhardt, 1996, pp. 135ff.

15 According to the British Medical Journal, the United Kingdom has granted its first embryo research licenses. As Mayer documents, human embryonic stem cells are useful because they are very primitive – they have the potential to develop into any type of cell in the body. Stem

cell therapy is believed to be effective in treating diseases such as diabetes and Parkinson's, but it has been difficult to produce enough cells to treat even one patient (Mayor, 2002).

The American Academy of Pediatrics Committee on Pediatric Research and the Committee on Bioethics have also recently endorsed human embryo research.

> Recently, several investigators have successfully isolated and cultured pluripotent stem cells from frozen human embryos donated by couples who had previously undergone in vitro fertilization and whose additional embryos were no longer clinically needed. Concrete benefits for children resulting from pluripotent stem cell research with human embryos are anticipated, including treatments for spinal cord and bone injuries, diabetes, primary or acquired immunodeficiencies, cancer, metabolic and genetic disorders, and a variety of birth defects. Research with human embryos that involves drug or toxin testing could benefit children suffering from toxicities of drug treatment and environmental pollutants as well as prenatal drug use disorders, such as fetal alcohol syndrome. Research using material derived from embryos also could be used in the study of normal and abnormal differentiation and development, which could benefit children with birth defects, genetically derived malignancies, and certain genetic disorders.
>
> An important long-term benefit of research using human embryos can be found in the field of teratology. Experiments that involve exposing pregnant mice to a teratogen at specific times after mating and observing the resulting defects have demonstrated that early exposure can result in very specific developmental defects. Other research on mouse embryos has advanced the ability to evaluate gene function in the early embryo. In the future, it may be possible to combine these approaches to obtain important insights into teratogenesis in humans. Specifically, there is the future prospect of studying the expression of specific genes in embryonic cell lines exposed in vitro to teratogens. Such research could potentially provide insights into the approximately 40% of anatomic defects in infants for which there are currently no explanations (2001, p. 814).

[16] Blackstone, reflecting on the common law of England, argued: "There is nothing which so generally strikes the imagination and engages the affections of mankind, as the right of property; or that sole and despotic dominion which one man claims and exercises over the external things of the world, in total exclusion of the right of any other individual in the universe (1803, book 2, p. 1). The nature of property rights, their character, scope, and form, was drawn from the nature of persons. Under the traditional law of torts, the person includes any part of the body as well as anything attached to it and practically identified with it. Violation of a person included nonconsensual contact with the individual's "… clothing, or with a cane, a paper, or any other object held in his hand …" (Prosser, 1971, p. 34). Interest in the integrity of the person included his body and all the things intimately associated with it. As such, property is an extension of the person and is protected as part of the individual's forbearance rights against battery, unauthorized touching or use.

[17] Note, such an account is consistent with understanding persons as free to choose to participate in insurance schemes which create welfare rights for the poor, ill, or disadvantaged, however "disadvantaged" is defined. One could imagine Atheistcare as including rights to third-party assisted reproduction, human cloning, abortion, organ vending for transplantation, and assisted-suicide, to protect those "disadvantaged" is such areas of life, while members of Vaticare might accept lower standards of care in deference to providing more care or equal care for the poor. State authority would not exist to force insurance plans to offer compatible comprehensive levels of coverage. In general, it would be

an illicit use of force to compel either participation or taxpayer financing of any such scheme, even through majority democratic rule. The moral authority to interfere with such rights is limited to peaceable consent among persons and communities.

18 As Locke notes, governments which use the property of their citizens without permission are conceptually no different than thieves: "Wherever law ends, tyranny begins, if the law be transgressed to another's harm; and whosoever in authority exceeds the power given him by the law, and makes use of the force he has under his command to compass that upon the subject which the law allows not, ceases in that to be a magistrate, and acting without authority may be opposed, as any other man who by force invades the right of another. This is acknowledged in subordinate magistrates. He that hath authority to seize my person in the street may be opposed as a thief and a robber if he endeavours to break into my house to execute a writ, notwithstanding that I know he has such a warrant and such a legal authority as will empower him to arrest me abroad. And why this should not hold in the highest, as well as in the most inferior magistrate, I would gladly be informed. Is it reasonable that the eldest brother, because he has the greatest part of his father's estate, should thereby have a right to take away any of his younger brothers' portions? Or that a rich man, who possessed a whole country, should from thence have a right to seize, when he pleased, the cottage and garden of his poor neighbour? The being rightfully possessed of great power and riches, exceedingly beyond the greatest part of the sons of Adam, is so far from being an excuse, much less a reason for rapine and oppression, which the endamaging another without authority is, that it is a great aggravation of it. For exceeding the bounds of authority is no more a right in a great than a petty officer, no more justifiable in a king than a constable. But so much the worse in him as that he has more trust put in him, is supposed, from the advantage of education and counsellors, to have better knowledge and less reason to do it, having already a greater share than the rest of his brethren" (1690, §202).

REFERENCES

___ (2000). 'A church of women', editorial, *America*, June 17-24.

___ (2000). 'Protestant pastors support death penalty.' *Christian Century*, September 27-October 4, 948-949.

121st General Assembly of the Presbyterian Church in the United States (1981). 'The nature and value of human life.' In: *In Life and Death We Belong to God*, Christian Faith and Life Area, Congregational Ministries Division, PC (USA). Louisville: Presbyterian Distributions Services.

Acton, L. (1988). *Essays in Religion, Politics, and Morality.* J. Rufus Fears (Ed.). Indianapolis: Liberty Classics.

Alora, A. and J. Lumitao (Eds.) (2001) *Beyond a Western Bioethics: Voices from the Developing World.* Washington, D.C.: Georgetown University Press.

American Academy of Pediatrics Committee on Adolescence (1993). 'Homosexuality and adolescence.' *Pediatrics* 92, 631-634.

American Academy of Pediatrics Committee on Pediatric Research and Committee on Bioethics (2001). 'Human embryo research.' *Pediatrics* 108 (3), 813-817.

Atkinson, G. and A. Moraczewski (Eds.) (1980). *Genetic Counseling, the Church & the Law; A Task Force Report of the Pope John Center.* St. Louis: Pope John XXIII Medical-Moral Research and Education Center.

Bay, E. (1995). 'The Christian faith and euthanasia.' In: *In Life and Death We Belong to God,* Christian Faith and Life Area, Congregational Ministries Division, PC (USA). Louisville: Presbyterian Distributions Services.

Bell, N. (1991). 'Ethics issues in AIDS education.' In: F. Reamer (Ed.). *AIDS & Ethics.* New York: Columbia University Press.

Blackstone, W. (1803). *Commentaries on the Laws of England.* G. Tucker (Ed.). New York: Augustus M. Kelley Publishers. South Hckensack, N.J.: Rothman Reprints, Inc.

Bobrow, M. and E. Manners (1994). 'The social consequences of advances in the clinical applications of genetics.' In: I. Robinson (Ed.), *Life and Death Under High Technology Medicine.* Manchester, UK: Manchester University Press.

Calhoun, J. C. (1992). *Union and Liberty: The Political Philosophy of John C. Calhoun,* R. Lence (Ed.). Indianapolis: Liberty Classics.

Cherry, M. (2000a). 'Is a market in human organs necessarily exploitative?' *Public Affairs Quarterly* 14(4), 337-360.

Cherry, M. (2000b). 'Polymorphic medical ontologies: Fashioning concepts of disease.' *The Journal of Medicine and Philosophy* 25, 519-538.

D'Antonio, W.V. (1999). 'Trends in U.S. Roman Catholic attitudes, beliefs, behavior.' *National Catholic Reporter* October 29.

Engelhardt, H.T., Jr. (1996). *The Foundations of Bioethics.* New York: Oxford University Press.

Engelhardt, H.T., Jr. (1998). 'Generic chaplaincy: Providing spiritual care in a post-Christian age.' *Christian Bioethics* 4(3), 231-238.

Engelhardt, H.T., Jr. (2000). *The Foundations of Christian Bioethics.* Lisse: Swets and Zeitlinger.

Frasen S. and J. Walters (2000)., 'Death – Whose decision? Euthanasia and the terminally ill.' *Journal of Medical Ethics* 26(2), 121-126.

Gunderson, M. and D. Mayo (2000). 'Restricting physician-assisted death to the terminally ill.' *Hastings Center Report* 30 (6), 17-23.

Gutmann, A. (1995). 'Civic education and social diversity.' *Ethics* 105, 557-579.

Habermas, J. (1999). 'From Kant to Hegel and back again – The move towards detranscendentalization.' *European Journal of Philosophy* 7(2), 129-157.

Habermas, J. (2000). 'From Kant to Hegel: On Robert Brandom's pragmatic philosophy of language.' *European Journal of Philosophy* 8(3), 322-355.

Harrison, B. (1983). *Our Right to Choose: Toward a New Ethic of Abortion.* Boston: Beacon Press.

Hegel, G.W.F. (1967[1821]). *Philosophy of Right.* T.M. Knox (Trans.). New York: Oxford University Press.

Heisig, J. (2002). 'Catholicizing health.' In: H.T. Engelhardt and M.J. Cherry (Eds.), *Allocating Scarce Medical Resources: Roman Catholic Perspectives.* Washington, D.C.: Georgetown University Press.

Hoshino, K. (1995a). 'Gene therapy in Japan: Current trends.' *Cambridge Quarterly of Healthcare Ethics* 4, 367-370.

Hoshino, K. (1995b). 'HIV+ /AIDS related bioethics issues in Japan.' *Bioethics* 9 (3/4), 303-308.

Hoshino, K. (ed.) (1997a). *Japanese and Western Bioethics: Studies in Moral Diversity.* Dordrecht: Kluwer Academic Publishers.

Hoshino, K. (1997b). 'Bioethics in the light of Japanese sentiments.' In: K. Hoshino (Ed.), *Japanese and Western Bioethics: Studies in Moral Diversity* (pp. 13-24). Dordrecht: Kluwer Academic Publishers.

John Paul II (1993). *Veritatis Splendor*. Vatican City: Libreria Editrice Vaticana.

John Paul II (1995). *Evangelium Vitae*. Vatican City: Libreria Editrice Vaticana.

Lebacqz, K. (1991). 'Reflection.' In: R. Hamel (Ed.), *Active Euthanasia, Religion and the Public Debate*. Philadelphia: Trinity Press International. Reprinted in S. Lammers and A. Verhey (Eds.), *On Moral Medicine*, 2nd ed., Grand Rapids, MI: Eerdmans.

Locke, J. (1980 [1690]). *Second Treatise of Government*. C.B. Macpherson (ed.). Indianapolis: Hackett Publishing Co.

Maguire, D. and J. Burtchaell (1998). 'The Catholic legacy and abortion: A debate.' In: S. Lammers and A. Verhey (Eds.), *On Moral Medicine*, 2nd ed. Grand Rapids, MI: Eerdmans.

Mayor, S. (2002). 'United Kingdom grants first embryo research licenses.' *British Medical Journal* 324 (7337), 562.

Milunsky, A. and G. Annas (1976). 'Prenatal diagnosis of genetic disorders: An analysis of experience with 600 cases.' *Journal of the American Medical Association* 230, 232.

Namihira, E. (1997). 'The characteristics of Japanese concepts and attitudes with regard to human remains.' In: K. Hoshino (Ed.), *Japanese and Western Bioethics: Studies in Moral Diversity* (pp. 61-72). Dordrecht: Kluwer Academic Publishers.

National Academy of Sciences (1986). *Confronting AIDS: Directions for Public Health, Health Care, and Research*. Washington, D.C.: National Academy Press.

Nuffield Council on Bioethics (1995). *Human Tissue: Ethical and Legal Issues*, London: Nuffield Council.

Poppema, S. T. (1996). *Why I am an Abortion Doctor*. Amherst: Prometheus Books.

Prosser, W. (1971). *Law of Torts*. St. Paul: West Publishing Co.

Rawls, J. (1993). *Political Liberalism*. New York: Columbia University Press.

Rawls, J. (1999). *A Theory of Justice*. Cambridge: Belknap.

Rawls, J. (2001). *Justice as Fairness: A Restatement*. E. Kelly (Ed.). Cambridge: Harvard University Press.

Sadegh-Zadeh, K. (2000). 'Fuzzy health, illness, and disease.' *The Journal of Medicine and Philosophy* 25, 605-638.

Scott, R. (1981). *The Body as Property*. New York: Viking Press.

Scott, R. (1990). 'The human body: Belonging and control.' *Transplantation Proceedings* 22, 1002-1004.

Singer, P. (1993). 'More on euthanasia: A response to Pauer-Studer.' *Monist* 76 (2), 158.

Singer, P. and P. Ratiu (2001). 'The ethics and economics of heroic surgery.' *Hastings Center Report* 31 (2), 47-48.

Skrabanek, P. (1994). *The Death of Humane Medicine and the Rise of Coercive Healthism*. Suffolk: The Social Affairs Unit.

Spong, J. (1996). 'In defense of assisted suicide.' *The Voice of the Diocese of Newark*, January/February, 3-4.

Task Force on Pediatric AIDS (1993). 'Adolescents and the human immunodeficiency virus infection: The role of the pediatrician in prevention and intervention.' *Pediatrics* 92, 626-630.

Transplantation Society (1970). 'Statement of the committee on morals and ethics of the Transplantation Society.' *Annals of Internal Medicine* 75, 631-633.

West, R. (1990). 'Taking freedom seriously.' *Harvard Law Review*, 104-143.

Whitmore, T. (1994). 'Notes for a "new, fresh compelling" statement.' *America* 171 (10), 14.

World Health Organization (1991). 'Human organ transplantation. A report on the developments under the auspices of the WHO.' *International Digest of Health Legislation* 42, 389-396.

RUIPING FAN

RECONSTRUCTIONIST CONFUCIANISM AND BIOETHICS: A NOTE ON MORAL DIFFERENCE

I. TAKING A CUE FROM KAZUMASA HOSHINO: MORAL REFLECTION IN THE PACIFIC RIM HAS A CHARACTER OF ITS OWN

At the threshold of the 21st century, despite the cultural catastrophes of the 20th century, China, Japan, and the Pacific Rim generally have a sense of moral deportment, medical ethics, and health care policy radically different from that undergirding the bioethics of America and Western Europe. This difference can be traced to numerous sources. In this note, I address one of these sources: Confucianism. Most particularly, I argue how Confucianism properly understood can not only explain these differences, but show how these differences can serve as a cultural resource. They can supply the basis for a vigorous new bioethics with ancient roots in the Pacific Rim. I approach this challenge through a proposal for the reinvigoration of Confucian thought under the title of "Reconstructionist Confucianism". By this I mean to bring together a number of sentiments and insights drawn from the Confucian tradition, which are regaining a voice around the Pacific Rim not only in China, but also in South Korea, Singapore, and Japan. These have focused on the goal of recapturing an authentic understanding of Confucian life, drawing out its implications for bioethics and health care policy.

Reconstructionist Confucianism is a constructive response to anti-Confucian thought of various types. Following the Opium War in the mid-19th century, Chinese intellectuals increasingly laid the blame for the failure of China in dealing with the aggression of Western industrialized countries at the feet of Confucianism. The anti-Confucian passion found its expression in the May Fourth Movement in 1919 in the notorious slogan – "down with the Confucian house." This slogan continued to have force throughout the century. In the first part of the 20th century, all newly introduced fashionable "isms" in Chinese society – such as Darwinism, positivism, pragmatism, anarchism, Nietzschism, and Marxism – construed Confucianism as a reactionary ideology grounded in

H.T. Engelhardt, Jr. and L.M. Rasmussen (eds.), Bioethics and Moral Content: National Traditions of Health Care Morality, 281–287.

China's feudalistic past that should be abandoned as a whole. The anti-Confucian movement reached its peak in the Chinese Marxists' cultural revolution in the latter part of the 20th century. Not only have almost all social institutions based on Confucian values been ruthlessly destroyed; Confucian symbolism has taken on a character of ill repute. Meanwhile, the efforts of a small group of Neo-Confucian scholars to defend a recast account of Confucianism have achieved little success (Alitto, 1986).

Reconstructionist Confucianism is committed to the recapturing of authentic Confucian community in the Pacific Rim. Reflecting on the Confucian way of life after its being marginalized and ridiculed for more than a century in China, Reconstrunctionist Confucianism finds its ideals and values nevertheless worth cherishing and reconstructing for contemporary society. Unlike traditional Confucianism, Reconstructionist Confucianism recognizes that it is being articulated in a moral and political environment in many ways hostile to Confucianism. It notices as well that contemporary Neo-Confucianism is increasingly adept at retranslating the commitments of Confucianism so as to reshape them in non-Confucian, modern Western terms. More specifically, contemporary Neo-Confucianism has reshaped Confucianism in terms of the requirements of modern Western liberal social-democratic theory.

Unlike Neo-Confucianism, Reconstructionist Confucianism affirms the following five points as cardinal to understanding and pursuing the truth of Confucian views. These five points lie at the foundations of a Confucian morality and bioethics.

1. Reconstructionist Confucianism considers any attempt to read into classical Confucianism social-democratic concerns with liberty, equality, and human rights as a form of naive presentism. Such attempts involve an illicit reconstruction of the past.
2. Reconstructionist Confucianism also judges any attempt to recast core Confucian commitments in liberal social-democratic concerns as incompatible with the fundamental commitments of Confucianism. Cardinal Confucian concepts (such as *ren* and *li*) presuppose understandings of morality and justice that are not reducible without loss of meaning to social-democratic concerns with equality, justice, and human rights.
3. Reconstructionist Confucianism holds that it provides a more ample account of human flourishing and morality than that offered by other accounts including social-democratic moral and political

theory. It is family-oriented, *junzi*-oriented, and virtue-oriented. The individual is encouraged to living out a Confucian way of family life through cultivating virtue and becoming a *junzi*, an exemplary person of good character and moral integrity.

4. Reconstructionist Confucianism recognizes Confucian thought not as a return to the past but as an approach for the realization of the future. Confucianism is not an antique stage of human development, but an answer to the social and political problems associated with so-called modernization.
5. Reconstructionist Confucianism calls for reconstructing social institutions through reformulating public policy in accordance with fundamental Confucian concerns and commitments.

These five points frame a moral perspective structured around philosophical, normative and metaethical commitments different from those underpinning the liberal social democratic moral-political accounts of the West.

II. THE CHARACTERISTICS OF A RECONSTRUCTIONIST CONFUCIAN BIOETHICS

A bioethics grounded in a Reconstructionist Confucianism in a number of important points differs in its commitments from a bioethics lodged within the dominant liberal Western European and American paradigm. Three points deserve special attention.

1. Reconstructionist Confucian bioethics is family-oriented. Confucians take the family as their primary moral community in society. There is a familialist focus on health care as well as health care decision-making.
2. Reconstructionist Confucian bioethics is *junzi*-oriented. The term *junzi* is used from the Chinese because, as with all of the cardinal concepts in Confucianism, there is no exact equivalent in Western concepts. Though *junzi* has some family resemblances with the Western notion of a gentleman, its meaning is distinctly different. The character of being a *junzi* encourages scholars, physicians, and all health care providers to play a role of noble character and moral integrity in guiding health care policy, practice and decision-

making. In particular, they ought to pursue the Confucian ideal of sagehood.

3. Reconstructionist Confucian bioethics is virtue-oriented. It understands that the moral life, including correct bioethical action, is embedded in an encompassing way of life that nurtures human character and function. The Confucian virtues are those excellent human traits that manifest harmonious human relationships as well as appropriate human conduct. Particular moral goods and moral principles are understood in terms of these virtues, which are in turn understood in terms of an integrated way of life (Confucius, 1971; Mencius, 1970).

These commitments of a Confucian moral account are grounded in the claim that it is only in this way of life that true human flourishing can be realized. In other moral accounts, cardinal human goods are either illicitly reduced to instrumental values or treated in a way that distorts their significance. Thus, for example, liberal individualist accounts of human flourishing reduce the communal good of the family to the good of the individuals who constitute the family. In this circumstance, one loses a true understanding of a common good, in that common goods are in the end reduced to goods that particular individuals realize in collaboration with other individuals. The common good is no longer appreciated as a good realized only within the common communal structure of the family. In contrast, the good of the family is understood by liberal individualist theories as a special good for individuals. The family as an irreducible social category of meaning and locus for virtue is denied.

In order to understand the important balance between family and family member, one should note an important element of the familist view: both individuals and their families possess intrinsic good and have a standing of their own. The family is not reduced to its constituting members. Nor is the standing and worth of the individual members denied. Instead, it is recognized that family members realize their virtue and human flourishing within families. Therefore, the presumption must always be that patients are to be treated within the context of their families.

III. SOME IMPLICATIONS OF A RECONSTRUCTIONIST CONFUCIAN BIOETHICS: THE CASE OF INFORMED CONSENT AND THE ROLE OF PHYSICIANS

Because of the recognition of the family as the primary locus for human social life and flourishing, as well as the acknowledgement that not only illness and suffering, but also the complex decisions of health care are difficult if confronted alone, the family becomes the central source of authority for treatment. This prima facie presumption that it is families who will consent to ordinary treatment, as well as choices regarding withholding and withdrawing treatment, is enough to distinguish a Reconstructionist Confucian bioethics from those of the established Western individualistic bioethics (Fan, 1997; Fan, 2002). In the absence of an explicit act of exit from the family, it is the family who should frame health care decisions in collaboration with the physician. Although the traditional big family no longer exists in most places, Confucian familialism is still at home in the Pacific Rim, though its typical model of shared family-determination on health care issues is frequently in tension with the liberal individualist pattern of self-determination in contemporary legislature and policy formulation.

It is important to appreciate this role of family determination in health care practice. It is also practically unfruitful as well as morally problematic to impose an individualistic mode of decision making in societies with a Confucian ethical background. In gaining consent for treatment, the goal should not be to approach the patient in isolation from the family, but instead, to approach the patient through and within the family. As already mentioned, the presumption should be that the patient is a member of his family, unless he explicitly exits. Thus, unlike the presumption of liberal individualistic bioethical theory, the burden is on the patient to demand to be treated as an isolated, atomic individual. The patient in a Confucian bioethical understanding should not be required to shoulder the burden to be treated within the authority of the family as it is required in the West. In the Western individualistic model, a competent patient must take formal steps to establish the authority of the family for decisions on his behalf. In the Confucian model, this burden is taken from the shoulders of the patient.

As a further example of the Confucian understanding of the family authority, one might consider the issue of organ donation. When governments in the Pacific Rim have attempted to develop the individualistic advance directives for the donation of organs, they find that the families often hinder the acquisition of organs from family members even after they have signed such agreements. The prima facie locus of authority for Confucians remains familist. From the Confucian view, the whole family has a legitimate interest and authority to decide how their family member's body is appropriately to be handled. Physicians usually support and act in terms of the family's wishes. People still hold that this familist understanding of shared human life is more appropriate than the individualistic vision of a human right to decide whatever one prefers. Without seriously taking into account this familialistic perspective, public policy formulation cannot be effective. Moreover, such policy is at odds with cardinal values and norms affirmed by Confucianism.

Another crucial point must be underscored: the recognition of the moral authority of physicians. Confucians understand medicine as "the art of humanity." Traditional Confucian physicians practice medicine as the way of realizing their Confucian life and pursuing their Confucian ideal of virtue-cultivation. It is the health and well-being of people that constitute the end of Confucian medicine. The true physician, as the great Confucian physician Sun Si Miao (541-680) stated, must possess professional and moral features: proficiency in techniques and sincerity in ethics (Gan, 1995). They should not only treat diseases, but also provide appropriate guidance in health care decision making. This understanding of the role of the physician differs from today's increasingly influential social ethos of the so-called patients' rights and self-determination. This social ethos appears to enlarge the patient's autonomy, but it in fact downplays the physician's virtues and harms the patient's well-being. It takes the physician as no more than a businessman who provides services based on voluntarily-made contracts. This is not good news for patients and families. In order to regain the pursuit of the true moral ends of medicine, people must recognize the necessity of cultivating the virtues of physicians in their medical practice, and families should seek virtuous physicians for their health care. Moreover, they will expect to follow the guidance of virtuous physicians in confronting diagnostic and therapeutic decisions.

It is important to recognize that the proper role of the Confucian physician is not that of an arrogant paternalism. Instead, the physician is required to act out of commonly affirmed Confucian understandings of value and virtue shared by physician, family, and patient. In particular, the physician is required to respect the place of the family and to honor its authority. The model is one of an interaction involving physician, family, and patient embedded in a way of life focused on nurturing character and virtue. Given the centrality of the concern for harmony, health care choices must attend to the harmony of physician, family, and patient in the treatment of disease. The special place of the physician is realized insofar as the physician achieves a preeminence of virtue, that is, become *junzi* – a person who appreciates and fulfills the special requirements for character in the context of health care.

IV. CONCLUSIONS

Kazumasa Hoshino's support for a bioethics and health care policy grounded in authentic Asian moral philosophical commitments finds its realization in a Reconstructionist Confucian account. His concerns and insights have proven true. As has been argued, this leads to rejecting the radically individualist assumptions of Western bioethics regarding health care decision-making. The focus falls not on the individual, but on the family as a corporate decision-maker. This quite different focus of Confucian bioethics can help provide a balance to global bioethical discussions. Aspirations to a global bioethics notwithstanding, there is no consensus regarding the appropriate content and structure of bioethics. Contemporary moral and bioethical debate is defined by real moral difference.

City University of Hong Kong
Kowloon, Hong Kong SAR, PRC

REFERENCES

Alitto, Guy S. (1986). *The Last Confucian*, 2nd ed. Berkeley: University of California Press.

Confucius (1971). *Confucian Analects, the Great Learning & the Doctrine of the Mean*. James Legge (Trans.). New York: Dover Publications.

Fan, Ruiping (1997). 'Self-determination vs. family-determination: Two incommensurable principles of autonomy.' *Bioethics* 7, 309-322.

Fan, Ruiping (2002). 'Reconsidering surrogate decision making: Aristotelianlism and Confucianism on ideal human relations.' *Philosophy East & West* 52, 346-372.

Gan, Zhuwang (1995). *Sun Si Miao Ping Zhuan*. Nanjing: Nanjing University Press.

Mencius (1970). *The Works of Mencius*. James Legge (Trans.). New York: Dover Publications.

NOTES ON CONTRIBUTORS

Kurt Bayertz, Ph.D., is Professor, Department of Philosophy, University of Münster, Münster, Germany.

Jonathan Chan, Ph.D., is Assistant Professor, Department of Religion and Philosophy, Hong Kong Baptist University, Kowloon Tong, Hong Kong, SAR, People's Republic of China.

Ho Mun Chan, Ph.D., is Associate Professor of Philosophy, Department of Public and Social Administration, City University of Hong Kong, Hong Kong, SAR, People's Republic of China.

Mark J. Cherry, Ph.D., is Assistant Professor, Department of Philosophy, St. Edward's University, Austin, Texas, USA.

Marion Danis, MD, is Head, Section on Ethics and Health Policy, Department of Clinical Bioethics, National Institutes of Health, Bethesda, Maryland, USA.

Corinna Delkeskamp-Hayes, Ph.D., is Director, European Programs, International Studies in Philosophy and Medicine, Freigericht, Germany.

H. Tristram Engelhardt, Jr., M.D., Ph.D., is Professor, Department of Philosophy, Rice University, and Professor Emeritus, Baylor College of Medicine, Houston, Texas, USA.

Ruiping Fan, Ph.D., is Assistant Professor, Department of Social and Public Administration, City University of Hong Kong, Hong Kong, PRC.

Michael D. Fetters, M.D., is Assistant Professor, Department of Family Medicine, University of Michigan Health System, and Fellow in Bioethics at the University of Michigan, Ann Arbor, Michigan, USA.

Fabrice Jotterand, MA, is Co-Managing Editor, *The Journal of Medicine and Philosophy*, and Co-Managing Editor, *Christian Bioethics*.

Maurizio Mori, Ph.D., is Professor of Bioethics, Turin University, Turin, Italy.

Lisa M. Rasmussen, MA, is Co-Managing Editor, *The Journal of Medicine and Philosophy*, and Managing Editor, *Philosophical Studies in Contemporary Culture* book series.

Hans-Martin Sass, Ph.D., is Professor, Kennedy Institute of Ethics, Georgetown University, Washington, D.C., USA, and Professor, Zentrum für Medizinische Ethik Bochum, Ruhr-Universität Bochum, Bochum, Germany.

Kurt W. Schmidt, Ph.D., is Professor, Zentrum für Ethik in der Medizin am St. Markus-Krankenhaus, Frankfurt, Germany.

David Thomasma, Ph.D., was The Fr. Michael I. English, S.J., Professor of Medical Ethics, and Director of the Medical Humanities Program, Loyola University Chicago, Stritch School of Medicine, Maywood, Illinois, USA. He passed away in April, 2002.

Robert M. Veatch, Ph.D., is Professor, Kennedy Institute of Ethics, Georgetown University, Washington, D.C., USA.

Tangjia Wang, Ph.D., is Professor, Department of Philosophy, Fudan University, Shanghai, People's Republic of China.

INDEX

Philosophy and Medicine

1. H. Tristram Engelhardt, Jr. and S.F. Spicker (eds.): *Evaluation and Explanation in the Biomedical Sciences.* 1975 ISBN 90-277-0553-4
2. S.F. Spicker and H. Tristram Engelhardt, Jr. (eds.): *Philosophical Dimensions of the Neuro-Medical Sciences.* 1976 ISBN 90-277-0672-7
3. S.F. Spicker and H. Tristram Engelhardt, Jr. (eds.): *Philosophical Medical Ethics.* Its Nature and Significance. 1977 ISBN 90-277-0772-3
4. H. Tristram Engelhardt, Jr. and S.F. Spicker (eds.): *Mental Health.* Philosophical Perspectives. 1978 ISBN 90-277-0828-2
5. B.A. Brody and H. Tristram Engelhardt, Jr. (eds.): *Mental Illness.* Law and Public Policy. 1980 ISBN 90-277-1057-0
6. H. Tristram Engelhardt, Jr., S.F. Spicker and B. Towers (eds.): *Clinical Judgment.* A Critical Appraisal. 1979 ISBN 90-277-0952-1
7. S.F. Spicker (ed.): *Organism, Medicine, and Metaphysics.* Essays in Honor of Hans Jonas on His 75th Birthday. 1978 ISBN 90-277-0823-1
8. E.E. Shelp (ed.): *Justice and Health Care.* 1981 ISBN 90-277-1207-7; Pb 90-277-1251-4
9. S.F. Spicker, J.M. Healey, Jr. and H. Tristram Engelhardt, Jr. (eds.): *The Law-Medicine Relation.* A Philosophical Exploration. 1981 ISBN 90-277-1217-4
10. W.B. Bondeson, H. Tristram Engelhardt, Jr., S.F. Spicker and J.M. White, Jr. (eds.): *New Knowledge in the Biomedical Sciences.* Some Moral Implications of Its Acquisition, Possession, and Use. 1982 ISBN 90-277-1319-7
11. E.E. Shelp (ed.): *Beneficence and Health Care.* 1982 ISBN 90-277-1377-4
12. G.J. Agich (ed.): *Responsibility in Health Care.* 1982 ISBN 90-277-1417-7
13. W.B. Bondeson, H. Tristram Engelhardt, Jr., S.F. Spicker and D.H. Winship: *Abortion and the Status of the Fetus.* 2nd printing, 1984 ISBN 90-277-1493-2
14. E.E. Shelp (ed.): *The Clinical Encounter.* The Moral Fabric of the Patient-Physician Relationship. 1983 ISBN 90-277-1593-9
15. L. Kopelman and J.C. Moskop (eds.): *Ethics and Mental Retardation.* 1984 ISBN 90-277-1630-7
16. L. Nordenfelt and B.I.B. Lindahl (eds.): *Health, Disease, and Causal Explanations in Medicine.* 1984 ISBN 90-277-1660-9
17. E.E. Shelp (ed.): *Virtue and Medicine.* Explorations in the Character of Medicine. 1985 ISBN 90-277-1808-3
18. P. Carrick: *Medical Ethics in Antiquity.* Philosophical Perspectives on Abortion and Euthanasia. 1985 ISBN 90-277-1825-3; Pb 90-277-1915-2
19. J.C. Moskop and L. Kopelman (eds.): *Ethics and Critical Care Medicine.* 1985 ISBN 90-277-1820-2
20. E.E. Shelp (ed.): *Theology and Bioethics.* Exploring the Foundations and Frontiers. 1985 ISBN 90-277-1857-1

Philosophy and Medicine

21. G.J. Agich and C.E. Begley (eds.): *The Price of Health.* 1986
ISBN 90-277-2285-4
22. E.E. Shelp (ed.): *Sexuality and Medicine.* Vol. I: Conceptual Roots. 1987
ISBN 90-277-2290-0; Pb 90-277-2386-9
23. E.E. Shelp (ed.): *Sexuality and Medicine.* Vol. II: Ethical Viewpoints in Transition. 1987 ISBN 1-55608-013-1; Pb 1-55608-016-6
24. R.C. McMillan, H. Tristram Engelhardt, Jr., and S.F. Spicker (eds.): *Euthanasia and the Newborn.* Conflicts Regarding Saving Lives. 1987
ISBN 90-277-2299-4; Pb 1-55608-039-5
25. S.F. Spicker, S.R. Ingman and I.R. Lawson (eds.): *Ethical Dimensions of Geriatric Care.* Value Conflicts for the 21th Century. 1987 ISBN 1-55608-027-1
26. L. Nordenfelt: *On the Nature of Health.* An Action-Theoretic Approach. 2nd, rev. ed. 1995 SBN 0-7923-3369-1; Pb 0-7923-3470-1
27. S.F. Spicker, W.B. Bondeson and H. Tristram Engelhardt, Jr. (eds.): *The Contraceptive Ethos.* Reproductive Rights and Responsibilities. 1987
ISBN 1-55608-035-2
28. S.F. Spicker, I. Alon, A. de Vries and H. Tristram Engelhardt, Jr. (eds.): *The Use of Human Beings in Research.* With Special Reference to Clinical Trials. 1988
ISBN 1-55608-043-3
29. N.M.P. King, L.R. Churchill and A.W. Cross (eds.): *The Physician as Captain of the Ship.* A Critical Reappraisal. 1988 ISBN 1-55608-044-1
30. H.-M. Sass and R.U. Massey (eds.): *Health Care Systems.* Moral Conflicts in European and American Public Policy. 1988 ISBN 1-55608-045-X
31. R.M. Zaner (ed.): *Death: Beyond Whole-Brain Criteria.* 1988
ISBN 1-55608-053-0
32. B.A. Brody (ed.): *Moral Theory and Moral Judgments in Medical Ethics.* 1988
ISBN 1-55608-060-3
33. L.M. Kopelman and J.C. Moskop (eds.): *Children and Health Care.* Moral and Social Issues. 1989 ISBN 1-55608-078-6
34. E.D. Pellegrino, J.P. Langan and J. Collins Harvey (eds.): *Catholic Perspectives on Medical Morals.* Foundational Issues. 1989 ISBN 1-55608-083-2
35. B.A. Brody (ed.): *Suicide and Euthanasia.* Historical and Contemporary Themes. 1989 ISBN 0-7923-0106-4
36. H.A.M.J. ten Have, G.K. Kimsma and S.F. Spicker (eds.): *The Growth of Medical Knowledge.* 1990 ISBN 0-7923-0736-4
37. I. Löwy (ed.): *The Polish School of Philosophy of Medicine.* From Tytus Chałubiński (1820–1889) to Ludwik Fleck (1896–1961). 1990
ISBN 0-7923-0958-8
38. T.J. Bole III and W.B. Bondeson: *Rights to Health Care.* 1991
ISBN 0-7923-1137-X

Philosophy and Medicine

39. M.A.G. Cutter and E.E. Shelp (eds.): *Competency.* A Study of Informal Competency Determinations in Primary Care. 1991 ISBN 0-7923-1304-6
40. J.L. Peset and D. Gracia (eds.): *The Ethics of Diagnosis.* 1992 ISBN 0-7923-1544-8
41. K.W. Wildes, S.J., F. Abel, S.J. and J.C. Harvey (eds.): *Birth, Suffering, and Death.* Catholic Perspectives at the Edges of Life. 1992 [CSiB-1] ISBN 0-7923-1547-2; Pb 0-7923-2545-1
42. S.K. Toombs: *The Meaning of Illness.* A Phenomenological Account of the Different Perspectives of Physician and Patient. 1992 ISBN 0-7923-1570-7; Pb 0-7923-2443-9
43. D. Leder (ed.): *The Body in Medical Thought and Practice.* 1992 ISBN 0-7923-1657-6
44. C. Delkeskamp-Hayes and M.A.G. Cutter (eds.): *Science, Technology, and the Art of Medicine.* European-American Dialogues. 1993 ISBN 0-7923-1869-2
45. R. Baker, D. Porter and R. Porter (eds.): *The Codification of Medical Morality.* Historical and Philosophical Studies of the Formalization of Western Medical Morality in the 18th and 19th Centuries, Volume One: Medical Ethics and Etiquette in the 18th Century. 1993 ISBN 0-7923-1921-4
46. K. Bayertz (ed.): *The Concept of Moral Consensus.* The Case of Technological Interventions in Human Reproduction. 1994 ISBN 0-7923-2615-6
47. L. Nordenfelt (ed.): *Concepts and Measurement of Quality of Life in Health Care.* 1994 [ESiP-1] ISBN 0-7923-2824-8
48. R. Baker and M.A. Strosberg (eds.) with the assistance of J. Bynum: *Legislating Medical Ethics.* A Study of the New York State Do-Not-Resuscitate Law. 1995 ISBN 0-7923-2995-3
49. R. Baker (ed.): *The Codification of Medical Morality.* Historical and Philosophical Studies of the Formalization of Western Morality in the 18th and 19th Centuries, Volume Two: Anglo-American Medical Ethics and Medical Jurisprudence in the 19th Century. 1995 ISBN 0-7923-3528-7; Pb 0-7923-3529-5
50. R.A. Carson and C.R. Burns (eds.): *Philosophy of Medicine and Bioethics.* A Twenty-Year Retrospective and Critical Appraisal. 1997 ISBN 0-7923-3545-7
51. K.W. Wildes, S.J. (ed.): *Critical Choices and Critical Care.* Catholic Perspectives on Allocating Resources in Intensive Care Medicine. 1995 [CSiB-2] ISBN 0-7923-3382-9
52. K. Bayertz (ed.): *Sanctity of Life and Human Dignity.* 1996 ISBN 0-7923-3739-5
53. Kevin Wm. Wildes, S.J. (ed.): *Infertility: A Crossroad of Faith, Medicine, and Technology.* 1996 ISBN 0-7923-4061-2
54. Kazumasa Hoshino (ed.): *Japanese and Western Bioethics.* Studies in Moral Diversity. 1996 ISBN 0-7923-4112-0

Philosophy and Medicine

55. E. Agius and S. Busuttil (eds.): *Germ-Line Intervention and our Responsibilities to Future Generations.* 1998 ISBN 0-7923-4828-1
56. L.B. McCullough: *John Gregory and the Invention of Professional Medical Ethics and the Professional Medical Ethics and the Profession of Medicine.* 1998 ISBN 0-7923-4917-2
57. L.B. McCullough: *John Gregory's Writing on Medical Ethics and Philosophy of Medicine.* 1998 [CiME-1] ISBN 0-7923-5000-6
58. H.A.M.J. ten Have and H.-M. Sass (eds.): *Consensus Formation in Healthcare Ethics.* 1998 [ESiP-2] ISBN 0-7923-4944-X
59. H.A.M.J. ten Have and J.V.M. Welie (eds.): *Ownership of the Human Body.* Philosophical Considerations on the Use of the Human Body and its Parts in Healthcare. 1998 [ESiP-3] ISBN 0-7923-5150-9
60. M.J. Cherry (ed.): *Persons and Their Bodies.* Rights, Responsibilities, Relationships. 1999 ISBN 0-7923-5701-9
61. R. Fan (ed.): *Confucian Bioethics.* 1999 [APSiB-1] ISBN 0-7923-5853-8
62. L.M. Kopelman (ed.): *Building Bioethics.* Conversations with Clouser and Friends on Medical Ethics. 1999 ISBN 0-7923-5853-8
63. W.E. Stempsey: *Disease and Diagnosis.* 2000 PB ISBN 0-7923-6322-1
64. H.T. Engelhardt (ed.): *The Philosophy of Medicine.* Framing the Field. 2000 ISBN 0-7923-6223-3
65. S. Wear, J.J. Bono, G. Logue and A. McEvoy (eds.): *Ethical Issues in Health Care on the Frontiers of the Twenty-First Century.* 2000 ISBN 0-7923-6277-2
66. M. Potts, P.A. Byrne and R.G. Nilges (eds.): *Beyond Brain Death.* The Case Against Brain Based Criteria for Human Death. 2000 ISBN 0-7923-6578-X
67. L.M. Kopelman and K.A. De Ville (eds.): *Physician-Assisted Suicide.* What are the Issues? 2001 ISBN 0-7923-7142-9
68. S.K. Toombs (ed.): *Handbook of Phenomenology and Medicine.* 2001 ISBN 1-4020-0151-7; Pb 1-4020-0200-9
69. R. ter Meulen, W. Arts and R. Muffels (eds.): *Solidarity in Health and Social Care in Europe.* 2001 ISBN 1-4020-0164-9
70. A. Nordgren: *Responsible Genetics.* The Moral Responsibility of Geneticists for the Consequences of Human Genetics Research. 2001 ISBN 1-4020-0201-7
71. J. Tao Lai Po-wah (ed.): *Cross-Cultural Perspectives on the (Im)Possibility of Global Bioethics.* 2002 ISBN 1-4020-0498-2
72. P. Taboada, K. Fedoryka Cuddeback and P. Donohue-White (eds.): *Person, Society and Value.* Towards a Personalist Concept of Health. 2002 ISBN 1-4020-0503-2
73. J. Li: *Can Death Be a Harm to the Person Who Dies?* 2002 ISBN 1-4020-0505-9

Philosophy and Medicine

74. H.T. Engelhardt, Jr. and L.M. Rasmussen (eds.): *Bioethics and Moral Content: National Traditions of Health Care Morality*. Papers dedicated in tribute to Kazumasa Hoshino. 2002 ISBN 1-4020-6828-2

KLUWER ACADEMIC PUBLISHERS – DORDRECHT / BOSTON / LONDON

MIX
Papier aus verantwortungsvollen Quellen
Paper from responsible sources
FSC® C105338

If you have any concerns about our products,
you can contact us on
ProductSafety@springernature.com

In case Publisher is established outside the EU,
the EU authorized representative is:
Springer Nature Customer Service Center GmbH
Europaplatz 3, 69115 Heidelberg, Germany

Printed by Libri Plureos GmbH
in Hamburg, Germany